THE THERAPIST'S GUIDE TO PSYCHOPHARMACOLOGY

Also Available

Clinician's Guide
to Research Methods in Family Therapy:
Foundations of Evidence-Based Practice
Lee Williams, JoEllen Patterson,
and Todd M. Edwards

Essential Assessment Skills
for Couple and Family Therapists
Lee Williams, Todd M. Edwards,
JoEllen Patterson, and Larry Chamow

Essential Skills in Family Therapy:
From the First Interview to Termination,
Third Edition
JoEllen Patterson, Lee Williams, Todd M. Edwards,
Larry Chamow, and Claudia Grauf-Grounds

Religion That Heals, Religion That Harms:
A Guide for Clinical Practice
James L. Griffith

The Therapist's Guide to Psychopharmacology

WORKING WITH PATIENTS, FAMILIES, AND PHYSICIANS TO OPTIMIZE CARE

THIRD EDITION

JoEllen Patterson
James L. Griffith
Todd M. Edwards

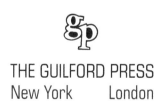

THE GUILFORD PRESS
New York   London

As with every work dealing with science, the contents of this book are subject
to evolving standards and advancements. Being apprised of such changes and
advancements is an important part of the informed consent to which patients are
entitled. In addition, any summary treatment of a subject so complicated can omit
details such as rare or newly discovered but unconfirmed contraindications. Because
medications should only be administered according to the most current guidelines
available, practitioners are strongly reminded to consult and review carefully the
product information sheets that accompany each drug administered, in light of the
patient's history.

The authors have checked with sources believed to be reliable in their efforts to
provide information that is complete and generally in accord with the standards of
practice that are accepted at the time of publication. However, in view of the possibility
of human error or changes in medical sciences, neither the authors, nor the editor and
publisher, nor any other party who has been involved in the preparation or publication
of this work warrants that the information contained herein is in every respect accurate
or complete, and they are not responsible for any errors or omissions or the results
obtained from the use of such information. Readers are encouraged to confirm the
information contained in this book with other sources.

Library of Congress Cataloging-in-Publication Data

Names: Patterson, JoEllen, author. | Griffith, James L., 1950– author. |
  Edwards, Todd M., author.
Title: The therapist's guide to psychopharmacology : working with patients,
  families, and physicians to optimize care / JoEllen Patterson, James L. Griffith,
  Todd M. Edwards.
Description: Third edition. | New York : The Guilford Press, [2021] |
  Includes bibliographical references and index.
Identifiers: LCCN 2021022843 | ISBN 9781462547661 (paperback) |
  ISBN 9781462547678 (hardcover)
Subjects: LCSH: Psychopharmacology. | Psychotropic drugs. | Psychotherapy. |
  BISAC: MEDICAL / Psychiatry / Psychopharmacology | MEDICAL / Nursing /
  Psychiatric & Mental Health
Classification: LCC RC483 .T454 2021 | DDC 615.7/8—dc23
LC record available at *https://lccn.loc.gov/2021022843*

About the Authors

JoEllen Patterson, PhD, LMFT, is Professor in the Marital and Family Therapy Program at the University of San Diego. She is also Associate Clinical Professor of Family Medicine, Global Health, and Psychiatry at the University of California, San Diego, School of Medicine. Dr. Patterson has published five books that have been translated into multiple languages, and has served on the editorial boards for journals including *Families, Systems, and Health; Family Process;* and the *Journal of Marital and Family Therapy.* Dr. Patterson received a Rotary International Scholarship to work at Cambridge University, as well as three Fulbright Awards to work in Norway, Hong Kong, and New Zealand. Her global work includes initiatives in Jordan and Ecuador.

James L. Griffith, MD, is the Leon M. Yochelson Professor and Chair in the Department of Psychiatry and Behavioral Sciences at the George Washington University (GWU) School of Medicine and Health Sciences. As a psychiatric educator, Dr. Griffith developed GWU psychiatry residency training distinguished for its excellence in cultural psychiatry, global mental health, and psychosocial care for medically ill patients. Dually trained in psychiatry and neurology, Dr. Griffith for three decades has taught psychiatry residents a curriculum that integrates humanistic psychiatry with psychopharmacology, now published in *Academic Psychiatry* as a model curriculum for psychiatry residencies.

Todd M. Edwards, PhD, LMFT, is Professor in the Marital and Family Therapy Program at the University of San Diego. He is also Voluntary

Assistant Clinical Professor in the Department of Family Medicine and Public Health at the University of California, San Diego, and Visiting Professor at NOVA University in Lisbon, Portugal. Dr. Edwards is a clinical member and approved supervisor in the American Association for Marriage and Family Therapy and an editorial board member for the *American Journal of Family Therapy* and the *Journal of Family Psychotherapy.*

Preface

Many years ago, we were supervising student therapists working in community clinics. During the students' case presentations, they would frequently mention, almost as an afterthought, that their patients were taking medication X. Being therapists, we knew little about **psychotropic medication.**[1] It was not our domain, after all. Instead, we refocused the discussion onto the "important" material—the topics we understood.

At that time, "important" material could include the patient's presenting concerns and diagnosis, family problems, stressors, previous mental health history, or therapeutic relationships. As clinicians, however, we prided ourselves on not being wedded to one particular model, theory, or treatment protocol. We were open to almost all material, as long as it pertained to the patient's psychological, relational, or social experiences.

At the same time that we were ignoring information about psychotropic medication usage or biological treatments, there were increasing references to biological influences and biological treatments in the mental health literature. Research from neuroscience, genetics, and epigenetics provided evidence for the critical importance of having a rudimentary understanding of biological etiologies and treatments. Reading scientific literature, having friends and family members who began taking antidepressants, and having our own patients ask about medications, we

---

[1] Terms in **boldface** type are included in the Glossary at the end of the book.

soon realized that psychotropic medication and other biological treatments were burgeoning approaches to treatment. To stay current, we had to gain a rudimentary knowledge about neuroscience, genetics, and psychotropic medications (Patterson & Magulac, 1994). A fair amount of research has been published on these topics since the revised edition of this book was released over a decade ago. We have incorporated a careful selection of recent research relevant to the topics in this edition. A summary of some of the most important changes in this edition are outlined at the end of this preface.

EMBRACING THE "BIO" IN BIOPSYCHOSOCIAL

While espousing the biopsychosocial model in our work as therapists in primary care medical settings, we did not have enough knowledge of human biology, genetics, and neuroscience to consider our patients' biological influences and needs. Regardless of our knowledge or interest, neurobiological research was creating a revolution by offering treatments for psychological disorders that sometimes involved simply taking a pill every morning. These new treatments were often less intrusive than traditional, weekly psychotherapy, and they were frequently being delivered by primary care physicians, not psychiatrists. In addition, research suggested that psychotherapy could affect biological systems such as the brain (Kandel, 1995, 1998, 2006; Barsaglini, Sartori, Benetti, Pettersson-Yeo, & Mechelli, 2014). These combined research initiatives demonstrated that cause and effect within the biopsychosocial model is a multidirectional process.

The biopsychosocial model was originally created for physicians to help them have a more balanced view of patients' needs. Engel (1980) suggested that the biomedical model was flawed because it ignored the patient's context and even the patient herself. Instead, Engel suggested that the organized whole (the patient), as well as the component parts (the patient's brain, immune system, family, environment, etc.), should be considered. According to systems theory, every unit is at the same time both a whole and a part. Nothing exists in isolation. Thus, physicians must take into account not only the patient's physical body and the disease but also the patient's reported inner experiences (feelings, sensations, memories) as well as his or her reported and observable behavior.

Similar to a physician's myopic, biological view, we as therapists were equally short-sighted. We were psychosocially fixated: We focused on our patients' experiences and feelings to the extent that we ignored their biological systems. Not acknowledging or understanding the importance of these systems meant that we ignored possible treatment options that targeted them—that is, we failed to consider psychotropic medications. And by failing to consider psychotropic medications in treatment, we were possibly failing our own patients.

Realizing that our therapeutic knowledge had to expand if we were going to truly follow a biopsychosocial model, we learned everything we could about medications and started encouraging our students to do the same. Textbooks for nonphysicians about psychotropic medications were published (Beitman, Blinder, Thase, Riba, & Safer, 2003; Gitlin, 1996; Riba & Balon, 1999; Sammons & Schmidt, 2001; Miklowitz & Gitlin, 2014). Courses about neurobiology, medications, and genetics were added to mental health training programs. A paradigm shift was occurring: the dissolving of mind–body dualism.

However, this revolution in the academic mental health community did not necessarily lead to better patient care. Although we could explain the basic neurobiological mechanisms of medications, we could not get our patients to keep taking them if their spouses did not like the way the patients' sex drives were affected, if the medications made the patients gain weight, or if the medications were taken off an insurance company's reimbursed medications list. The books we collectively read on combining psychotherapy and medications or simply educating nonphysicians and patients about medications has led us to believe that providing knowledge to mental health professionals would be enough to create change. This assumption was not true. In addition, there was virtually no communication between the prescribing physician—regardless of his or her medical discipline—and the therapist. Also, family members, who may be most affected by patients' responses to medication, were completely ignored. The impact of payers, employers, health care system providers, and others was never mentioned along with the discussion of the neuromechanisms of the medications. But these impediments were the everyday challenges that we faced with our patients. Even if our patients were open to the idea of medication, structural impediments, especially the lack of communication between the prescribing physician and the therapist, limited the medications' effectiveness.

Engel (1980) had originally focused on the biological, psychological, and social systems of his patients. But we were discovering that other systems were also affecting the care we could offer. The organizational and financial structures of the health care systems, as well as the divisions among the different mental health disciplines, meant that patient care was often fragmented and uncoordinated.

THE COLLABORATIVE CARE MOVEMENT

At the same time that we were struggling with these issues, there was a growing movement in health care that had as its goal the collaboration of physicians and therapists in assessing, planning, and providing patient care. A growing group of health professionals had been attempting to repair both the fragmentation in health care services and the conceptual split between mind and body. In fact, there were already several organizations and groups devoted to this model of care, especially in the United States, Canada, Europe, Australia, and the United Kingdom. In recent years, the World Health Organization has also created a program for low- and middle-income countries, the Mental Health Gap Action Program (Mh-Gap), focused on principles of collaborative care (World Health Organization, 2019).

Defining Collaborative Care

Collaborative care (more recently referred to as **integrated care**) has many definitions. It does not refer to **split care** or colocated care, which usually implies that the physician treats the biological part of the patient by prescribing medication, and the therapist does the rest. Although split care may be attractive in terms of cost and ease for the provider, it is inadequate care. Patients need their therapist and physician to communicate, particularly in the creation and maintenance of a treatment plan. Although it's ideal if the communication occurs within an integrated care setting (mental health services integrated into the medical setting), most therapists don't share space with physicians and will contact the physician via phone, letter, or electronic communication (under a signed release of information).

Collaboration also differs from consultation. Consultation implies an event rather than a process. It is possible that a psychiatrist, for example, could conduct an evaluation and offer suggestions without prescribing medication, which may negate the need for ongoing contact. However, in most cases, the physician ideally becomes a treatment team member, not simply a consultant who offers expert advice and disappears.

One definition of collaboration is "the concurrent use of medical and mental health services" (Roesler, Gavin, & Brenner, 1995). Although this definition is absolutely correct, it obscures the diversity in how collaborative treatment is delivered. Collaboration can include phone calls, hallway discussions, exchanges of emails, participation by a physician—primary care or otherwise—in part or all of a therapy session, and meetings that involve all professionals, the patient, and his or her family. Nor does this definition suggest the difficulty in practicing collaboratively. Even with good intentions to "work together" and "share care," good collaboration is hard work.

Collaborative Care: An Integrated Conceptualization

As clinicians, we began to understand that a collaborative care model addresses gaps and fragmentation in the health care delivery system. It means that we do not have to know every fact about every system that might affect our patient's care. Instead of viewing ourselves as the sole deliverers of treatment, we have become the purveyors of possibilities in a system that extends beyond our own personal limitations, in addition to offering the patient our clinical expertise.

All treatment options are equally plausible, regardless of whether we can deliver the treatment ourselves. We might provide the treatment, or we might serve as a conduit of information and resources so that our patient can receive the best possible care. When psychotropic medications are used, we consider their impact beyond the patient's biological system. In a collaborative care model, it has become our job to understand the impact that psychotropic medications could have on patients and their families, at home or in their work environment, even though as therapists we do not provide the medication ourselves.

PREPARING THE NEXT GENERATION OF THERAPISTS

Despite our immersion in medical settings and the collaborative/integrated care movement, we were doing training as usual. That is, we were training future therapists to work independently, using the tools that we gave them, including theory and popular treatment techniques. At best, working with other colleagues meant providing a referral for some specialized treatment, such as psychological testing.

Eventually we realized that our training models would no longer work. Using the ideals of the collaborative care movement, we began creating new treatment goals. Believing that psychotropic medication might be an essential treatment and that many of our patients would be obtaining medication from their physicians, we considered what new knowledge future therapists (our students) would need.

This book is the result of our collective search for better ways to care for patients with mental health problems. Its purpose is to provide the information a non-MD therapist needs to know about psychotropic medication and collaborative care. It is intended for nonprescribing clinicians who work in outpatient mental health settings as well as therapists seeing patients in medical settings. We wrote it with two objectives in mind: to give readers a basic knowledge of pharmacotherapy for various mental health disorders, and, equally important, to provide a conceptual framework, a mind-set, and specific approaches for working in a collaborative care environment with medical professionals who *do* prescribe psychotropics.

Our goal in this book is to provide basic scientific information about psychotropic medications and, even more important, to offer pragmatic advice on helping patients benefit from these medications. Although there are many potential concerns, such as a family's response and insurance issues, we believe collaboration—with patients, family members, and prescribing physicians—is the cornerstone of efficacy.

This book focuses on a non-MD therapist and a physician working together to care for their common patient. However, the non-MD therapist could be a psychologist, a social worker, a marriage and family therapist, a nurse, or a counselor. When we refer to physicians, we generally mean a family physician, a psychiatrist, an internist, a pediatrician, an obstetrician-gynecologist, or, more recently, a nurse practitioner. Although communication is easiest when therapists share space with physicians, we recognize that most therapists will collaborate at a distance. This book is primarily intended for therapists who want to build collaborative relationships and learn the biological information they need to communicate with physicians.

In writing this book, we made a few assumptions:

1. We want this book to be theory-neutral. Each model and every therapist makes unique contributions to the therapeutic process. You might be an expert in cognitive-behavioral therapy, family systems theory, interpersonal psychotherapy, or another model; your expertise is a critical component of healing. However, because we assume that you already have expertise in some type of psychotherapy—that is not the focus of this book.

2. Rather, we assume you want to improve your collaborative relationships with physicians. We suggest you can do this by knowing more about psychotropic medications, biological systems, and how biological treatments affect the human body and brain.

3. In addition to promoting more collaboration with physicians, we also advocate for more family involvement in health care. We urge you

to think about not only your individual patient but also his family. This need became strikingly clear to us when a seriously depressed mother went to her primary care doctor because she "didn't know what else to do." She had seen several mental health professionals during the past year, yet none of their treatments had helped her. The physician enlisted the aid of an on-site therapist, and they interviewed the patient together. Fifteen minutes into the interview, it became clear that the patient was a single mother of a 6-year-old and an 8-year-old. She tearfully reported that the 8-year-old had taken on all household responsibilities: walking her younger brother to and from school, preparing all meals, and doing all the shopping and other "parenting" responsibilities that the mother could not do—given that she could not get out of bed most days. The patient reported that she had never given this information to any other health care professionals simply because none had asked. Often, health care professionals are focused only on the individual patient who is present during the interview. As a result, they can miss important information about other family members and the repercussions of the problem throughout the entire family.

4. Some readers, particularly those already trained in neuroscience and biological treatments, may find specific parts of this book too simplistic. We have tried to write the book so that you can skip the parts that are not helpful and turn instead to the sections that offer new information. You may find the chapters on collaboration especially useful.

5. We assume you are pressed for time, the physicians you work with are pressed for time, and the payers (including employers and insurance companies) want the patient to get better as quickly as possible. The physicians you work with might have little knowledge or interest in your contribution to the shared treatment—namely, the therapy. They may even have little time or interest in working or communicating with you. Although it is helpful if both professionals share a commitment to collaborative care, it is not essential. Some physicians will be enthusiastic about collaborating; others will express ambivalence or disinterest.

6. Biological treatments are changing at a rapid pace, and this book can quickly become dated. Thus, we have tried to write in terms of general ideas or principles. Often, we talk about classes of medications, not specific drugs. We know you need to find your own methods of staying abreast of trends in psychopharmacology and collaborative care. We hope this book serves as one foundation for the ongoing process of learning about biology, neuroscience, epigenetics, psychotropic medications, and collaborative care.

WHAT'S NEW IN THE THIRD EDITION

As mentioned earlier, we made several changes to this edition of the book. Below are highlights of some new features.

• We have made clearer distinctions between *distress* and *disorder.* That is, psychotherapists most commonly work with mental health problems that are best understood and addressed as normal emotional responses to adverse life circumstances. Medication has little or no role in treatment of such "normal" distress. However, both normal stress responses and psychiatric illnesses produce symptoms of anxiety and depression, so it is important to distinguish between "normal" distress and a psychiatric illness for which medications may be needed. This, of course, is a major diagnostic responsibility of a psychiatrist if one is involved in the care, but it is valuable for a psychotherapist to understand how a psychiatrist operates.

• New vignettes have been added to illustrate collaborative care in the treatment of both psychiatric illnesses and normal syndromes of distress, such as demoralization.

• We have included many of the "rules of thumb" that psychopharmacologists utilize in diagnosis and treatment. These are general principles that have exceptions in individual cases but are accurate most of the time. For example, *All serotonin reuptake inhibitors can be used to treat all anxiety disorders* (Chapter 5) and *Antidepressants have no role to play in care for grief or demoralization* (Chapter 3) are generally true as rules of thumb, but can have exceptions. It is useful for a psychotherapist to be aware of what is usually the case, while also realizing there can be exceptions. Discerning these exceptions is usually the task for a psychiatric consultant.

• Our aim is to help a psychotherapist to understand how a psychiatrist thinks when diagnosing psychiatric disorders and utilizing medications to treat or prevent episodes of anxiety, depression, psychosis, or other psychiatric illnesses. Increasingly, it has been shown that effective treatment of such major disorders as major depressive disorder, bipolar disorder, or schizophrenia depends upon a well-implemented, multimodality treatment program, not just prescribing a medication. Effective multidisciplinary treatment programs require each member of the team to have a basic understanding of the role of medications, both what medications can and cannot accomplish and side effects that must be monitored. The role of the psychotherapist often is an important one for patient education, monitoring adherence to medication regimens, and monitoring both responses to treatment and medication side effects.

• We have expanded information about the therapeutic relationship in a new Chapter 11. This discussion also focuses on principles of evidence-based practice (EBP), shared decision making among all stakeholders, and conducting a critical appraisal of all treatment possibilities.

A WORD ABOUT LANGUAGE

Since we assume our readers have differing foundations of knowledge about medications, we have tried to make the book helpful to any reader. One way we do this is by putting words that might be unfamiliar in boldface. These words can be found in the Glossary or they can be referenced online for more information.

We used generic names of medications throughout the text. Since psychotherapists are often more familiar with trade names for some medications, we inserted commonly utilized trade names in parentheses as well. We do not endorse preferential use for any trade-name medication versus its generic form.

Additionally, there are several case illustrations throughout this book. These cases describe clinical experiences with our patients but in each case either the identity of the patient is disguised or a composite patient is created to illustrate a point.

CONCLUSION

We have narrowed our focus to the information you need to effectively collaborate with your medical colleagues. That information includes the following:

- Basic neuroscience information on how the brain works and how drugs affect the brain.
- Biomedical information that you need to understand about psychotropic medications, one of the key treatments the physician might utilize. This is organized by specific disorders.
- An action plan for building collaboration.

We discuss what a therapist might consider when deciding to refer a patient to a generalist physician or a psychiatrist. The basic tenets of collaborative care are covered, including but not limited to collaboration around the patient's psychotropic medication. Whether you are currently in a private practice or in a hospital-based interdisciplinary team, this section provides tools to enhance collaboration.

We recognize that your professional experiences may be significantly different from ours. But we surmise that you share some of our frustrations as we try to provide excellent care in a rapidly changing health care world. Your training may not have provided all of the tools you need for optimal care, and you may be frustrated with the limits of your work setting. We hope this book supplies some knowledge and ways to help you overcome the limits you have faced in caring for your patients.

Acknowledgments

We express deep appreciation to Anuj (AJ) Jenveja, whose meticulous attention to detail and gentle encouragement made writing this book a pleasure. In addition to supporting the authors, AJ managed several other graduate students who worked on this book, and he served as a role model for his classmates. He also worked with staff at The Guilford Press to make sure that all the details of producing a book were completed.

While working on this book, AJ completed his clinical training in the Family Medicine Residency at the University of California San Diego. AJ is both a strong clinician and a competent editor. He was chosen as the Outstanding Graduate of the 2020 class of Marriage and Family Therapy students at the University of San Diego. We consider it an honor to have worked with him during the past 2 years.

Contents

PART I

THE MIND–BODY CONNECTION

Should psychotherapists learn about psychiatric medications? Psychotherapy originated at the start of the 20th century as Sigmund Freud's "talking cure." As the 20th century ended, however, treatment of mental health problems was becoming dominated by medications—psychopharmacology, not psychotherapy. Prescribing medications was primarily a task for psychiatrists and primary care physicians, who held medical licenses for prescribing. As time passed, however, it became evident that many patients benefited from a combination of both psychotherapy and psychopharmacology. Psychotherapists and physicians then began partnering with "split treatment" arrangements, although confusion often persisted as to how best to interface these fundamentally different treatment approaches. Some psychotherapists showed active disinterest in psychiatric medications as "not my job." Likewise, some psychopharmacologists showed little interest in or regard for their patients' psychotherapies (Luhrmann, 2000).

This text makes a strong argument that the most effective care for mental health problems occurs when physician and psychotherapist work in close collaboration. In a collaborative relationship, the physician conveys to a patient the need for a program of treatment, not just a medication. In addition to medication, the psychotherapist will provide psychotherapy and help guide needed lifestyle changes for effective treatment. Similarly, the psychotherapist, working collaboratively, emphasizes the importance of adherence to a medication regimen, while providing education and monitoring both treatment effects and side effects (Sparks, Duncan, Cohen, & Antonuccio, 2011). There are specific reasons why

1

psychotherapists should be knowledgeable about psychiatric medications, how they work, what are expectable positive treatment effects, and what are common negative side effects:

1. To facilitate communication with physicians. Physicians have a detailed understanding of treatment options using medications. Psychotherapists can best understand and talk with physicians if they are familiar with terms like *neurotransmitter, serotonin,* and *anticholinergic.*

2. To help explain the need for medications to patients and family members. Patients and family members can feel stigmatized when a psychiatric medication is prescribed, fearing they will be labeled as "mentally ill" by their families, coworkers, or community. Patients may feel more comfortable taking their medications when they have some understanding of why medications are helpful and how they work in the body. Although the prescribing physician is the ideal person to provide this information, not all physicians have the time or inclination to discuss it in any detail with their patients. It will often strengthen your relationship with your patients and their confidence in your collaboration with their physicians if you can answer some of their questions and help them understand the information their physicians give them (within the limits of your professional scope of practice and personal knowledge). You may also find that educating your patients about their brain's biology can provide them with more productive ways to think about their medications—for example, by replacing "I must be crazy if I need to take drugs" with "My brain systems that manage stress can operate more effectively with support from medication."

3. To use an understanding for how the brain processes information as a guide to doing psychotherapy or family therapy. For example, trauma-focused psychotherapy and psychotherapies that strengthen emotion regulation rely upon a neurobiological model for guidance in helping clients to stay in a "zone of tolerance" for emotional arousal (Rothschild, 2017; van der Kolk, 2014). Mindfulness approaches to psychotherapy rely upon an understanding of top-down neural regulation of bottom-up processing of sensory information, as discussed in Chapter 1 (Andre, 2011).

CHAPTER 1

How the Brain Works
A BASIC SKETCH

In order to understand how medications work, it is important to have a basic understanding of the nervous system as well as an understanding of how it normally operates so a person can flourish. This is a bit like journeying to a new country and starting by learning where the largest cities and major roadways are on a map (see Figure 1.1). Our analogous list of major sites in the human nervous system will involve only the following components:

1. The **prefrontal cortex** and the **executive functions** and **social cognition** networks that it supports.
2. The **salience network** and its components—most important of which are the **amygdala, insula,** and **ventral anterior cingulate gyrus.**
3. The **autonomic nervous system** and its two divisions, the **sympathetic nervous system** and the **parasympathetic nervous system.**
4. The **monoamine systems,** three of which we will discuss in detail based upon their utilization of **norepinephrine, serotonin,** or **dopamine** as their primary **neurotransmitters.**

In this chapter, we will discuss how all these components work together to enable a human being to live and thrive in an ever-changing environment that regularly poses challenges and threats. This discussion will help you understand how most mental health problems are problems of **dysregulation** for which strengthening **top-down regulation**

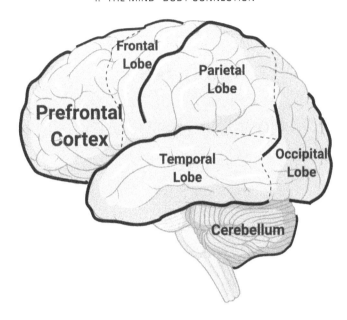

FIGURE 1.1. The parts of the brain.

of **bottom-up information processing** is often the needed solution. This paradigm underpins not only how medications work, but also how psychosocial interventions work by strengthening emotion regulation. These include such treatment programs as dialectical behavioral therapy, acceptance and commitment therapy, and the incorporation of yoga, mindfulness practices, or exercise into treatment programs.

If you do not have familiarity with the functional organization of the human nervous system, it may be helpful to read in more detail about each of the bolded terms as you encounter them. We begin by discussing how our biological evolution reshaped the architecture of the human brain into a social brain built for relationships (see Figure 1.2).

THE HUMAN BRAIN AS A PRODUCT OF EVOLUTION

Both psychotherapy and psychopharmacology rely upon brain circuits that evolved long ago and helped *Homo sapiens* to thrive in competition with other early hominids, such as the Neanderthals. Over the course of evolution, the human brain underwent two notable increases in size: 1.5–2.0 million years ago, and again 200,000–500,000 years ago (Mithen, 1996). These expansions in overall brain size were largely due to enlargement of the human prefrontal cortex. The prefrontal cortex is small in most mammals, even among higher primates, such as macaque monkeys. In human beings, however, it has expanded to constitute about 20% of the entire brain. This large prefrontal cortex has mostly served the development of executive functions (planning, organizing, prioritizing, using self-talk to regulate one's behavior) and social cognition (noticing social cues, organizing into groups, making psychological sense of other people, feeling empathy for others).

In a social group where individuals cooperate, compete, and create alliances and coalitions, individuals with an ability to predict the behavior of others will achieve the greatest reproductive success. Social intelligence—powers of social forethought and understanding—is essential for maintaining social cohesion so that practical knowledge can be shared within the group. This "social brain" provided humans with capabilities for making psychological sense of each other, that is, to accurately imagine the contents and logic of each other's minds.

Not surprisingly, psychiatric disorders have their most disabling effects when they alter a person's capacities for social relatedness with others, such as an inability to notice social cues or to show empathy for another person's distress. All serious mental illnesses involve dysfunction in how the prefrontal cortex can effectively regulate other brain systems.

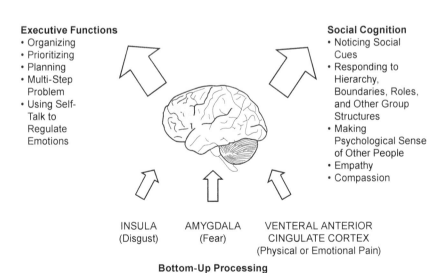

Executive Functions
- Organizing
- Prioritizing
- Planning
- Multi-Step Problem
- Using Self-Talk to Regulate Emotions

Social Cognition
- Noticing Social Cues
- Responding to Hierarchy, Boundaries, Roles, and Other Group Structures
- Making Psychological Sense of Other People
- Empathy
- Compassion

INSULA (Disgust)   AMYGDALA (Fear)   VENTERAL ANTERIOR CINGULATE CORTEX (Physical or Emotional Pain)

Bottom-Up Processing

FIGURE 1.2. The evolution of the prefrontal cortex and the ascent of *Homo sapiens*.

NEURONS, NEUROTRANSMITTERS,
AND NEUROTRANSMITTER RECEPTORS

Understanding how psychiatric medications work begins with a basic understanding of how the brain works. The human brain is made up of 100 billion cells called **neurons.** In addition, there are a similar number of **glial cells** that give a physical architecture to the brain and provide metabolic support for the neurons. Neurons in the brain differ from other cells in the body in that they are primarily designed for communicating with each other. Neurons are designed to pass an electrical charge along their surface from one end to the other, then to transfer the electrical charge to the next neuron, then to the next (see Figure 1.3). Transfer of the electrical charge from one neuron to the next is accomplished by dumping a molecule called a neurotransmitter into the cleft between neurons, called a **synapse.** The neurotransmitter drifts across

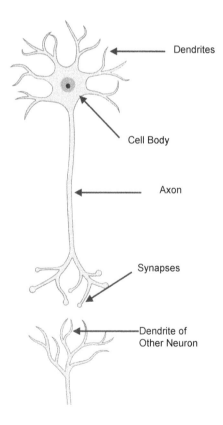

FIGURE 1.3. The neuron, or nerve cell.

the synapse to attach to a neurotransmitter receptor on the next post-synaptic neuron, where it activates another electrical charge that travels the length of the neuron to the next neuron, and so forth (see Figure 1.4). Often the traveling electrical charge is simply called an electrical impulse. An electrical impulse serves as the most fundamental unit of information in the nervous system.

At a physiological level, most psychiatric medications exert their effects by blocking access of neurotransmitters to receptors on postsynaptic neurons. Some medications strengthen the binding of neurotransmitters to receptors. Other medications block the **reuptake** for future reuse of neurotransmitters after their release into synaptic clefts. Each type of neurotransmitter will react with one specific type of receptor site and no other, similar to a lock and key. There are at least 40 different chemicals that have been shown to act as neurotransmitters; some of the most common are listed in Table 1.1.

Most synapses in the central nervous system (CNS) will conduct an impulse (usually via a neurotransmitter) in one direction only; that is, from the **axon** of the presynaptic neuron to the **dendrite** or cell body

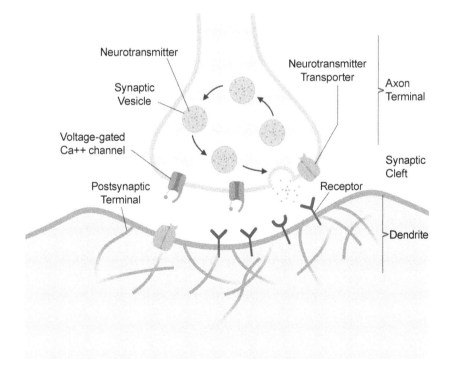

FIGURE 1.4. The nerve synapse.

TABLE 1.1. Some of the Most Common Neurotransmitters

Neurotransmitter	Function/biology	Disorder if malfunction	Medications used to influence this neurotransmitter
Acetylcholine	Usually excitatory, except for some parasympathetic nerve endings where it is inhibitory (such as the effect on the heart by the vagus nerve). Secreted by many neurons, including those in the motor area of the brain, basal ganglia, skeletal muscle motor neurons, all preganglionic autonomic nervous system neurons, all postganglionic parasympathetic neurons, and some postganglionic sympathetic neurons.	Complex, diffuse symptoms affecting all bodily systems. This is a complex, widespread neurotransmitter, the receptor sites of which are affected (usually adversely) by some psychotropic medications (anticholinergic side effects).	Very diffusely affected by many medications. In particular, antihistamines, anti-Parkinsonian drugs, and medications for dementia affect this system, as do numerous medications for general medical conditions. Many psychiatric medications have side effects that occur because of their influence on the acetylcholine receptors.
Dopamine	Usually inhibitory. Secreted by neurons in substantia nigra onto neurons of the basal ganglia, both subcortical areas of the brain.	Disorder in the dopamine system has been hypothesized to be important in psychotic disorders, and many antipsychotic medications work on dopamine receptors, of which there are several subtypes. Affects cardiovascular system and has other widespread effects.	Diffusely affected by many medications. Antipsychotic medications and some antidepressants have some dopaminergic effects; certain medications, used for general medical conditions also affect dopamine receptors.

GABA (gamma-aminobutyric acid)	Inhibitory. Secreted by neurons in the cerebral cortex, subcortical area, and spinal cord.	Anxiety states, also involved in chemical dependency.	Diffusely affected by many medications. Many antianxiety medications work on GABA receptor sites, especially in the frontal lobe of the brain. Alcohol, benzodiazepines, and barbiturates all affect GABA receptors, as do other drugs.
Norepinephrine	Mostly excitatory, but inhibitory in some areas. Secreted by neurons in the locus ceruleus (subcortical area) to widespread areas of the brain, controlling wakefulness, overall activity, and mood. Also diffusely secreted in the sympathetic nervous system.	Diffuse and widespread symptoms, including depression, changes in blood pressure, heart rate, and diffuse physiological responses, among many others. An important transmitter in the sympathetic branch of the autonomic nervous system.	Diffusely affected by many medications. Several antidepressants work specifically on this neurotransmitter and its receptor sites. Many medications for general medical conditions affect this neurotransmitter as well.
Serotonin	Usually inhibitory; helps control mood, influences sleep, and inhibits pain pathways in the spinal cord. Secreted by subcortical structures into hypothalamus, brain, and spinal cord. There are many subtypes of serotonin receptors.	Diffuse and widespread symptoms: depression, headache, diarrhea, constipation, sexual dysfunction, and other medical symptoms.	The selective serotonin reuptake inhibitors (SSRIs), the most commonly used antidepressants, work specifically on this neurotransmitter system.

(**soma**) of the postsynaptic neuron. A particular postsynaptic neuron will have anywhere from 10,000 to 200,000 terminals, or receptor sites, that interact with presynaptic neurons via release of neurotransmitters.

FUNCTIONAL BRAIN CIRCUITS

The neuron is the fundamental anatomical unit of the brain. However, the fundamental functional unit is not an isolated neuron but rather an entire circuit of interconnected neurons. A **functional brain circuit** can be thought of as a "family" of neurons that are interconnected. Like a medieval village family where Smiths are carpenters, Joneses are blacksmiths, and Kellys are tailors, each functional brain circuit carries out a specific sensory, cognitive, or behavioral action. Functional brain circuits are the building blocks of behaviors that involve thoughts, feelings, and actions. Functional brain circuits govern how the brain senses its surrounding world, processes information, and expresses adaptive actions in response.

A **signaling pathway** is the organized transfer of information between and within neurons so that the brain can sense changes in its environment, interpret those sensory stimuli, generate complex motor and behavioral responses, and store the information in memories. A signaling pathway can involve sensory receptors in body tissues that link to release of neurotransmitters that activate a sequence of brain circuits, which, in turn, prompt secretion of hormones that exert effects upon body tissues. Each of these steps serves as a link in a chain of command that connects sensing one's environment, to acting upon that environment to ensure survival and well-being of the species. For example, many mothers who nurse their newborn infants are familiar with the breast milk "let down" reflex. Sometimes just hearing the sound of her crying baby causes milk to be secreted from the mother's breast. How the sound of the baby can exert such an immediate effect upon the mother's body is an example of a signaling pathway. Its steps are as follows:

- The baby's crying sound is detected by the cochlea of the mother's ear.
- The cochlea activates nerve fibers that enter her brainstem to end within the nucleus of her eighth cranial nerve.
- The eighth cranial nerve nucleus activates a neural pathway that travels upward and, after several relays, activates neurons in the hypothalamus.

- The hypothalamic neurons release a small protein, oxytocin, into the bloodstream.
- When oxytocin travels to the mother's breast through the bloodstream, it causes contraction of the muscles surrounding the milk ducts, causing milk to be secreted.

Signaling pathways for specific human behaviors involving multiple functional brain circuits are linked together for a single common purpose. Some of the steps of a signaling pathway can involve types of tissues other than neurons, such as sensory receptors; release of hormones; or muscle contractions.

Intrinsic Connectivity Networks: Our "Clans" of Functional Brain Circuits

Complex domains of behavior, such as executive functions or detection of emotionally salient events, are subserved not by simple functional brain circuits, but by large networks that combine many different functional neural circuits into an integrated whole. **Intrinsic connectivity networks** (**ICNs**) are large-scale networks of brain circuits that have characteristic functions and behavioral correlates, such as executive functions, social cognition, or memory.

In comparison to single circuits, these ICNs might be likened to clans, or "families of families," of functional neural circuits (Laird et al., 2011). The prefrontal cortex on the left side of the brain houses ICNs that support executive functions, while the prefrontal cortex on the right side houses ICNs that support social cognition.

Executive Functions

Executive functions is an umbrella term for a number of cognitive processes, such as planning, organizing, prioritizing, selective focusing of attention, multistep problem solving, verbal reasoning, inhibiting impulses, mental flexibility, multitasking, and initiation and monitoring of actions. Executive functions represent the evolutionary achievement of functional brain circuitry anatomically located within the prefrontal cortex of the brain's hemisphere that is also dominant for language (usually the left hemisphere).

Executive functions enable humans to override responses that might otherwise be automatically elicited by environmental stimuli. Some of these executive functions include:

1. Planning for an envisioned future and decision making
2. Correcting or troubleshooting errors
3. Acting in situations requiring novel, unrehearsed solutions
4. Navigating technically difficult or high-risk situations
5. Managing situations that require overriding a strong habitual response or resisting temptation

Frank McCourt (1996), in *Angela's Ashes,* described his Ireland childhood, half-starved, disheveled, chronically ill, and lacking any adult encouragement; he nevertheless determined to go to the United States and gain an education. He made plans and backup plans. He secretly created a post office savings account where he could save a few pence at a time. Utilizing creativity and ingenuity, he worked from one odd job or money-making scheme to another. At age 19, he purchased a steamer ticket to the United States. Such pathways thinking and agency thinking is emblematic for how executive functions operate (Snyder, 2000): "Here I am, there is where I want to be, these are steps I can take to get there." Despite a childhood of extraordinary poverty and neglect, Frank McCourt's executive functions kept finding pathways to a future he could only envision with his imagination. His memoir won a Pulitzer Prize.

Social Cognition

Social cognition is the broad set of skills that enable a person to utilize relationships to cope with life's challenges. It includes perceptual skills for noticing social cues and patterns of interaction, as well as social processes such as rules of hierarchy or group boundaries. Social cognition enables emotional awareness of others and oneself. Whereas the dominant (for language) hemisphere houses the infrastructure for executive functions, the nondominant hemisphere provides the infrastructure for social cognition. The dorsomedial prefrontal cortex supports **mentalization** as the cognitive capacity to make psychological sense of other people, while the ventromedial prefrontal cortex supports the emotional perspective-taking of empathy. Executive functions and social cognition can be coordinated to enable the most sophisticated problem solving, strategic planning, and collaboration skills in all the animal kingdom.

Salience Network

The brain's salience network detects meaningful stimuli in a person's surrounding environment and generates appropriate emotions in response.

These emotions provide needed direction and motivation for taking action—to feel fear readies both mind and body for flight; to feel anger readies mind and body to fight; to feel shame readies mind and body to hide from sight; and so forth. The salience network operates both within and outside of conscious awareness. Brain circuits that constitute the salience network include those organized around the amygdala (to detect threatening stimuli), insula (to detect distasteful or disgusting stimuli), and ventral anterior cingulate cortex (to detect emotionally or physically painful stimuli).

The salience network alerts the prefrontal cortex that "there is work to be done." The salience network also sets in simultaneous motion two other systems whose roles are to get the body and mind ready for action:

1. The autonomic nervous system (ANS), which readies the various body organ systems for whatever path of action will be required. The sympathetic division of the ANS prepares for a fight-or-flight response—racing the heart, elevating blood pressure, releasing extra glucose into the bloodstream. The sympathetic nervous system is thus an accelerator that puts the entire body into crisis mode. The parasympathetic nervous system is a decelerator that puts a brake on the sympathetic system in order to fine-tune behavioral responses to environmental demands. The parasympathetic division readies the body for one of three options when facing adversity: to freeze death-like, to fight or flee, or to "tend and befriend," bonding with others to meet adversity together (Porges & Dana, 2018). For example, an unexpected loud explosion would immediately activate the sympathetic nervous system—speeding heart rate, raising blood pressure, shifting blood flow away from the visceral body organs to the muscles—readying the body for a possible need to flee. Simultaneous activation of the parasympathetic nervous system might lead a few people to freeze immobile, others to flee, and still others to seek other people who could help. Which parasympathetic action would be largely determined by the person's behavioral genetic history; by the extent to which the person did, or did not, feel both frightened and trapped; as well as by any personal history of past traumatic events (Levine, 2010; Porges & Dana, 2018).

2. The monoamine systems, which utilize serotonin, norepinephrine, or dopamine as neurotransmitters, prime the CNS for a rapid response (norepinephrine, serotonin) or more sharply targeted response (dopamine) when facing an adversity. For example, a mouse unexpectedly scurrying across the floor of one's office would likely produce

activation of norepinephrine into the cerebral cortex. For the next 20 minutes or so, information processing would be speeded within the cerebral cortex and a shift termed a *heightened signal-to-noise ratio* would occur in the brain's perceptual systems for how quick-moving objects are perceived. This bias also creates risks for overinterpretation of moving shadows as possible mice, when the same shadows would never previously have attracted attention.

The ANS and the monoamine systems typically activate in concert. Their dual mission is to prepare both mind and body to act upon plans put forward by the prefrontal cortex as it responds to the salience network's alert.

EMOTION REGULATION AND TOP-DOWN/BOTTOM-UP INFORMATION PROCESSING

In its quest for survival, *Homo sapiens* faced a dilemma. Safety meant staying in close touch with changing conditions in the environment. This awareness entailed letting sensations from seeing, hearing, touching, tasting, and smelling course freely into the nervous system. This was termed bottom-up information processing (Gross, 2007; McRae, Misra, Prasad, Pereira, & Gross, 2012).

However, the prefrontal cortex, for all its wonderful capabilities, was also the part of the brain most vulnerable to stress. When flooded with too much stimulation, the prefrontal cortex would stop functioning, leaving the person too frazzled to think or function. A method was needed to dampen arousal from incoming stimuli so that executive functions and social cognition could perform optimally. The solution was top-down regulation by the prefrontal cortex. The prefrontal cortex would send its descending fibers into the major components of the salience network (amygdala, insula, anterior cingulate cortex) to inhibit their transmission of sensory information into the brain. By deactivating these transmission centers, this top-down regulation could preserve a relatively quiet environment for the prefrontal cortex to focus on its work.

Emotion regulation refers to a person's ability to find the best balance between the brain's "need to know" (bottom-up processing) and its "need to think" (top-down regulation). Emotion regulation is the focus of clinical intervention both with medications and psychosocial interventions that strengthen top-down regulation.

Achieving Emotion Regulation through Attention Reallocation

The brain's attention systems enable awareness to be concentrated upon discrete stimuli in the environment while screening out extraneous "noise." Attention systems involve three different anatomic regions in the brain that subserve three different types of attention—alertness, vigilance for emotionally salient events in the environment, and "spotlight" executive attention that enables a person to focus on one target in the environment while screening out awareness of all else.

In the brain, "attention trumps emotion." That is, wherever attention is focused determines whether or not an emotional response can be generated in response to an environmental event. This fact underpins much of psychotherapy, particularly hypnosis, such that shifting focus of attention shifts a person's emotional state. For example, the old adage of athletes in training, "No pain, no gain," implicitly shifts focus of attention from the pain of training to the pleasure of winning in competition. In the American classic *The Adventures of Tom Sawyer,* Tom says a single sentence to his friends laughing at him for having to work on a Saturday morning: "Does a boy get a chance to whitewash a fence every day?" Soon his friends are joyfully whitewashing the fence, while Tom heads out to go fishing (Twain, Fishkin, Doctorow, & Stone, 1997). Interventions that reassign focus of attention are particularly valuable in enabling emotion regulation.

In summary, the brain's salience network conducts surveillance over the ever-changing environment, detecting meaningful stimuli and generating emotional responses to them. These emotional responses provide a direction and level of motivation for executive functions and social cognition to act. The ANS and monoamine systems are simultaneously activated to ready both the body organs and brain information-processing systems to align with the kind and intensity of emotion.

However, regulation of the emotional response is necessary. The prefrontal cortex is the part of the brain most sensitive to stress. An excess of stimulation can overwhelm the prefrontal cortex, leaving a person feeling "frazzled," flooded, unable to think clearly or to utilize relationships effectively. Top-down regulation from the prefrontal cortex and reallocation of attention by the dorsal cingulate cortex can dampen, or even suppress entirely, the initial emotional response. This top-down regulation of bottom-up information processing balances needed sensitivity of awareness for the environment with long-term commitments and social desirability. It enables humans to pause and think, rather than to respond immediately when something happens that is emotionally upsetting. As Howard Thurman has stated: "The test of life is how much pain and disturbance we can absorb without spoiling our joy" (Thurman, 2010).

CONCLUSION

Functional brain circuits are the shared target for both medications and psychotherapeutic interventions. Psychotherapeutic interventions use language and relationship to shift focus of attention or to reframe meaning so that emotional activation changes. Medications produce changes in emotional activation through a different means. Generally, psychiatric medications do not intervene directly in the complex operations of prefrontal cortex ICNs for executive functions and social cognition. Rather, they alter functioning of the regulatory systems—sometimes the ANS, more often the monoamine systems—that ready the mind and body to respond to stressors. In subsequent chapters, we will examine how medications can modify regulatory symptoms in a manner that relieves the suffering of anxiety and depression.

CHAPTER 2

How Psychotropic Drugs Work

Why does suddenly stopping some antidepressants result in withdrawal symptoms, yet stopping others does not? Why should some medications be taken on an empty stomach? Why is the status of the liver important for some medications, whereas kidney function is relevant for others? Why do some psychotropic medications have noticeable effects minutes to hours after ingestion (e.g., the antianxiety benzodiazepines), whereas others (e.g., antidepressants) take days or weeks for their effects to become apparent? The answers to these questions lie in several pharmacology factors, especially (but not restricted to) **pharmacokinetics** and **pharmacodynamics.** Medications differ in the ways they are processed once inside our bodies. They also differ in the ways they affect our bodies. These differences confer unique pharmacological "profiles" that make medications produce a unique set of clinical characteristics. When physicians—who more often than not have several medications to choose from for a particular disorder—select a drug, they consider all these characteristics and attempt to match them to the specific needs, sensitivities, and preferences of each individual patient. The purpose of this deliberate decision-making process is to offer the patient an optimal **risk–benefit ratio.** That is, the goal is to select a medication that will produce the strongest possible therapeutic effect with the fewest possible negative side effects.

HOW THE BODY HANDLES DRUGS: PHARMACOKINETICS

The ultimate target for psychotropic drugs is the brain—in fact, specific areas in the brain. Ideally, clinicians would be able to deliver a drug to the desired target and only to that target. This, of course, is not possible, at least not at the current level of clinical biotechnological development. Drugs must use a rather nonspecific method of "public transportation" to reach the brain: the bloodstream. Drugs transported by our blood-stream do make it to the intended targets. Unfortunately, they also reach many unintended areas in the brain, as well as elsewhere in the body. This process, known as **distribution,** will be affected by various factors, including characteristics of the drug. Side effects usually result from this lack of specificity in the delivery system. But first, drugs must reach the bloodstream, and they do so through a process called **absorption.** Dif-ferent routes can be used: Swallowing a pill is the most common. The pill is dissolved in the stomach or in the intestines, a phenomenon mediated by specific "juices" that prepare the drug to cross the microscopic pores that allow entry into the bloodstream. Certain properties of a particular drug will result in faster or slower absorption and, as a result, increase or decrease the time required to reach an appropriate **concentration** of the medication in the bloodstream. The presence of food in the stomach may, in some cases, interfere with the speed of absorption. Conversely, certain drugs have an irritating effect on the lining of the stomach that may lead to adverse consequences, namely, inflammation and pain. Thus, some drugs have instructions to "take with food" and others have instructions to "take on an empty stomach."

In certain clinical situations, we want the beneficial effect of the drug to occur as quickly as possible. For example, an acutely agitated or anxious patient must be given relief very quickly, so getting the drug into the bloodstream quickly would be of great benefit. For these situations, certain drugs may be given **parenterally**—that is, via routes other than the digestive system, such as **intramuscular** injections of antianxiety or antipsychotic drugs. Intravenous injection of a drug delivers it directly into the bloodstream, causing an immediate effect.

Another way to get a drug into the bloodstream quickly is inha-lation. In fact, the short time between the inhalation and the desired effect can sometimes be exploited, frequently with hazardous conse-quences, as with recreational drugs. For example, nicotine and cocaine, which are very quickly absorbed through the nasal mucosa and the lung tissue, reach the brain in a matter of seconds. Other routes and tech-niques may be used to deliver drugs to the brain in a controlled fashion. Injections directly into the spinal fluid may be used for certain neuro-logical conditions. Other drugs, after being administered, are released slowly over a period of days or weeks. Certain antipsychotic prepara-tions (i.e., haloperidol [trade name Haldol], fluphenazine [trade name Prolixin], and risperidone [trade name Risperdal or Consta]) can be injected intramuscularly, and they are formulated to release the drugs over a period of several weeks. This "**depot**" method of administration can provide an essential, consistent baseline concentration of medication for patients who otherwise would not take their medications reliably on a daily basis. Slow-release patches applied to the skin also enable the gradual absorption of certain medications. Nicotine patches, for example, have become useful aids for smoking cessation programs. Selegiline (trade name Emsam), a patch-based antidepressant, is also available for clinical use.

Once a drug is in the bloodstream, it is subjected to various factors that can influence how much of it will get into the brain. Some drugs have great affinity for fatty tissue and will be retained in areas of the body where such tissue is in abundance. Such medications need to be taken in higher doses in order to achieve therapeutic concentrations in the blood. Some drugs become tightly bound to proteins found in the bloodstream. The protein-bound fraction is kept inert, and only the small amount of free drug is available for reaching the brain.

If a second medication is added—whether for psychiatric purposes or for a concurrent medical problem—there is always the possibility of drug interactions. If the new medication is highly protein-bound, it can compete for the proteins occupied by the first medication and in fact displace some of it, which then becomes free in the bloodstream. Effectively, the concentration of the first medication is now larger, so more of it reaches the brain, with potentially toxic results.

If, following absorption, medications were undisturbed by the body, we would need to take only one dose for an eternal effect. Of course, this is not the case. As soon as drugs enter the bloodstream, the process of **metabolism** ensues. The body recognizes the drug as a foreign substance and eliminates it outright (say, via the kidneys, as in the case of lithium) or transforms it chemically, using a complex enzyme mechanism located in the liver. This chemical transformation enables the medication to be eliminated through the urine. In some cases, the chemical transformation produces a new compound that may also have therapeutic effects (or, in some rare instances, a toxic effect). For example, fluoxetine (trade name Prozac) is transformed into norfluoxetine, which is also an antidepressant. A similar situation occurs with the old tricyclic antidepressants (amitriptyline [trade name Elavil] to nortriptyline; the latter, in fact, is "transformed" in the laboratory and marketed as a separate antidepressant, with the trade name Pamelor).

All these different factors—absorption, distribution, metabolism, and **excretion**—interact with each other and determine together various pharmacological parameters that have clinical significance:

• **Peak concentration:** the time required for the drug, once it is administered, to reach maximum concentration in the bloodstream. For those medications that have an "immediate" effect and in which the magnitude of the effect is proportional to the dose (curiously, this is not the case with all medications), knowing the peak concentration will enable us to predict, approximately, the time required for maximum intensity of the desired effect (i.e., how long it will take to feel better).

• **Trough level:** the point at which the concentration of the medication in the bloodstream is at its lowest. Trough levels that are very low, say, because of lengthy intervals between doses, may actually result in a loss of benefit or may even result in withdrawal symptoms.

• **Half-life:** the time required for the concentration of a medication to decrease by 50% in relation to its peak level. This is the result of metabolism and excretion.

• **Steady state:** the amount of time required for a drug to reach a stable concentration level in the bloodstream. This means that the amount entering the body (repeated doses) matches the amount being eliminated (metabolism and excretion). Typically, for most drugs this time is estimated to be about five half-lives for the medication in question (assuming, of course, no interactions with other medications and other phenomena). So a medication with a half-life of 24 hours will take 5 days to reach steady state. The range of half-lives for psychotropic medications is quite wide, measured from hours (e.g., some benzodiazepines) to many days (norfluoxetine, the active metabolite of fluoxetine). The concepts of steady state and half-life are critical when evaluating clinical results (including the assessment of need for dose adjustments), adverse events, and medication discontinuation phenomena.

• **Plasma level:** for some psychotropic medications, certain correlations have been established between plasma level (the concentration of a drug in the liquid portion of the blood) and therapeutic benefit. Using this method, the prescribing physician can make adjustments to the doses with the goal of reaching drug concentrations in the blood that are associated with optimal response. In a few instances—for example the antiobsessional clomipramine (trade name Anafranil) and the antidepressant nortriptyline (trade name Pamelor)—clinical research and experience have established a **therapeutic window,** that is, the boundaries of a minimum concentration that must be reached and a maximum concentration that must not be exceeded for the drug to work well. If a patient's blood level is outside the window, in either direction, the benefit is often diminished.

HOW DRUGS AFFECT THE BODY: PHARMACODYNAMICS

What are the effects of the medication on our systems, in particular, on the intended targets? Given our current understanding, the intended targets are usually the receptors found on the surfaces of the neurons in the brain. For example, some antidepressants interact with norepinephrine and/or serotonin receptors; some antipsychotics exert their effects on dopamine receptors. These effects may either enhance the function normally carried out by the receptor or inhibit it. Other, more complex interactions can also occur in the neuron. Pharmacodynamics describe the therapeutic and adverse effects of medication. An effect on the desired target will result in symptom relief, but it may produce side effects on unintended targets. Ideally, one would want a medication with high selectivity, that is, affecting the desired target with no or minimal effects on other systems. However, often, the negative effects of a medication are the first changes a patient experiences. You may refer a patient for a medication evaluation who is ambivalent about taking medication for his psychiatric symptoms. The first changes he notices are negative symptoms such as dry mouth, constipation, or change in sexual functioning. As a result of these physiological changes, the patient stops the medication before experiencing the positive effects such as remission of his depressive symptoms. To avoid this scenario, the therapist and physician should educate the patient about what to expect and urge him to keep taking the medication until a positive response is achieved. If the therapist is concerned about a patient's response to the medication, she should contact the physician or urge the patient to contact the physician.

In some cases, a desirable drug will produce a therapeutic benefit at a dose substantially less than the higher dose that produces serious side effects. This is often referred to as the drug's **therapeutic index.** Lithium is an example of a psychotropic drug with a low therapeutic index; small amounts in excess of the doses needed to control manic symptoms may produce serious or even life-threatening side effects.

Throughout these medication processes of pharmacokinetics and pharmacodynamics, the body's organ systems are reacting by working to maintain homeostasis. For example, the kidneys detect the lithium as an excess salt in the blood, and they strive to eliminate it. There is a tremendous orchestration of activity going on everywhere in the body (not just the brain) in response to any psychotropic medication, as this is added to the daily physiology of health or disease in that person. Every time a medication is taken, those mechanisms of homeostasis come immediately into play: Every time one neurotransmitter is altered, it sets off a string of counterreactions throughout the body. All of the neu-rotransmitters affect functions throughout the body and, at the current level of biotechnological development, it is simply impossible to give a medication that creates only one change in one area of the body.

DIVERSE POPULATIONS

To make things a little more complex, different population subgroups with unique pharmacokinetic and pharmacodynamic profiles may require adjustments in dosing and scheduling in order to achieve opti-mal risk–benefit ratios with certain medications. Children and older adults are common examples. During their training, many physicians have been admonished to "start low and go slow" when prescribing for geriatric patients. Older adults have absorption, distribution, metabolic, and excretion rates that often differ significantly from those of younger adults. In addition, older adults often suffer from a number of other medical problems, which in some cases may affect the way they respond to and tolerate medications. Moreover, treatments that they may be receiving for these other medical conditions may interact with the psy-chotropic medications being prescribed.

An emerging area in clinical pharmacology that promises to pro-duce some clinically meaningful guidelines is **ethnopharmacology.** It has been suspected for a long time that different ethnic groups metabo-lize and respond to medications differently. These differences appear to be primarily genetically determined. However, other factors, such as dietary predilections, may be at work as well. This means that "stan-dard" doses for specific medication might require adjustments when pre-scribed for members of specific ethnic groups. For example, some data suggest that tricyclic antidepressants are metabolized differently among African Americans (higher blood levels, more side effects, and faster response), Asians (longer elimination times), and native Puerto Ricans (similar response with lower doses and increased side effects) (Preskorn, Feighner, Stanga, & Ross, 2004) from how they are metabolized among European Americans. Differential responses among some ethnic groups have been reported also for SSRIs, lithium, clozapine (trade name Clo-zaril), risperidone (trade name Risperdal), and olanzapine (trade name Zyprexa), to name a few.

The clinical clue that ethnic differences may be affecting drug metabolism is either that a patient cannot tolerate a medication at even small doses due to side effects or that usual doses of a medication produce neither treatment effects nor side effects. Awareness of populations at high risk for **rapid metabolizers** or **slow metabolizers** helps a clinician stay vigilant. Some side effects are both common and serious, requiring vigilance whenever the medication is prescribed. For example, as many as 50% of African Americans and Central Americans develop metabolic syndrome (weight gain, high serum lipids, type 2 diabetes) when atypical antipsychotic medications, such as olanzapine, are prescribed.

Future research should result in recommendations for specific dose adjustments or, better yet, specific tests that will serve as guidelines for dosing and monitoring the use of psychotropic medications in different populations. Considering all of these factors in psychotropic medication management often constitutes some of the most complex challenges in the practice of medicine.

CONCLUSION

Medications differ in the ways they are processed, from their absorption into the bloodstream to their degradation and excretion by the liver and kidneys. The pharmacokinetic and pharmacodynamic profile of each drug describes these differences that confer its unique clinical properties. Physicians select a drug in part based upon these characteristics. They attempt to match these profiles to the specific needs, sensitivities, and preferences of each individual patient. This decision attempts to offer the patient an optimal risk–benefit ratio, in which a medication produces the strongest possible therapeutic effect with the fewest possible negative side effects.

PART II

PSYCHIATRIC DISORDERS AND THEIR TREATMENT

In this section, we discuss the various psychiatric disorders and the medications that have proven effective in treating them. Each chapter focuses on a specific category of disorder and includes the following:

- a definition of the disorder and a summary of the symptoms it gives rise to;
- how to distinguish the psychiatric disorder from normal syndromes of distress that produce similar symptoms;
- the neurobiology of the disorder;
- medications that are commonly used to treat the disorder; and
- issues related to the disorder that may be important in therapy with the patient and/or collaboration with the physician.

To establish a relationship and join with a physician–collaborator, you should understand her worldview and ways of thinking and talking about patients. Depending on your theoretical orientation, making a diagnosis according to *Diagnostic and Statistical Manual of Mental Disorders* ("DSM") criteria may play a greater or lesser role in how you ordinarily conceptualize your patients' difficulties. For the physician, accurate diagnosis based on criteria in the DSM is the linchpin of treatment. The physician will usually be appreciative if you can assist her by communicating your working diagnosis and the symptoms that led you to it in terms of DSM criteria.

Often the target symptoms are just as important as the diagnosis in deciding which medication would be most helpful. The target symptoms are those symptoms that are interfering with the patient's life and functioning. They are often (but not always) part of the diagnostic criteria, such as insomnia, poor concentration, and fatigue. Although the diagnosis is important, the target symptoms will assist the physician in deciding which medication within a class would be the best choice.

Distinguishing psychiatric disorders from normal syndromes of distress can be a difficult diagnostic challenge. There is a wide range of normal emotional responses to losses, threats, and predicaments that life can bring. However, it is important to distinguish "normal" demoralization, grief, loss of dignity, and spiritual anguish from depression as a mental illness, as we will subsequently discuss. An inability to distinguish normal syndromes of distress from mental illness can result in excessive use of medications and underutilization of psychosocial interventions in clinical practices (Horwitz & Wakefield, 2007, 2012).

These chapters will also help you understand any therapeutic effects and unwanted side effects your patients have when they are taking psychotropic medications. Because you will usually see the patient more often than the physician does, you may be the first professional to whom the patient brings these issues. Although these concerns should be communicated to the physician—and any medication changes must be made by the physician—your knowledge can often reassure the patient—for example, that it is normal for many antidepressant medications to take a few weeks to begin alleviating symptoms. We have designed these chapters to provide you with the basic information you will need to discuss medications in terms your patients will find relevant and useful, to discuss your patients in terms physicians will be familiar with, and to alert you to therapeutic issues that may arise in the process of diagnosis and medication.

CHAPTER 3

Depression

Mr. King was a depressed middle-aged man who had been consistently successful in the business world until a recent venture failed. Now he was embarrassed at the modest lifestyle in which he and his wife could afford to live. As he lapsed further into depression, she began resenting the minimal help he provided in maintaining the household, as well as his unending criticism of her efforts. He reluctantly agreed to begin individual therapy to help him develop better coping strategies and to grieve his losses. He and his wife were also treated in marital therapy to foster mutual empathy and communication and to resurrect lost passion. During the ensuing months, there was little improvement. At some point, Mr. King, having read an article on depression in one of the airline trade magazines, began asking for antidepressant medication. Initially, his therapist resisted, referring him to a psychiatrist because a chemical solution seemed to represent obvious avoidance of painful, but necessary, changes. Eventually, though, she relented. Mr. King was referred to a psychiatric consultant who noted from his evaluation that Mr. King scored 21 on the **Hamilton Depression Scale (HAM-D)**, which was in the severe range of major depressive disorder (MDD; Hamilton, 1960). The psychiatric consultant elicited from Mr. King the history of a previous depression for which he had not sought professional treatment. Further, prior to the failed business venture Mr. King had been experiencing a low mood, poor sleep, high anxiety, and loss of enjoyment in usual recreational activities, suggesting that depression may have contributed to the business failure rather than the other way around. A month after starting an antidepressant medication prescribed by his psychiatrist, Mr. King was brighter, more optimistic, less critical of his wife, and carrying through with some of the never acted upon ideas that they had discussed in therapy. Mrs. King, in response, showed more compassion and less detachment. Their fighting diminished. Individual therapy and marital therapy that had not been working suddenly seemed to begin working.

In all of mental health, *depression* is probably the most familiar term to most people. Yet how to treat depression—whether with psychotherapy or antidepressant medications—can be confusing. Over the course of a lifetime, many people experience losses, traumatic experiences, betrayals, and disappointment; low moods seem an expectable part of the fabric of life. Psychotherapy focused upon coping more effectively with life's adversities makes sense. What has distinguished modern psychiatry, however, has been the identification of depression as a mood disorder in large part determined by problems in functional brain circuits and signaling pathways that regulate mood. Depression is not simply a normal response to harsh adversities but is a mental illness. This understanding of depression became critically important as new somatic treatments were developed for depression as a mood disorder—antidepressant medications, **electroconvulsive therapy** (ECT), and new neuromodulation treatments. As might be expected, these new somatic therapies proved to be of no use when depressive feelings simply arose in response to life's harsh adversities.

DISTRESS OR DISORDER?: WHY ACCURATE DIAGNOSIS IS IMPORTANT

Distinguishing between a low mood as a **normal syndrome of distress,** such as demoralization, grief, loss of dignity, alienation (feeling that "I don't belong"), or spiritual anguish, and as depression as a mood disorder is vitally important (Griffith & Gaby, 2005). There are specific psychotherapeutic interventions that can relieve suffering from different normal syndromes of distress, but the same approach that may help demoralization or grief often has no effect in the throes of a severe depressive disorder. For example, one of the clearest accounts of the differences between grief and depression comes from a chapter in Kay Jamison's (2009) *Nothing Was the Same: A Memoir.* Jamison, coauthor of both scientific and lay audience books on bipolar disorder, wrote about her husband's death, contrasting it with her personal experiences of bipolar depression (Jamison, 2009, pp. 169–170):

Richard's death stirred up such a darkness in me that I was forced to examine those things that depression and grief hold in common and those they do not. The differences were essential, the similarities confounding.

I did not, after Richard died, lose my sense of who I was as a person, or how to navigate the basics of life, as one does in depression. I lost a man who had been the most important person in my life and around whom my future spun. I lost many of my dreams, but not the ability to dream. The loss of Richard was devastating, but it was not deadly.

I knew depression to be unrelenting, invariable, impervious to event. I knew its pain to be undeviating. Grief was different. It hit in waves, caught me unaware. It struck when I felt most alive, when I thought I had moved beyond its hold. . . . Pain brought so often into one's consciousness cannot maintain the same capacity to wound. Grief conspires to ensure that it will in time wear itself out. Unlike depression, it acts to preserve the self. Depression is malignant, indiscriminately destructive. Grief may bear resemblance to depression, but it is a distant kinship.

The role of diagnosing depression as a mood disorder belongs to general physicians and mental health professionals. Regrettably, the DSM diagnostic system on which most U.S. psychiatric practices operate has limited capabilities for distinguishing normal distress from mood disorders. Also, many physicians move quickly by trying medications first, rather than waiting to see the outcome of psychotherapy. For a variety of reasons, antidepressant medications appear to be prescribed far more frequently than rigorous diagnostic assessments might indicate they should. This may explain in part why recent meta-analyses of treatment outcome studies have found antidepressant medications to show minimal benefits when compared to placebos (Kirsch, Moore, Scoboria, & Nicholls, 2002). Diagnostic criteria on which medication treatment is commonly based may be too broadly inclusive, intermixing other kinds of human distress with depression as a mental illness, thereby "washing out" beneficial effects that would be evident if distress and disorder were more precisely distinguished. For example, increased mortality risks for heart attack patients became an issue of concern 2 decades ago for psychiatrists, primary care physicians, and cardiologists. Of patients with cardiovascular disease, 20% suffered from depression, and death rates were significantly increased when patients with heart attacks were also depressed. A randomized controlled study was conducted to determine if administering the antidepressant sertraline to depressed patients with heart attacks might mitigate this risk. However, sertraline produced no detectable reduction in morbidity or mortality. Only a subgroup of patients with well-defined mood disorders (high depression scale scores, history of severe depressions, depressed mood prior to the heart attack) benefited from sertraline. We can surmise that heart attacks produce grief and demoralization as a normal response to a threatening, potentially disabling, possibly lethal life event. Those with such a normal syndrome of distress failed to benefit from medication. Those with a well-defined primary mood disorder did benefit (Joynt & O'Connor, 2005; Glassman et al., 2002).

Distinguishing distress from disorder matters in another way that directly touches the work of psychotherapy. When the problem is a normal syndrome of distress, the message to the patient is "What you are feeling is what anyone else would feel given your circumstances. Life feels hard because it is hard" (Slavney, 1999). Depression is viewed as a normal emotional response to adversity. Psychotherapy then focuses upon unburdening stressors, mobilizing strengths and relational support, and empathy that honors the patient's struggle while avoiding attribution of psychopathology as cause of suffering. If the problem is clinical depression, however, the message is that symptoms are due to a mental illness, and the underlying pathology requires diagnosis and treatment. The framing of the problem matters.

> Ms. Winslow was diagnosed with colon cancer, an illness that had ended the life of her mother. While she was being treated for the cancer, her family became alarmed when she began neglecting care of the family home, withdrew from friends, stopped attending church, and spoke of discontinuing chemotherapy treatments. Her family convinced her to see a psychiatrist for treatment of depression. The psychiatrist, however, concluded that Ms. Winslow was primarily demoralized, not depressed. She showed only a modest elevation in score on the HAM-D, and she was able to enjoy pleasurable things. She felt afraid, overwhelmed, and worn down by her illness, and she was losing hope. The psychiatrist recommended that she begin individual and family therapy with a therapist experienced in the care of medically ill patients. Ms. Winslow regained her footing as she coped emotionally with a life-threatening illness, and her family organized a plan to provide the support she needed. Ms. Winslow's mood lifted. The psychiatrist never prescribed medication.

> On the other hand, Mr. Warren was a middle-aged man who sought psychiatric treatment for depression. This was the third episode since his 20s when he "felt awful every day," slept poorly, felt continuously apprehensive, lost interest in his hobbies, and had little libido. A successful entrepreneur, he was widely admired for his business

successes. He was in a long-term relationship with a woman he loved. He commented, "I love my work, I love my girlfriend, and I have everything I could want. But all I can think about is that I would rather be dead." A diagnosis of recurrent MDD was made, and Mr. Warren was immediately engaged in a treatment program that included antidepressant medication, cognitive-behavioral therapy (CBT) for depression, an exercise program, and psychoeducation on treatment and prevention of mood disorders. His depressive symptoms showed dramatic improvement by the fourth week.

Criteria used to distinguish depression from normal distress are less than perfect (see Table 3.1). By examining multiple criteria, however, it is usually possible to establish a preponderance of evidence that a low mood is one or the other. Demoralization is an example of a common normal syndrome of distress. Demoralization is the "helplessness, hopelessness, confusion, and subjective incompetence that people feel when sensing that they are failing their own or other's expectations for coping" (Frank & Frank, 1991, p. 14). Demoralization and depression share many features—both produce low mood, poor sleep, low energy, loss of appetite, and poor concentration. However, there are some criteria that distinguish the two (Griffith & Norris, 2012):

1. Demoralization occurs in immediate proximity to a stressful event, with severity that correlates roughly with severity of stressor, and remits when the stressor remits. Depression waxes and wanes without a necessary connection to a specific stressor (Horwitz & Wakefield, 2007).

2. **Hedonia** is lost with depression; that is, pleasurable activities fail to bring pleasure, while a demoralized person can feel better when there is good news or something to take pleasure in.

3. Guilty ruminations, loss of self-worth, and suicidal ideation are common in depression. They can occur but are uncommon with demoralization.

4. For depression, there commonly is a history of past similar episodes lasting weeks to months.

5. Depression, but not demoralization, often has a family history of mood disorder.

6. When examined with a standardized, quantified assessment instrument, such as the HAM-D, scores are only mildly elevated by demoralization but severely elevated by depression.

7. Depression, but not demoralization, commonly shows improvement with antidepressant medications, either currently or in the past.

Psychotherapists would be wise to read two scholarly but readable texts: *Loss of Sadness* (Horwitz & Wakefield, 2007), which makes the case against overmedicalization of normal sadness, and *Against Depression* (Kramer, 2005), which makes the case against underdiagnosis of depression as psychiatric illness. Their juxtaposition argues strongly for the importance of accurate distinctions between normal syndromes of distress and psychiatric disorders (see Table 3.1). Contrasting case illustrations for treatment of demoralization and MDD show how these diagnostic distinctions matter throughout a collaborative care course of treatment.

CASE ILLUSTRATIONS: CONTRASTING DEMORALIZATION WITH MDD

Ms. Allen: Coping with Major Stressors While Also Depressed

Ms. Allen, 45 years old, called Ms. Daley, a licensed professional counselor, seeking a psychotherapy appointment for "feeling overwhelmed." Ms. Allen had been skeptical about any value to come from psychotherapy. However, she had been repeatedly urged by her best friend who said she had been greatly helped by sessions with Ms. Daley. Ms. Allen told Ms. Daley that she was constantly tired and sleeping poorly since her recent divorce. She was engaged in an ongoing custody battle with her former husband over their two teenage children. Ms. Daley listened

TABLE 3.1. Distinguishing Demoralization from Depression

	Demoralization	Depression
Onset, severity, and time course coincident with specific stressor	Common	Possible, but uncommon
Hedonia (capacity to feel pleasure)	Intact	Impaired
Self-condemnation and self-loathing	Absent	Common
Suicidal ideation	Rare	Common
Elevated scores on standardized depression assessment instruments (such as Hamilton Depression Scale)	Absent (or mild)	High
Symptom reduction with antidepressant medication	Absent	Common

Note. Data from Griffith and Norris (2012), Griffith and Gaby (2005), and Slavney (1999).

as her client detailed her story from beginning to end. Ms. Allen told how she and her husband fell in love, married, and partnered closely through graduate school. While his career had advanced rapidly in a start-up health care data management company, she had stepped back in her career to work part-time jobs that accommodated her role as primary parent for their young children. Their lives became increasingly separate worlds. Her husband then had an affair with a coworker that ended their marriage. Ms. Allen recently received a poor performance review in her workplace and now worried about her job security. She blamed her work problems on the stress of her divorce. Her therapist listened empathically to this story and validated Ms. Allen's experience of loneliness and feeling overwhelmed, while expressing concern over Ms. Allen's self-judgment that she "should be handling this better." Ms. Daley also expressed concern over Ms. Allen's fatigue, insomnia, and lack of physical and emotional self-care. She asked Ms. Allen to take a PHQ-9 Depression Scale, which showed a high score of 15. She told Ms. Allen, "I want you also to see Dr. Phillips, my psychiatric colleague, to see whether antidepressant medication also may be helpful. The challenges you are facing are daunting, you are facing all this alone, and it will be hard to do that with little energy or sleep." Ms. Allen initially resisted the idea, feeling that taking psychiatric medication would be "the final insult to my life." However, she eventually accepted her psychotherapist's framing of the issue as: "The obstacles you face are hard ones, and you are doing it alone. You need to be at your best both for your sake and for your children."

When Ms. Allen met with Dr. Phillips, she noticed that, unlike her therapist, she asked more about Ms. Allen's symptoms than her personal story. She focused particularly upon Ms. Allen's feelings of worthlessness and inability to take pleasure in anything. She learned that Ms. Allen had to force herself to stay engaged in her children's activities, as well as other interests that she used to enjoy. Ms. Allen felt that she was "just going through the motions." Dr. Phillips inquired about a similar episode after the birth of Ms. Allen's second child that lasted several months. She learned that Ms. Allen's mother had episodes of depression. She told Ms. Allen, "When making decisions about medications, we need to attend to the pattern of depression symptoms, their severity and duration, and how much these things are affecting your life. It helps to utilize an assessment instrument that has research support for being able to distinguish depression from other kinds of distress in a person's life." She then administered the HAM-D, which showed a score of 19, in the severe range of MDD. She explained that depression of this severity usually requires medication because its symptoms interfere too much with the concentration, energy, and reflective thought that psychotherapy requires in order to be effective. Ms. Allen's family history and past history of depressive episodes strengthened this conclusion. The psychiatrist recommended escitalopram as an antidepressant medication with few expectable side effects. Ms. Allen agreed to take it for a 1-month trial basis.

By the second week of escitalopram treatment, Ms. Allen felt a notable increase in her energy. She began feeling as if there was "a floor to my despair." Her sleep and ability to experience enjoyment in her children improved. She began a productive psychotherapy with her therapist focused upon engaging in supportive relationships, practicing emotional self-care, and launching an assertive legal defense in her custody struggle with her ex-husband. She experienced no significant side effects from her once-daily dose of escitalopram. She felt that the antidepressant medication was simply one more modality of her recovery program that had multiple arms.

Mr. Ford: Demoralized by Chronic Pain

Mr. Ford was a 45-year-old man with severe degenerative spinal disk disease who came to the hospital emergency department seeking help for his pain, but also acknowledging that he was having suicidal impulses. The emergency medicine physician consulted a psychiatric colleague, Dr. Smith, to assess Mr. Ford's level of suicide risk and to determine whether psychiatric hospitalization was needed.

Mr. Ford described to Dr. Smith his history of chronic pain and disability. He was taking a complex regimen of antidepressant, psychostimulant, and multiple analgesics that only partially relieved his chronic pain. In addition, he recently had gone on disability status and was financially stressed. He wondered now whether life could be still worth living. He denied having a plan for suicide but acknowledged spending a recent evening on the Internet looking at suicide websites. In her assessment, Dr. Smith noted that Mr. Ford still could experience pleasure and enjoyment of some activities—movies, reading, watching baseball games—and that he had normal energy and appetite with no self-deprecatory ruminations. His HAM-D score was only 12 (mildly elevated). She concluded that Mr. Ford's diagnosis was primarily demoralization with despair about ending his physical pain, rather than a mood disorder.

"Would you wish to die if you did not have to live with so much pain?" Dr. Smith asked.

"No," Mr. Ford responded. "I'm not depressed. I just can't live with this much pain every day."

"What held you back from acting on one of the suicide methods that you read about on the Internet?" Dr. Smith asked.

"The efforts that my doctors and a few other people have made to get me as far as they've been able," he responded. "I don't want to let them down." He named four people who had most helped him rally after becoming despondent.

Then he added, "I've always spent my time helping other people." Dr. Phllips asked what he meant.

"All my work has been for other people—nonprofit organizations, public service. I've always worked in the government." He told how he not only had worked long hours in his government job but also had volunteered his time for community service projects and nonprofit advocacy groups.

"It sounds like your sense of purpose from your work has been important," Dr. Smith commented. "For you it has mattered a lot to know that what you do makes a difference in people's lives."

Mr. Ford agreed, adding that it had been a mistake to stop working. Then he described his current dilemma—his last remaining volunteer role in an organization had been serving as secretary in a nonprofit organization. He had been under pressure to resign because he had not kept good track of its records during his illness. While he agreed that his performance in that position had been erratic, he worried about what it would be like to feel that he had nothing useful to offer. This had in part precipitated his current crisis.

Listening to how strongly Mr. Ford relied upon relational coping and altruism as his strengths, the Dr. Smith proposed to Mr. Ford that (1) they could work together to see if his pain management program could be strengthened, either through another revision of medications or addition of physical therapy and other nonpharmacological pain management methods; (2) a counselor, Ms. Daley, who worked with Dr. Smith, could meet regularly with Mr. Ford in psychotherapy; (3) they could work to organize a meeting with Mr. Ford and some supportive friends to seek ideas for how Mr. Ford could continue using his knowledge and skills to make a contribution to the lives of others; and (4) both Dr. Smith and Ms. Daley could continue to monitor any recurrent impulses toward self-harm.

Questions for Consideration

1. *Ms. Allen presented her psychotherapist with a narrative of sorrow and loss for which psychotherapy would seem ideally fitted. Why did her psychotherapist so quickly request psychiatric consultation?*

Three symptoms—anhedonia, sense of worthlessness, and suicidal impulses—are common in MDD but rare in demoralization or grief. *Anhedonia* is the inability to enjoy or feel pleasure in usual activities or relationships that should bring enjoyment or pleasure. Most symptoms of depression—poor sleep, low energy, difficulties concentrating—are nonspecific and seen with any kind of life stress. They don't discriminate depression as a mental illness from the "normal suffering" from life's adversities. Anhedonia as seen with Ms. Allen is a strong indicator for a diagnosis of major depression and consideration of antidepressant medication. In addition, Ms. Allen showed a high score on a PHQ-9 depression scale, and her low mood was impacting her functioning in both parenting and work roles, all of which weigh in favor of an MDD diagnosis.

2. *Both the psychiatrist and the psychotherapist listened to Ms. Allen's and Mr. Ford's stories, but how did they listen in different ways?* It was important that both psychiatrist and psychotherapist hear fully each of these two patients' stories and respond to each with acknowledgment, empathy, and compassion. However, the psychotherapist shifted her focus of attention onto "experience-near" elements—her patient's despair, loneliness, and self-judgment and how these affected her patient's coping responses and relationships. The psychiatrist shifted her focus to "experience-distant" elements of her patient's story, such as symptoms of depression as a diagnostic category—What were the most prominent symptoms? What was their pattern of occurrence? What were any associated risk factors for depression? She administered the HAM-D, whose 17 questions about depression symptoms produce a score that predicts accurately which patients are likely to respond to medication.

TREATING DEPRESSION WITH ANTIDEPRESSANTS: GENERAL PRINCIPLES

Most commonly, a physician makes a diagnosis of MDD using the DSM-5 (American Psychiatric Association, 2013) or the most recent *International Statistical Classification of Diseases and Related Health Problems* (ICD-11; World Health Organization, 2019) diagnostic criteria. Some individuals have dysthymic disorder (persistent depressive disorder) as a milder but chronic form of depression in which some of the symptoms of MDD last for at least 2 years.

A diagnosis of MDD does not necessarily give guidance as to whether antidepressant medications or psychotherapy, or both, should be employed. Psychotherapy and antidepressants have equivalent treatment outcomes for most patients with mild to moderate MDD (Hansen, 2005). A diagnosis of MDD does not tell a prescriber which drug to employ from a list of 21 different antidepressant medications that are considered "evidence-based" (Cipriani et al., 2018) (see Table 3.2). Since the U.S. Food and Drug Administration does not require head-to-head trials assessing one antidepressant against the others, we don't have data to support choosing one as the most effective one. Instead, the prescribing physician usually chooses from among the 21 evidence-based antidepressants one whose expectable side effects, as derived from research studies, are likely to be tolerable for the patient (e.g., avoids a sedating medication when the patient already complains of excessive sleepiness).

Regardless which antidepressant medication is chosen, there are basic principles about antidepressant medications that are important for both patients and clinicians to be aware of.

1. Antidepressants are effective, but their beneficial effects can be overridden if the depressed person remains subject to severe or uncontrollable daily life stressors, such as relationship conflicts, loneliness, or a nongratifying work life. They also can be limited by use of alcohol, marijuana, or other recreational drug use.

TABLE 3.2. Meta-Analyses of 21 Antidepressant Medications Considered Evidence-Based for Treatment of Major Depressive Disorder

Most effective	Least effective
• Agomelatine	• Fluoxetine
• Amitriptyline	• Fluvoxamine
• Escitalopram	• Reboxetine
• Mirtazapine	• Trazodone
• Paroxetine	
• Venlafaxine	

Most accepted/tolerable	Least accepted/highest dropout rates
• Agomelatine	• Amitriptyline
• Citalopram	• Clomipramine
• Escitalopram	• Duloxetine
• Fluoxetine	• Fluvoxamine
• Sertraline	• Reboxetine
• Vortioxetine	• Trazodone
• Venlafaxine	

Note. Data from Cipriani et al. (2018).

2. Antidepressants typically take 2–4 weeks to become effective, and their beneficial effects may not be experienced fully until 6 weeks. Side effects, unfortunately, occur right away, making adherence to treatment an important topic for psychotherapists to help address.

3. Antidepressants are not addictive or abusable, and their effectiveness continues long term. Patients with recurrent depressions have fewer episodes while continuing to take full doses daily, year after year.

It is perhaps most accurate to think of antidepressants as belonging to the family of medications called anodynes—medications that are palliative painkillers, such as aspirin or steroids. Antidepressants appear to not target specific disorders so much as bolster the stability of brain systems responding to threat or alarm. When a depressed or anxious patient takes these medications, fewer symptoms of depression or anxiety are expressed.

Despite their name, antidepressants, with few exceptions, are as effective, or more so, at relieving anxiety symptoms as they are depression symptoms (Lewis et al., 2019; Schatzberg & DeBattista, 2015, p. 431). As a general principle, all commonly utilized selective serotonin reuptake inhibitor (SSRI) antidepressants are also effective for all anxiety disorders (Kavan, Elsasser, & Barone, 2009; Ravindran & Stein, 2010). Of commonly used antidepressants, only bupropion [trade name Wellbutrin] is ineffective for treatment of anxiety disorders (Schatzberg & DeBattista, 2015, p. 431). We will next examine some of the mechanisms through which antidepressants act to produce these palliative effects.

HOW ANTIDEPRESSANTS WORK

Asking how antidepressants "work" is a complex question. It has different answers depending upon the goal—at the personal level of the individual interacting with others in society, or at the body organ level of functional brain circuits, or at the cellular level of neurons making synaptic connections with other neurons.

At the whole-person level, antidepressant medications facilitate assertive coping strategies when adversities are encountered. As discussed in Chapter 1, mammals have three patterns of response to threats or adversities—to freeze as if dead, to avoid or submit, or to move forward and strive to prevail. Perhaps the most important impact of antidepressant treatment is its shifting a depressed person behaviorally from an avoidant coping style to an assertive coping style.

At the functional brain circuitry level, antidepressants have multiple effects that can be best discussed jointly with events happening at the cellular level.

● First, chronic stimulation of norepinephrine and serotonin receptors by antidepressant medications activates a sequence of enzymatic reactions within postsynaptic neurons that ultimately strengthen synaptic connections with other neurons. This enzyme cascade prompts the DNA within the neuron to build additional stores of a protein, cyclic AMP response element binding protein (CREB). CREB initiates the repair and rebuilding of synapses, facilitating future communication between neurons. This production of CREB may serve as one final common pathway for antidepressants that regulates the serotonergic and noradrenergic systems (Blendy, 2006).

● Antidepressant medications, electroconvulsive therapy (ECT), and physical exercise each stimulate synthesis of a tiny protein, called **brain-derived neurotrophic factor (BDNF)**. BDNF activates receptors inside the cytoplasm of neurons that in turn activate protective enzymatic cascades, called MAP-kinase and PI3K cascades (Bjorkholm & Monteggia, 2016). These intracellular enzymatic cascades prompt the DNA to build BCL-2 proteins. When excessive excitatory stimulation causes too many calcium ions to enter a neuron, the excess of calcium can activate apoptotic enzyme sequences that end in cell death. BCL-2 proteins block such **apoptotic pathways** from killing the neuron. Lithium at therapeutic serum levels increases BCL-2 in the cerebral cortex of experimental animals.

● The hippocampus, which is at the center of signaling pathways for forming and retrieving new memories, is also the only place in the brain where new neurons are routinely produced. The dentate gyrus of the hippocampus is fully repopulated with new neurons over a 4- to 8-month period. This **neurogenesis** in the hippocampus is dependent upon adequate levels of BDNF. Reduced hippocampal neurogenesis may be associated with some of the cognitive effects of depression on working memory and new learning. Chronic stress and depression markedly diminish BDNF. Antidepressants and ECT increase levels of BDNF and the rate of neurogenesis (Rotheneichner et al., 2014).

At a cellular level, **tricyclic** and **heterocyclic** antidepressants, **SSRI (selective serotonin reuptake inhibitor)** antidepressants, and **SNRI (serotonin–norepinephrine reuptake inhibitor)** antidepressants all inhibit reuptake of serotonin and/or norepinephrine after they have been released into the synaptic cleft. This action causes the serotonin and norepinephrine neurotransmitters to accumulate within the synapse. These pools of neurotransmitters stimulate a serotonin or norepinephrine autoreceptor, whose job it is to slow down the discharge rate of the neuron when excessively stimulated, that is, to act as a "brake" on how fast the neuron fires. At first the braking effects slow down **neurotransmission** in the serotonin or norepinephrine systems. This slowing down correlates behaviorally with the low mood and irritability that sometimes occurs during the first days after an antidepressant is prescribed. After 10–14 days, however, excessive stimulation of the autoreceptor desensitizes the autoreceptor, analogous to wearing out the brakes in an automobile when overused. Unrestrained, the firing rate of the neuron then rises to a higher than normal rate. This elevated neurotransmission of the monoamine systems produces the effects outlined in the section above. These longer term changes correlate with amelioration of dysphoric mood and recovery of hedonia, energy, sleep, and depressive symptoms, usually 2–4 weeks after initiating antidepressant treatment. Elevated neurotransmission within the monoamine systems strengthens emotion regulation, so that the prefrontal cortex can exert more effective top-down control over bottom-up processing by amygdala, insula, and ventral anterior cingulate systems. Alarm responses are dampened and body arousal drops.

Looking across these three levels of description, we can see how antidepressants act at multiple sites at a cellular level to have dual effects at a brain circuitry level: First, they amplify neurotransmission in serotonin and norepinephrine monoamine systems, with the downstream effect of strengthening synaptic connectivity between neurons, rendering emotion regulation by prefrontal cortex more effective; second, they initiate intracellular processes that protect stressed, vulnerable neurons, such as BCL-2 synthesis, and processes that rebuild synapses, such as BDNF and CREB synthesis. These changes are manifested behaviorally in a shift from avoidant coping to assertive coping in the person's daily life. With the lifting of depression, a person becomes more able to feel motivated by desire, to seek goals, and to strive to overcome obstacles.

THE DOWNSIDES OF ANTIDEPRESSANT USE: SIDE EFFECTS

As mentioned earlier, there are now 21 different antidepressants that can be regarded as evidence-based for treatment of depression (Cipriani et al., 2018). Since we have limited data to guide choices based upon which antidepressant is most effective, selection is more often based upon side-effect profile. After all, nothing could be worse for a depressed person than to take a medication that makes them feel worse than they felt without the medication. Selecting medications with tolerable side effects is essential for patients to adhere to treatment.

Although a physician will prescribe an antidepressant medication, the psychotherapist may be in the best position to monitor side effects and treatment adherence. A therapist typically has more frequent patient encounters, longer encounters, and a better vantage point for observing directly a patient's well-being in daily life. It is important for a therapist to know her client's medications and their common side effects, since this is important information to relay to the prescribing physician. Some patients would feel stigmatized if a physician were to prescribe a medication for mood or anxiety symptoms. Some patients with diagnosable mood or anxiety disorders continue to require long-term maintenance medications even after acute symptoms improve, in order to reduce future risks for relapse. Patients often feel confused about why they should take an antidepressant or mood stabilizer after acute symptoms dissipate. In such cases, the therapist can have a crucial role in helping a patient accept the need for medication and understand its rationale.

Most antidepressant side effects are due to the medication-blocking neurotransmitter receptors other than those associated with mood improvement, as shown in Table 3.3. The older tricyclic antidepressants

TABLE 3.3. Tricyclic Antidepressants

Side Effects Due to Blockade of Neurotransmitter System Receptors	
1. Postsynaptic Alpha$_{-1}$ Receptors	Postural hypotension
2. Histamine Type 1 Receptors	Increased appetite and sedation
3. Histamine Type 2 Receptors	Reduced stomach acid secretion
4. Muscarinic M$_{-1}$ Receptors	Dry mouth, constipation, blurry vision, tremor, rapid pulse, confusion (in overdose)

Side Effects Due to Excessive Activation of Neurotransmitter Receptors	
1. Serotonin 5HT$_{-3}$ Receptors	Cramping, nausea, diarrhea
2. Serotonin 5HT-2A Receptors	Agitation, sexual side effects
3. Serotonin 5HT-2C Receptors	Increased appetite, weight gain

No Side Effects from Either Activation or Blockade of Neurotransmitter Receptors	
1. Dopamine Receptors	No effects of significance

have most of these side effects. The SSRI, SNRI, and other newer antidepressants have few or none of these side effects, as discussed in subsequent sections. The most common SSRI side effects are sexual side effects—diminished libido, erectile dysfunction, or anorgasmia—that may be due not to a neurotransmitter mechanism, but rather to a decrease in nitric oxide level that serves a normal physiological role in sexual arousal.

MANAGING ANTIDEPRESSANT SIDE EFFECTS

Waiting

Side effects are least disruptive to long-term treatment when they can be managed by adjusting the dose and administration schedule of the medication and waiting. A conservative approach waits for the passage of time, perhaps several weeks, to see if side effects, such as sexual side effects, disappear with habituation to the medication. Many side effects, such as nausea, slowly disappear for most patients during the first weeks of treatment. Spontaneous resolution of sexual side effects is not as common, but when it happens there is no need to change the medication or dose.

Reducing Dose

Reducing the dose of the antidepressant is also an alternative. Since most side effects are dose-related, a decrease in the dose would be expected to result in amelioration of side effects, and indeed, it often does. The problem with this approach is that there is an inherent risk of relapse with dose reductions, meaning clinicians who choose this approach will have to monitor patients closely.

Drug Holiday

A third conservative approach is the drug holiday. For example, a patient can skip taking the drug for a day or so before planned sexual activity. The sharp reduction in antidepressant blood levels sometimes results in temporary disappearance or at least reduction of the sexual dysfunction. This method has several limitations as well: It precludes spontaneous sexual activity; it may lead to relapse of depressive symptoms; it may produce antidepressant withdrawal symptoms (see Table 3.4), which can be severe enough to squelch the desire of even the most passionate of lovers; and it is restricted to patients on antidepressants with a short

TABLE 3.4. Symptoms That May Occur during Acute SSRI Withdrawal

Physical symptoms	Psychological symptoms
⊙ Lightheadedness	⊙ Anxiety/agitation
⊙ Headaches	⊙ Depression
⊙ Nausea, vomiting	⊙ Spontaneous, uncontrollable crying
⊙ Tremors	⊙ Irritability
⊙ Muscle pain	⊙ Restlessness
⊙ Sensations of electric shock	⊙ Decreased concentration
⊙ Insomnia, vivid dreams	⊙ Derealization, depersonalization
	⊙ Confusion
	⊙ Memory difficulties

half-life, such as paroxetine (trade name Paxil). Blood levels of long half-life compounds such as fluoxetine (trade name Prozac) would not drop quickly enough to create the planned holiday.

Substitution

Even in the presence of a robust antidepressant effect, the burden of side effects sometimes makes it impractical to continue with the same treatment. In these situations, the offending antidepressant is substituted by another one expected to have a much lower potential for causing side effects. This approach is also fraught with certain risks, as the response to one antidepressant does not guarantee a response to a different one, and thus relapse may occur. It is important to remember that not all antidepressants work with equal efficacy in all patients, and many times responses are idiosyncratic. Also, the introduction of a different antidepressant may result in the appearance of a new set of side effects— intolerable agitation, excessive sedation, or fatigue, to cite some common ones—that may turn out to be even more bothersome than the side effect that prompted the substitution.

Antidote Strategies

At least 30–40% of patients taking an SSRI or SNRI will report sexual side effects, such as delayed ejaculation, anorgasmia, impotence, or diminished libido. For sexual side effects, no single approach to management is consistently effective for all patients, but a series of countermeasures can be tried in sequence to determine which is most helpful for a specific patient (Balon & Segraves, 2008; Nurnberg et al., 2003; Schatzberg & DeBattista, 2015, pp. 70–72; Zajecka, 2001):

1. The half-life of paroxetine is sufficiently short that holding a dose for 24 hours before sexual activity can diminish adverse effects.
2. Bupropion at a dose of 150–300 mg daily can improve libido and sexual functioning for some patients when added to the original antidepressant.
3. Sildenafil (trade name Viagra) for some male patients significantly improves sexual functioning.
4. Cyproheptadine (trade name Periactin), a 5-HT$_2$ antagonist, has been reported effective in some cases when 4–12 mg is administered a few hours before sexual activity.
5. Amantadine, a dopamine agonist, has been reported effective in some cases at 100 to 300 mg daily doses.

When sexual side effects cannot be effectively managed, a switch to an antidepressant with few sexual side effects, such as bupropion, nefazodone, mirtazapine, or levomilnacipran may be warranted (Schatzberg & DeBattista, 2015, pp. 70–72).

Although it may be necessary to try more than one of these strategies before finding the one that will work for a particular patient, sexual dysfunction as a side effect must not be passively accepted during the treatment of individuals with depression. In fact, ignoring the importance of this side effect—or any others, for that matter—will greatly risk treatment nonadherence and the very real probability of relapse. Also, a clinician's indifference to the presence of sexual dysfunction is likely to affect the patient's self-esteem and relationship with his or her spouse or partner.

TYPES OF ANTIDEPRESSANT MEDICATIONS

There are five major classes of antidepressants. Medications that belong to the same class have similar therapeutic effects and side effects.

Monoamine Oxidase Inhibitors

Monoamine oxidase inhibitors (MAOIs) are the oldest antidepressants, yet they remain the most effective medications for some patients with mood and anxiety disorders. They were discovered through serendipity. Clinicians treating patients with tuberculosis noted that some patients stayed in more buoyant moods than might be expected given the loneliness of their isolation in sanitoriums and their often dire prognoses.

They identified isoniazid, an antituberculosis medication, as the factor that correlated with positive moods. Isoniazid proved to be a MAOI.

When **monoamines** serotonin, norepinephrine, and dopamine are secreted into synaptic clefts, they must be disposed of after the task of stimulating postsynaptic receptors has been accomplished. One mechanism, reuptake of the neurotransmitter, has already been discussed—a transporter molecule in the cell wall of the neuron attaches to the monoamine molecule and shuttles it back inside the neuron for reuse. A second mechanism is for an enzyme, monoamine oxidase, to degrade the monoamine enzymatically. Free-floating monoamine molecules can damage neurons, so monoamine oxidase acts as a scavenger to destroy free-floating monoamines within the cytoplasm of neurons.

Monoamine oxidase is also located in the lining of the intestines and in the liver to degrade any monoamines in the foods we eat. Tyramine, produced by fermentation in cheese, aged meats, beer, and many other foods, occurs commonly in most diets. Tyramine in the bloodstream can dangerously elevate blood pressure, so monoamine oxidase in the intestines and liver degrade it before it can do harm.

MAOIs work by deactivating monoamine oxidase. This permits serotonin, dopamine, and norepinephrine to remain longer and in larger quantities within their synapses, until the remaining mechanism, the reuptake transporter, can clean up. This has the effect of boosting neurotransmission in all three monoamine systems, with consequent reduction in anxiety and depressive symptoms. Some psychopharmacologists have argued that MAOIs are the most potent medications for treatment of panic disorder, and they have demonstrated particular efficacy for the subtype of atypical depression characterized by excessive fatigue, sleepiness, and increased appetite.

There are two MAOIs available as tablets for oral ingestion, **phenelzine** (trade name Nardil) and **tranylcypromine** (trade name Parnate). In addition, there is a **selegiline** transdermal patch (trade name Emsam), which a patient applies to his skin each day so that the MAOI selegiline can be absorbed directly through the skin into the bloodstream without entering the gastrointestinal tract (Schatzberg & DeBattista, 2015, pp. 134–149).

The challenge in using MAOIs is the requirement that patients adhere strictly to a diet that is free of tyramine (i.e., no aged or fermented foods) and also avoid medications that can impair serotonin reuptake. Foods that must be avoided include most foods in an Italian diet and many ethnic foods, such as sausages (Rappaport, 2007) (see Table 3.5). Parmesan and other sharp cheeses have extraordinarily high levels of tyramine, capable of producing dangerous levels of hypertension. Separately,

TABLE 3.5. Dietary Food Restrictions for Patients on MAOI Antidepressants

Foods to avoid	Foods permitted
• Aged or sharp cheeses • Fermented or dry sausage or pepperoni • Broad bean pods • Sauerkraut or soy sauce • Draft beer	• Fresh American cheese, mild cheeses • Fresh meat, poultry, fish • Bottled or canned beer (up to 2 glasses) • Red or white wine (up to 2 glasses)

Note. Data from Rappaport (2007).

medications that can inhibit serotonin reuptake can produce a sudden **serotonin syndrome** with hyperthermia, coma, seizures, and death. Such medications include all opioid medications other than morphine and codeine. Deaths have occurred when a MAOI-treated patient has been administered meperidine (trade name Demerol) in a hospital emergency room. Deaths have also occurred when a patient who has been on a MAOI has been inadvertently prescribed an SSRI antidepressant, such as **fluoxetine** (trade name Prozac). Despite these dangers, many patients fare best when treated with MAOIs rather than other antidepressants. Patients can improve provided they fully adhere to the dietary and medication restrictions.

An advantage of using the selegiline transdermal patch is that it leaves intact the monoamine oxidase in the gastrointestinal tract, eliminating the need for dietary food restrictions at the lower 6 mg or 9 mg daily dosages. Dietary restrictions are recommended at the higher 12 mg daily dosage. Drug–drug interactions remain a risk, however, so patients using the patch must remain vigilant in avoiding the medications in Table 3.6.

TABLE 3.6. Medication Restrictions for Patients Taking MAOIs

Serotonin syndrome risks	Hypertensive crisis risks
• Opioid analgesics (other than morphine or codeine, which are safe) • SSRI or SNRI antidepressants • Tricyclic antidepressants • Tryptophan • Dextromethorphan (in cough syrups)	• Cold tablets containing ephedrine, pseudoephedrine, or phenylpropanolamine • Psychostimulants (methylphenidate or amphetamine)

MAOIs, due to their lack of some side effects, such as dry mouth and sedation, are sometimes easier for patients to take than some other antidepressants are. But MAOIs have their own dangerous side effects, such as hypertensive crisis and serotonin syndrome, as well as list of "nuisance" side effects. Insomnia is the most common reason patients choose to discontinue MAOIs. Postural hypotension, experienced as dizziness on sudden standing from sitting or lying down, occurs at higher doses. Increased appetite with weight gain can occur. Reduced intensity of sexual orgasms at high doses, and difficulty with urination for older men with prostate hypertrophy can also occur (Schatzberg & DeBattista, 2015, pp. 134–149).

Tricyclic Antidepressants

Following discovery of the first antipsychotic medication, **chlorpromazine,** in 1950, researchers began testing similar compounds in a search for additional antipsychotic medications. A molecule characterized by its three-ring structure, **imipramine,** was found to have no antipsychotic properties, but it did produce behavioral activation and positive improvements in mood. Imipramine became the first tricyclic antidepressant. In 1962, imipramine was shown to be effective in stopping panic attacks in patients with panic disorder. In the late 1980s it was shown to produce notable reductions in generalized anxiety in patients with anxiety disorders. Today tricyclic antidepressants remain the most potent antidepressant medications, particularly in severe cases of depression, albeit with more side effects than the newer SSRIs and SNRIs.

Tricyclic antidepressants are reuptake inhibitors for both the serotonin and norepinephrine transporters. However, tricyclic antidepressants also block other neurotransmitter receptors. Blockade of these systems accounts for side effects of these medications, such as dry mouth, blurry vision, drowsiness, difficulty with urination, or dizziness when standing suddenly from postural hypotension (see Table 3.3). Generally, elderly patients have more severe side effects with tricyclic medications, but which ones and how severe otherwise varies greatly from one person to the next. Usually, side effects are maximal in the first few days after starting a medication, then attenuate over the next few weeks as the body accommodates. Newer SSRI and SNRI antidepressants are generally no more effective than tricyclics in diminishing depression symptoms, but they have less severe side effects for most people.

Tricyclic antidepressants repeatedly proved effective for MDD, panic disorder, and generalized anxiety disorder in research studies. The following brief vignette is typical for treatment of MDD with the tricyclic antidepressant, **amitriptyline.**

Ms. Woods was 40 years old when friends convinced her that she should consult a psychiatrist for her depression. She was ruminating on her life's failures and disappointments. She had become isolated at home and enjoyed no pleasurable activities. When asked directly she said she had no wish to keep living, although she had no plans for suicide. The psychiatrist found that she scored in a severe range on the HAM-D due to symptoms of low mood, severe insomnia, and mid-sleep awakenings, loss of interest in usually pleasurable activities, and a high level of anxiety. The psychiatrist suggested treatment with the tricyclic antidepressant, amitriptyline, since its sedative effects would also help her insomnia. In addition, she suffered from both migraine headaches and bouts of irritable bowel syndrome. Amitriptyline is an effective medication to prevent migraine headaches, and it often eases spasms of the gastrointestinal tract as a beneficial side effect. After the first week of treatment, Ms. Woods returned to the psychiatrist unhappy with her treatment due to daytime drowsiness, dry mouth, dizziness if standing too quickly, and blurry vision. The psychiatrist reassured her that these were typical side effects of the medication, and, on a positive note, their presence was evidence that her brain was being impacted by the medication. He assured her, "Side effects occur right away, symptoms improve in 2–4 weeks." Like clockwork, Ms. Wood's symptoms began to diminish by the second week. By the fourth week of treatment, she was sleeping well, enjoying reading and taking afternoon walks, with no anxiety. Her migraine headaches had diminished, and her irritable bowel symptoms had improved. "I feel more like me now," she said. Her amitriptyline side effects of sedation, dizziness standing, and blurry vision mostly disappeared over time, although dry mouth from diminished saliva persisted. Her psychiatrist suggested that she chew sugarless gum or sugarless mints to lessen this lingering problem.

Discovery of Nontricyclic Antidepressant Medications

While tricyclic antidepressants had potent therapeutic effects, the side effects of tricyclic antidepressants propelled a search for new drugs. The "nuisance side effects" of sedation, dry mouth, blurry vision, constipation, slow urination, increased appetite, impaired sexual functioning, and dizziness if standing too quickly (postural hypotension) led to high rates of treatment discontinuation. Many patients decided they would rather suffer depression than these side effects. Tricyclic antidepressants also proved dangerous for patients with heart electrical conduction abnormalities due to cardiac disease. Such patients could be at risk for sudden death. However, risks for lethal overdoses in suicide attempts spurred the greatest concern. Tricyclic antidepressants were rapidly absorbed into the bloodstream after oral ingestion. A typical daily dose of amitriptyline was 150 mg. Yet deaths from overdose suicide attempts often occurred with no more than 1,000 mg ingested at once—a 1-week supply of the medication.

A continuing search for safer antidepressants with few side effects continued. Pharmaceutical research programs were initially organized by a belief that the "antidepressant magic" of tricyclics lay in their three-ring molecular structure. Clinical researchers finally abandoned the three-ring criteria and began testing organic molecules with more, or less, than three rings. This search led to four nontricyclics that preserved most of the benefits of the tricyclics but with fewer side effects.

Trazodone, nefazodone, bupropion, and mirtazapine were new anti-depressants much safer in case of overdose, while still effective as anti-depressants. Nefazodone, trazodone, and bupropion were relatively free from weight gain as a side effect. All four medications were relatively free of sexual side effects, adding to their appeal. Trazodone proved less robust than the tricyclics as an antidepressant, but the potent sedation that it produced led to its most widespread use as a treatment for insomnia. Bupropion proved ineffective for anxiety symptoms, but still an effective and safe antidepressant, particularly for elderly or medically ill patients due to absence of cardiovascular system side effects. Mirtazapine had two major side effects adverse for many outpatients—increased appetite and sedation—but these same side effects were advantageous when patients had a chronic medical illness that produced appetite loss and disrupted sleep.

SSRI and "Dual-Action" SNRI Antidepressants

SSRI antidepressants were synthesized through a search for compounds that might have the antidepressant potency of tricyclic antidepressants but with minimal side effects. These efforts led first to fluoxetine, which was introduced in 1987, followed by fluvoxamine, sertraline, paroxetine, citalopram, and escitalopram.

Venlafaxine (trade name Effexor) is an SNRI. It was marketed in 1993, followed a decade later by duloxetine (trade name Cymbalta) and levomilnacipran (trade name Fetzima). As a general rule, all SSRI/SNRI antidepressants are effective for MDD, all anxiety disorders, and post-traumatic stress disorder. There is some evidence that tricyclic antidepressants are more potent in treating severe depression, such as patients with **melancholic depression,** or suicidal patients admitted to psychiatric inpatient units. Otherwise, tricyclics and SSRIs/SNRIs appeared to have equivalent efficacies.

The fact that SSRI and SNRI antidepressants were generally free of nuisance side effects, particularly dry mouth, blurry vision, urinary retention, and postural hypotension, expanded use of antidepressants to millions of Americans. SSRI and SNRI antidepressants are far safer in overdose than are tricyclic antidepressants. Almost no deaths have ever been recorded due to overdoses of SSRIs as the sole medication. A lethal dose of fluoxetine requires ingestion of an estimated 75 times a therapeutic daily dose. A lethal dose of venlafaxine requires approximately 30 times a therapeutic daily dose.

SSRI and SNRI antidepressants do have their own group of nuisance side effects. There are serotonin receptors in the gastrointestinal (GI) tract that when activated by SSRI or SNRI antidepressants produce significant rates of nausea, cramping, and diarrhea. Approximately 20% of patients will have significant GI side effects. Problematic for many, these antidepressants have high rates of sexual side effects, particularly delayed or absent orgasm. As discussed earlier, 30–40% of patients have some degree of diminished libido or anorgasmia.

While safe in overdose, SSRI and SNRI antidepressants can have a potentially lethal drug–drug interaction, serotonin syndrome, if inadvertently combined with medication that increases accumulation of synaptic serotonin in the brain. Serotonin syndrome can produce rigidity, extremely high body temperatures, seizures, coma, or death (Schatzberg & DeBattista, 2015, pp. 75, 114, 588). Serotonin syndrome can be precipitated by taking more than one antidepressant simultaneously or combining SSRI/SNRI antidepressants with drugs for medical conditions that nevertheless have serotonin-agonist properties. Chief among the latter are synthetic opioid medications (other than morphine or codeine) administered for pain management. Serotonin syndrome, with some deaths, has occurred when meperidine [trade name Demerol], fentanyl, or cough syrups containing dextromethorphan were given to patients already taking daily doses of SSRI, SNRI, or MAOI antidepressants.

Staying within their scope of practice, therapists can play important roles in educating patients about wise practices when utilizing antidepressant medications, such as the importance of taking medications as prescribed or risks from impulsive discontinuation of treatment. For example, sudden discontinuation of tricyclic, SSRI, or SNRI antidepressants produces an unpleasant, sometimes frightening, flu-like discontinuation syndrome, with malaise, nausea, headaches, dizziness, and agitation. The greatest risk for a discontinuation syndrome occurs with paroxetine, due to its short half-life. The physician can prevent a **discontinuation syndrome** simply by tapering the daily dose by 25% per week so that the antidepressant is slowly discontinued. The therapist's role can be important for facilitating an informed, collaborative relationship between patient and physician around medication decision making.

In summary, the six decades following serendipitous 1950s discoveries of tricyclic and MAOI antidepressants produced no game-changing advances in efficacy of antidepressant treatment, even though new generations of medications were developed. However, there were marked advances in reduction of side effects, expanding acceptability of medications. New drugs were safer in overdose. Several new antidepressants were free of sexual, weight gain, sedation, dry mouth, and other side effects that had led to discontinuation of tricyclics. Nevertheless, the new drugs had little new to offer the 15% of patients with treatment-**refractory** depression that had failed to respond to adequate doses and treatment duration with tricyclics or MAOIs. Psychopharmacology for mood disorders largely consisted of selecting the antidepressant medication whose side-effect profile best fit a particular patient's tolerances— not selecting medication based on evidence-based criteria for best efficacy.

A NOVEL TREATMENT: GLUTAMINERGIC MEDICATIONS AS ANTIDEPRESSANTS

The simplest explanation for the lack of progress in producing more efficacious medications is that each of the 21 evidence-based antidepressants still operated through the same physiological mechanism of enhancing efficiency of the monoamine systems. Since norepinephrine, serotonin, and dopamine account for less than 0.01% of all the brain's neurotransmitter synapses, researchers searched for other neurotransmitters that might regulate moods.

Ketamine, a medication that binds tightly to **NMDA glutamate receptors,** had been commonly utilized as an anesthetic for decades. However, researchers noted that in low doses it both relieved chronic physical pain and elevated the mood of research subjects. The mechanism through which ketamine exerts its mood-elevating effects has been unclear. Ketamine augments the actions of glutamate, the brain's major excitatory neurotransmitter. The prefrontal cortex exerts top-down regulation over the insula and ventral anterior cingulate circuits where bottom-up processing generates the suffering of physical or emotional pain. The most parsimonious explanation for ketamine's efficacy simply may be that it amplifies this top-down regulation by the prefrontal cortex.

Ketamine, in usual antidepressant doses, typically lacks adverse side effects. It is distinguished from other antidepressant medications by its rapid reversal of depressed mood within 4 hours of intravenous administration, peaking at 24 hours, and lasting up to 10 days. Unlike other antidepressant medications, ketamine can reverse the despair and suicidal ideation associated with stressful life circumstances, suggesting that it may have a specific role in acute care of patients who are suicidal due to life crises. An understanding for the appropriate niche for ketamine in the full scope of antidepressant therapies is still evolving (Sanacora et al., 2017).

Esketamine (trade name Spravato) is ketamine administered as a nasal spray. Esketamine has been approved for treatment-resistant depression by the U.S. Food and Drug Administration (FDA). However, FDA regulations require that administration occurs in the office of a physician registered in the FDA Risk Evaluation and Mitigation Program (REMS), where observation for adverse effects can be conducted over 2 hours postadministration. This limits use of esketamine in primary care settings. Since generic ketamine is commercially available as a veterinary anesthetic, there is a black market for self-administered ketamine. Self-administration is ill-advised due to possible hypertension or dissociative symptoms that can occur as side effects.

WHAT IF THE FIRST ANTIDEPRESSANT DOESN'T WORK?

Although antidepressant medications have made a dramatic difference in the outcome of depressive illness, they are by no means the panacea for which many had hoped. The overall *response* rate to antidepressants is thought to be in the vicinity of 60–70% after the first attempt. Response is defined as a 50% or greater reduction in the severity of symptoms, usually measured in research studies with the HAM-D (Hamilton, 1960) or the MADRS (Montgomery–Asberg Depression Rating Scale; Montgomery & Asberg, 1979).

Although this represents a considerable reduction in suffering and disability, it is not by any means the ultimate goal of treatment. If we apply the more stringent—and more logical—standard of *remission* (i.e., HAM-D scores of less than 7, more or less the equivalent to the feelings experienced by the average individual on a given Monday morning), then the efficacy of antidepressants drops to 35–50%. This limited performance leaves a considerable number of patients in need of supplemental or alternative treatment. Several factors are thought to be at play in those patients obtaining less than desirable clinical benefit (see Table 3.7).

TABLE 3.7. Considerations for Nonresponse to Treatment

- Reassessment of clinical status
- Reconsideration of the diagnosis
- Core residual symptoms or side effects
- Dose and duration
- Drug interactions
- Augmentation
- Substitution
- Treatment nonadherence

Wrong Diagnosis

Several subtypes of depression require specific treatment strategies that go beyond a simple course of conventional antidepressant therapy. These subtypes include **bipolar depression, major depression with psychotic features, seasonal depression, atypical depression,** "double depression" (major depression plus dysthymia), and depression **comorbid** with anxiety disorder, substance abuse, or persistent psychosocial stressors. When there is no significant improvement following an initial course of an antidepressant (nonresponse), the clinician will be well advised to reevaluate the patient for the presence of depressive subtypes or unique circumstances that require a specific approach.

Inadequate Treatment Trial

Even when the diagnosis is correct, certain minimal parameters of dose and time are necessary for satisfactory clinical outcomes. When tricyclic antidepressants were the mainstay of antidepressant treatment, their side effects required starting doses much lower than therapeutic doses. The physician had to increase doses slowly in order to minimize and manage the emerging side effects. It typically took 1–3 weeks to reach therapeutic doses. Because this requirement was not always understood, many patients failed to receive adequate doses, and nonresponse was an incorrect conclusion. Since the introduction of the SSRIs, physicians can quickly titrate up to full doses. Table 3.8 shows dose ranges for selected antidepressants. These ranges are for general reference only. Often, physicians will exceed FDA-approved doses when unique clinical situations so require.

A second important factor in nonresponse is insufficient duration of treatment. All antidepressant medications have a lag period between the time treatment starts and the time when a clinical response is readily

**TABLE 3.8. Dose Ranges
for Selected Antidepressants**

Drug name	Dose range (mg/day)
○ Amitriptyline	50–300
○ Bupropion	200–450
○ Bupropion SR	150–400
○ Citalopram	20–60
○ Clomipramine	50–250
○ Desipramine	100–300
○ Duloxetine	40–60
○ Escitalopram	10–20
○ Fluoxetine	20–60
○ Imipramine	75–300
○ Mirtazapine	15–60
○ Nortriptyline	75–150
○ Paroxetine	10–60
○ Paroxetine CR	12.5–62.5
○ Phenelzine	15–90
○ Sertraline	50–200
○ Tranylcypromine	30–60
○ Venlafaxine	75–300
○ Venlafaxine XR	75–225

apparent. One-third of patients who have shown no response at 2 weeks will experience substantial benefit if the same treatment is continued. When no response is seen after 4 weeks, a full fifth of these patients will still respond to treatment if continued to 6 weeks. As a practical point, it seems prudent to consider modifications to the treatment regime after 3–4 weeks if there has not been substantial improvement.

Once it has been determined that treatment response is unlikely, physicians have at their disposal a number of choices. These strategies— optimization (push the dose of the current drug to the maximum tolerable), substitution (change from one drug to another), and **augmentation** (keep the first drug but add another because the combination is often more effective than the first drug alone).

Unfortunately, clinical psychiatry has not yet validated systematic approaches to applying these techniques to treatment of refractory patients. The **STAR*D** project (Sequential Treatment Alternatives to Relieve Depression) has attempted to provide an answer to the question of what to do when a patient fails to benefit from the first antidepressant. This study tested the benefits and limitations of a sequential order of treatment strategies. Patients who did not respond to initial SSRI treatment (citalopram [trade name Celexa] was the SSRI used initially in all subjects) progressed to Level 1, where they were assigned to one of a number of treatment options. The options available at Level 2 included the addition of, or substitution of, CBT. If no response occurred at this level, patients then progressed to Level 3 and, as necessary, to Level 4, where more options were available (see Figure 3.1). The STAR*D protocol also provided for a minimum duration and dosages of each of the treatments utilized in order to avoid failures derived from insufficiency in these areas.

Initial results for the STAR*D study were published early in 2006, providing useful insights for the clinician (Rush et al., 2006; Trivedi, Fava, et al., 2006; Trivedi, Rush, et al., 2006). Level 1 patients treated with the citalopram showed only a 28% rate of remission. Level 2 results showed that patients who failed to benefit from SSRI treatment (citalopram) were good candidates for augmentation with sustained-release bupropion or with buspirone, or by switching to sustained-release bupropion or sertraline or sustained-release venlafaxine—three antidepressants with different mechanisms of action. One-third of the patients in each of these Level 2 groups reached remission. Thus, overall, after two

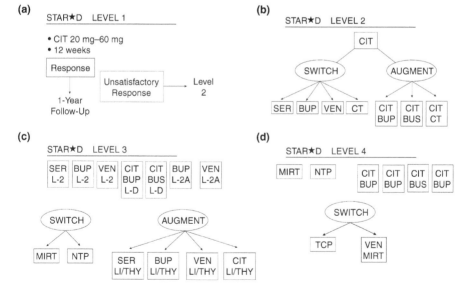

FIGURE 3.1. Protocol for the STAR*D project. (a) Level 1; (b) Level 2; (c) Level 3; (d) Level 4. CIT, citalopram; SER, sertraline; BUP, bupropion; VEN, venlafaxine; CBT, cognitive-behavioral therapy; BUS, buspirone; MIRT, mirtazapine; NTP, nortriptyline; LI, lithium; THY, thyroid hormone; TCP, tranylcypromine.

well-delivered (robust doses and sufficient duration) medication treatment courses only about 50% of the patients achieved full remission of symptoms. Level 3 results showed additional modest gains and comparable efficacy for lithium and thyroid augmentation (Lebowitz, Shores-Wilson, Rush, & STAR*D Study Team, 2006). Level 4 results also showed very modest treatment improvement in nonresponders (about 10%) and suggested that the extended-release venlafaxine–mirtazapine combination may be a better choice than MAOIs, based on ease of use.

Some Augmentation Strategies for Antidepressant Medications

As validated by the STAR*D study, augmentation agents can be added to boost the potency of an antidepressant when there has been a partial but insufficient response. This provides an alternative strategy to discontinuing the initial antidepressant and switching to a different one.

Lithium Augmentation

The augmentation strategy with the most evidence has been addition of lithium carbonate to the initial antidepressant (Bauer & Dopfmer, 1999). An estimated 50% of nonresponders to tricyclic antidepressants converted to responder status when low-dose lithium (300–900 mg daily) was added to the initial antidepressant. This low dose of lithium usually had no additional side effects. Moreover, about a third of patients for whom low-dose lithium is added to an antidepressant showed objective improvement in mood within the first 48 hours. However, most research studies on lithium augmentation were conducted with tricyclic and MAOI antidepressants, and the potency of lithium augmentation has appeared to be less with SSRIs.

Thyroid Augmentation

Addition of thyroid hormone to an initial antidepressant is an augmentation strategy supported by numbers of research studies, including the STAR*D. Either T4 (**thyroxine**) or T3 (**Cytomel**) can be added in small daily doses to the antidepressant.

Combining Antidepressant with Atypical Antipsychotic

Three atypical antipsychotic medications are FDA-approved as adjuncts (aripiprazole and quetiapine) or in combination (olanzapine–fluoxetine) with antidepressant medications. Meta-analyses of research studies have found adjunctive atypical antipsychotics to have a twofold higher odds of achieving remission compared to adjunctive placebo. Of these three strategies, aripiprazole augmentation has found greatest usage by far due to its minimal sedative and weight-gain side effects.

Addition of Second Antidepressant outside the Initial Class

Addition of a second antidepressant from a different drug class than that of the initial antidepressant has become common practice in community psychiatric practices but has not been studied in any systematic manner. No antidepressant is FDA approved for combination antidepressant treatment. Judiciously selected, however, combination regimens appear to be well tolerated with sustained benefits in some patients who have been unresponsive to **monotherapy.**

Some combination regimens that have at least a plausible rationale for use include:

- addition of low-dose tricyclic antidepressant to an SSRI;
- bupropion added to an SSRI or SNRI; and
- extended-release venlafaxine (in the morning) added to mirtazapine (at bedtime).

This combined regimen attempts to cross out each drug's side effects. Venlafaxine, an activating antidepressant, can counter the sedative side effects of mirtazapine in the morning. On the other hand, mirtazepine's antinausea side effect may counter gastrointestinal side effects of venlafaxine, and mirtazapine, taken at bedtime, can deepen sleep, while blocking sexual side effects that can occur with venlafaxine. (Schatzberg & DeBattista, 2015)

Addition of Buspirone

Several studies have found treatment-refractory patients to show improvement in depressive symptoms when buspirone is added for augmentation. Buspirone is most commonly prescribed for generalized anxiety disorder. Its use usually adds few side effects. (Schatzberg & DeBattista, 2015)

Addition of Omega-3 Fatty Acid Dietary Supplement

Addition of 2,000 mg daily doses of E-EPA (ethyl ester of eicosapentaenoic acid) to an antidepressant has been reported to decrease depressive symptoms for patients on chronic antidepressant treatment, but with "breakthrough depressions." Responses occurred in 2–3 weeks (Schatzberg & DeBattista, 2015).

Addition of Psychostimulant

Several negative studies have failed to show improvement in depressive symptoms when psychostimulants, such as methylphenidate (trade name Ritalin), or wakefulness medications, such as modafinil (trade name Pro-Vigil), were utilized as adjuncts to conventional antidepressant therapy. However, both medications can be effective for fatigue and **somnolence** that commonly persist as residual symptoms, even when other depression symptoms improved with antidepressant treatment. Patients with fatigue from chronic medical illnesses, such as AIDS, and elderly patients who are apathetic and anhedonic can be good candidates for psychostimulant or wakefulness augmentation. (Schatzberg & DeBattista, 2015).

ECT and Treatment-Resistant Depression

The long search for effective medications to treat depression has fallen short for many patients. The STAR*D study, for example, showed that only half of its patients achieved remission of symptoms after two trials of different antidepressant regiments. A review of multiple research studies found that between 29 and 46% of depressed patients fail to respond despite antidepressant treatment of adequate dose and duration. Of these, a third showed no response at all (Fava & Davidson, 1996). Depression that fails to respond to initial treatment becomes chronic in as many as 40% of elderly patients, a demographic group that is at highest risk for suicide (Rhee, Olfson, Sint, & Wilkinson, 2020; Unutzer & Park, 2012).

ECT has long stood as the most effective treatment for patients who show none or only partial responses to two or more antidepressant medication trials. ECT originated out of observations in German neuropsychiatric hospitals in the late 1800s that patients who had both epilepsy and severe mood disorders often showed remission of mood symptoms after a bout of seizures.

Use of ECT receded in the later 20th century as increasing numbers of antidepressant medications became available. However, antidepressant treatment outcomes have consistently fallen short of the 60–80% remission rates when ECT has been used as first-line treatment for severe or psychotic depression (Petrides et al., 2001). A meta-analysis of 18 randomized, controlled trials conducted by the United Kingdom ECT Review Group found ECT to be more efficacious than antidepressant pharmacotherapy, with an average effect size of 0.80 (Royal College of Psychiatrists, 2017). Speed of response with ECT was rapid—one-third of patients responded (HAM-D score <10) by the 6th session (2 weeks), and two-thirds of patients respond by the 10th session (3–4 weeks). For suicidal patients there was frequently cessation of suicidal impulses within the first week. ECT has been considered to be the treatment of choice for depression with psychotic features, such as delusions or hallucinations, in which suicide risk is high (Royal College of Psychiatrists, 2017).

There is a consensus among mood disorder specialists that ECT is underutilized due to the frequent need for hospitalization and societal stigma. Although its role diminished as antidepressant medications were developed, research on ECT has led to refinements that have substantially reduced its adverse side effects. Use of muscle relaxants, similar to surgical anesthesia, ended the physical jerking of seizures. Studies varying type and intensity of electrical shock and location of its contact with the brain have largely attenuated side effects of confusion or memory loss.

In an ECT treatment session, the electrical stimulus produces a generalized seizure in the patient's brain, lasting 30–90 seconds. This brain seizure activity is the variable responsible for ECT's therapeutic benefits. The patient gradually awakens from anesthesia a few minutes later. There is some cognitive confusion, which usually clears over the next 30–60 minutes. On average, depressed patients need 7–10 such treatments, usually given three times per week. A successful acute course of ECT will induce response and remission but it will not prevent relapse nor recurrences. Thus, once a response has occurred, the patient still must be started on antidepressant medications. In some cases, medications are ineffective in preventing relapses and/or recurrences, and thus ECT may be given as a continuation and/or maintenance treatment at weekly or monthly intervals, depending on the circumstances.

Several retrospective studies have confirmed the efficacy of ECT in bipolar disorder patients with **mania,** with approximately two-thirds of patients showing marked clinical improvement. **Catatonia,** a disturbance of motor behavior in patients with schizophrenia or psychotic depression, can be uniquely responsive to ECT (Petrides et al., 2001). ECT has long been regarded as a safe and effective treatment for severe depression in pregnancy, especially when the depressive disorder is life-threatening or has failed to respond to antidepressant medications. There is little evidence that it is harmful to the mother or fetus when both are carefully monitored (Yonkers et al., 2009). ECT is safe and effective even in elderly patients who have multiple medical comorbidities. It also has the advantage of administration with medically ill patients unable to take oral medications.

Neuromodulation

The effectiveness of ECT has led to a search for other ways to use electrical currents or magnetic fields to ameliorate depressive symptoms. Neuromodulation involves the use of magnetic fields or electrical stimulation to alter levels of activation of brain circuits that regulate mood.

Transcranial magnetic stimulation (TMS) is a noninvasive neuromodulation treatment in which an electromagnetic field is used to generate small electrical currents within the prefrontal cortex of a patient's brain. Treatments activate assertive coping behaviors and a more positive mood. TMS is FDA-approved for treatment of depression in adults who have failed one antidepressant medication trial.

Potential benefits of TMS over ECT are absence of a need for anesthesia, no electrical seizure induction, and no cognitive side effects. Unfortunately, the beneficial effects of TMS are much less robust than those of ECT, with a rate of depression symptom remission little better than with sham treatment. The main use of TMS is thus for mild to moderate depression in outpatient settings (Fox-Rawlings & Zuckerman, 2018).

Transcranial direct current stimulation (TDCS) delivers weak electrical currents across the prefrontal cortex of the brain via sponge electrodes placed on the scalp. Double-blind studies have reported mild efficacy in comparison to sham treatment (Loo et al., 2010). Advantages of the treatment are few adverse effects (tingling of skin commonly, rarely mild skin burns), low cost, and ease of administration. Its documented benefits thus far are insufficient to merit recommendation for treatment of MDD.

Vagal nerve stimulation (VNS) is a treatment developed initially for treatment-resistant epilepsy. A VNS device consists of an implanted pacemaker, akin to a cardiac pacemaker, that delivers low-frequency electrical pulses to the left cervical vagus nerve. Epileptologists had observed that some VNS patients reported improvements in mood, an effect subsequently shown to be independent of any benefits for the epilepsy. Response rates of 25–30% have been reported for depression symptoms, with improvement accruing slowly but then sustained over years. However, effectiveness in clinical practice remains uncertain. Surgery with general anesthesia is needed to implant the device. Rare occurrences of wound infection or hoarseness from vocal cord paralysis have been reported in 1% of cases. VNS is FDA-approved for chronic or recurrent depression (O'Reardon, Cristancho, & Peshek, 2006).

Deep brain stimulation (DBS) involves placement of depth electrodes into the brain, positioning them within the **subcallosal cingulate gyrus,** that is, the ventral anterior cingulate gyrus. This brain region serves a central role in generating the suffering component of emotional responses to noxious stimuli. Electrical stimulation of these electrodes deactivates the brain circuits of this region. During stimulation, some patients can verbally describe the receding of anguish, together with an opening of awareness to gratifying relationships and pleasurable life experiences. DBS is reserved for patients who have failed multiple medication trials. However, pilot trials have reported a long-term reduction of depression symptoms for over 60% of treatment-refractory patients (Anderson et al., 2012).

TREATING DEPRESSION AS A CHRONIC ILLNESS

It is useful to conceptualize drug treatment of depressive illness as occurring in phases. This approach is based on observations made in the natural course of the disorder and on the knowledge gained during the first decades after the introduction of antidepressant medications. Depression commonly is a chronic, episodic, remitting, and relapsing illness. Left untreated, episodes often will come and go over the years, with a general tendency to become more frequent and more severe with each subsequent relapse. The average length of a depressive episode— although there is great variability—is between 8 months and 2 years.

In general, it can take several weeks for the response to the medication to become apparent (as mentioned earlier, *response* is arbitrarily defined as a 50% reduction in the severity of symptoms, as measured by certain rating scales). Several more weeks may still elapse before full symptom **remission** occurs. This phase of treatment has been termed "acute treatment" (See Figure 3.2).

Once remission has taken place, many patients are naturally inclined to discontinue treatment. In fact, in the early days of antidepressant treatment, most physicians would discontinue medications as soon as remission occurred. It quickly became apparent that the risk of relapse was quite pronounced when medications were discontinued shortly after remission. To prevent this relapse, it is now standard to continue treatment for a period of time equivalent to the assumed natural duration of a typical depressive episode. Several time frames have been

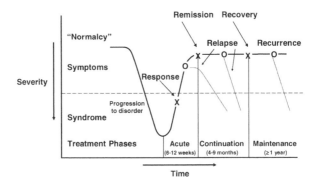

FIGURE 3.2. Phases of treatment for depression: The five R's. Data from Kupfer (1991) and Depression Guideline Panel (1993).

proposed for the duration of this second phase of treatment, termed the **continuation phase.**

Accordingly, treatment should last for at least about 9 months (up to 3 months to reach full symptom remission and 6 months to drastically reduce the risk of relapse). Dose reductions should be avoided during this period of treatment. In practical terms, most patients today receive antidepressant treatment at the same dose required to achieve remission for a total of 1 year before consideration is given to discontinuation.

The third phase of treatment is called the **maintenance phase.** As mentioned earlier, recurrence (the reappearance of symptoms reflecting a *new* episode) is the hallmark of many depressions. This pattern dictates the clinical strategy. If the patient has completed treatment for a first episode ever, there is a 50% likelihood that there will be no recurrence of a MDD. For such patients, many physicians will discontinue medication once a year has been completed after educating the patient on signs and symptoms that would signal a relapse.

When a patient has experienced two episodes of MDD, there is a 70% likelihood of future episodes. This presents a psychopharmacologist with a conundrum. Although most patients will continue to relapse, a large number will not, and it would be desirable to avoid unnecessary treatment. The physician must evaluate each patient's unique situation, with particular emphasis on factors that may pose a risk of recurrence. Shared decision making with the patient is often the most prudent course, considering cessation of antidepressant treatment while educating the patient and patient's family members to be aware of early signs of relapse and agree to return promptly should worrisome signs recur.

When patients have a history of three or more episodes—including the present one—the statistical likelihood of future episodes is over 90%. Continued full-dose maintenance treatment has been shown to reduce the number and severity of relapses. For this group of patients, it is best to continue maintenance medication treatment indefinitely. The risk of relapse, with consequent suffering, disability, loss of income, strained family relationships, potential need for hospitalization, and suicidal risk, greatly outweigh the burdens of side effects and the cost of maintenance treatment (Frank et al., 1990; Schatzberg & DeBattista, 2015, pp. 56–58).

Within these clinical guidelines, the unique characteristics of each patient will dictate the course to follow. Side effects, variations of clinical course, the presence of life stressors, economic considerations, relocation, concurrent illnesses, and other factors will affect the formulation of a specific plan that is suitable for a particular patient.

CONCLUSION

Problems involving depressed mood are likely the most common psychiatric problem that clinicians face in their practices. While low moods commonly occur due to losses, traumatic experiences, betrayals, and disappointments, they must be distinguished from depression as a mental illness. Psychotherapy, but not medications, can effectively relieve suffering from normal syndromes of distress. However, depression as a mood disorder often requires somatic treatments, such as antidepressant medications or ECT, and/or evidence-based psychotherapy, such as cognitive-behavioral or interpersonal psychotherapies, whose interventions target different processes than do psychotherapies for demoralization or grief.

Psychotherapists can serve a vital role when collaborating with a physician who prescribes antidepressant medication. Psychotherapists commonly have more frequent and longer clinical encounters with patients than do physicians. They can provide physicians with information from patients' daily lives that helps distinguish between depression as a mood disorder and demoralization as a normal response to life's adversities. Psychotherapists can serve important roles in patient education about depression symptoms, signs of possible relapse, and medication side effects. Depression is a problem optimal for collaboration between therapist and physician.

CHAPTER 4

Bipolar Disorder

Those affected with melancholia are not every one of them
affected according to one particular form; they are either
suspicious of poisoning or flee to the desert from misanthropy,
or turn superstitious, or contract a hatred of life. If at any time
a relaxation takes place, in most cases a hilarity supervenes . . .
the patients are dull or stern, dejected or unreasonably torpid,
without any manifest cause . . . they also become peevish,
dispirited, sleepless, and start up from a disturbed sleep.
Unreasonable fear also seizes them; if the disease tends to
increase . . . they complain of life, and desire to die.
—ARETAEUS DE CAPADOCCIA (2nd century C.E.)

This passage is perhaps the earliest documented clinical description of
bipolar disorder. Keen observers noticed not only that certain individuals suffered from depression but also that, seemingly inexplicably, their
mood would suddenly switch into the polar opposite: from dejection
to unbridled excitement, from profound despair to limitless optimism,
or from paralyzing fatigue to superhuman levels of activity and energy.
Bipolar disorder, as it is presently termed, historically has been called
manic–depressive insanity (as it was called in Kraepelin's [1919/1971,
1976] time) or manic–depressive illness. The term *bipolar* was coined
several decades ago in an effort to reflect the hallmark of the disorder:
two opposite poles of the affective continuum.

Diagnostically, there are different types and subtypes of bipolar
disorder that have different implications for course of illness and treatment (American Psychiatric Association, 2013). In addition to episodes
of depression, bipolar I patients have had at least one episode of mania
with symptoms of excessive energy, elevated mood, irritability, loss of

felt need for sleep, racing thoughts, and poor judgments involving spending money and social behavior that risk harm. When severe, acute mania can include psychotic symptoms, such as auditory hallucinations and delusional thinking. Bipolar II disorder has at least one past episode of **hypomania** in addition to depressive episodes. Hypomania consists of elevated mood, irritability, excessive energy, and impaired judgment but no psychotic symptoms. Cyclothymic disorder consists of episodes of hypomania alternating with minor depressive episodes. "Mixed state" describes a patient who appears to be experiencing mania and depression at the same time. In a mixed state, a patient can be in a high-energy, irritable state but with a dysphoric, agitated mood. Patients in mixed states can be at high risk for suicide.

Bipolar disorder affects about 1.2–1.5% of individuals over the course of their lifetimes. These figures cross cultural, economic, and ethnic boundaries (Goodwin & Jamison, 2007, p. 10). Bipolar disorder has a strong heritable component. Bipolar I disorder (defined below) appears to be equally common among females and males, whereas bipolar II disorder is more common in females.

Bipolar disorder is a lifetime disorder for which there is treatment but no cure. It has a profound impact on the patient and his or her family, coworkers, and friends and on society as a whole. Individuals with poorly controlled bipolar disorder have a high incidence of broken marriages and remarriages. Patients often find themselves unemployed, not infrequently having been fired from their jobs. Their friendships end, having been shallow and brief. Bipolar disorder is one of the most lethal among psychiatric disorders, with a lifetime risk of suicide between 8 and 20% (Goodwin & Jamison, 2007, pp. 249–251). For many, Kay Jamison's (1993) *Touched with Fire* has broadened our understanding of the twin faces of bipolar disorder as a "genius disease" that also can be disabling and lethal.

Although traditionally regarded as an illness with early-adulthood onset, bipolar disorder can begin in childhood, and is sometimes misdiagnosed as ADHD, oppositional defiant disorder, or **unipolar depression**. In rare instances, bipolar disorder can first appear late in life, after the age of 50. In such cases, the onset is usually due to strokes or other brain injury at the base of the brain's nondominant frontal or temporal lobe.

The natural course of bipolar disorder is episodic and highly recurrent. Initially, it can present with one or more episodes of depression before the first hypomanic or manic episode occurs. In many cases, manic and hypomanic episodes may precede or follow a depressive episode. Episodes usually last several months and may resolve spontaneously, without treatment. Recurrences every 2 years or so are not uncommon, and over time the frequency and intensity of episodes may actually worsen. In general, there is great variability in its course from patient to patient.

Bipolar I and bipolar II disorders are both mostly illnesses of depression. Both bipolar I and bipolar II patients spend threefold more days depressed than days manic during their lifetimes of illness. This predominance of depression is unfortunate in that it is the phase of the disorder that is most refractory to treatment. Bipolar II disorder is largely an illness of recurrent depressive episodes with only occasional hypomania, unlike bipolar I disorder. However, the predominance of depression, rather than mania, means that suicide attempts are more common in bipolar II disorder than in bipolar I disorder (Goodwin & Jamison, 2007, p. 251). Depressive episodes are responsible for most of global disability for bipolar disorder patients.

Bipolar disorder occurs in cycles. A cycle is measured from the beginning of one episode until the beginning of the next one. It includes both the symptomatic period (the "episode") and the intervening asymptomatic period that precedes the onset of the next episode. Some patients suffer from a rapidly cycling form of the disorder, with frequent, sometimes ultra-brief episodes that last a few days or even hours. "**Rapid cycling**" is defined as an individual who suffers four or more episodes (mania, hypomania, depressed, mixed, or a combination thereof) in the course of 1 year. The psychological and social scars resulting from episodes of mania and depression, which often require hospitalization, make it all but impossible for symptomatic patients to approach a modicum of stability and predictability in their daily activities. Mid- and long-term planning are a constant gamble.

CASE ILLUSTRATION: DAVID, NEW ONSET OF MANIA

David, a young leader of his sales force, was viewed as the future of a small company due to his extraverted enthusiasm and work ethic that captivated new customers. His coworkers were then shocked when they learned he was arrested for reckless driving and resisting arrest after aggressively forcing another car off the road. The arresting officer suspected he was driving while intoxicated, but David's blood alcohol level was in fact zero when measured at a nearby hospital emergency department, and his urine toxicology was negative. The emergency medicine physician who evaluated him requested psychiatric consultation. The psychiatric consultant diagnosed bipolar I disorder based upon David's current symptoms of mania—racing thoughts, irritability, impaired judgment, little sleep—and past history of two depressive episodes for which David did not seek treatment.

David's parents and siblings all opposed his admission to the inpatient psychiatric unit, stating that they "did not believe in psychiatry." Nevertheless, they supported his hospitalization when they realized that the alternative would be his arrest and confinement in jail. Following a diagnostic evaluation and stabilization of his mood with lithium carbonate, his psychiatrist began preparing David for discharge. David felt obligated to tell the truth about his diagnosis and treatment to his employer and family, both of whom asked to know the facts. However, David was anxious that his employer would not return him to roles of responsibility within his company. He also feared that his family would ridicule his taking lithium. His wife, however, was supportive of his treatment. The psychiatrist consulted a family therapist with whom he often collaborated to meet with David and his wife.

Meeting with the couple, the family therapist inquired both about the work culture of David's company and about David's family of origin. David explained that his company was not yet profitable but had a business plan that relied upon rapid expansion of its market share through recruitment of new customers. David's boss would have no opinion about David receiving psychiatric treatment, but he might be hesitant to rely again upon David's salesmanship should he hold doubts about David's reliability. David's family, on the other hand, embraced traditional values of self-reliance and personal spirituality. They felt that taking psychiatric medication was shameful and a moral failing. The family therapist told the couple: "There are different stories that you tell different people about the same set of facts. The stories of your daily lives that you tell each other are different from the stories you tell your children." The therapist then gave David and his wife an assignment to complete at home together before the next session. She asked them to compose one narrative for his employer and a different one for his family and church. When they returned, the therapist devoted the session to role plays in which David practiced presenting each of these narratives to the therapist, who role-played first his employer then his family members, while David's wife watched and critiqued his performance. For his employer, David attributed his disruptive conduct largely to sleep deprivation, which was factually true. He had slept little for days as he became increasingly manic. He made no mention of medication. David explained to his religiously adherent family that "My body is a temple of God" (I Corinthians 6:19) for which he had been given stewardship. David told them that his body was deficient in lithium, a salt similar to table salt, and that he would be taking no medication that was addictive. This explanation quieted their questions. David returned to a productive career at work. He and his wife read educational materials on bipolar disorder, as well as Kay Jamison's *Touched with Fire,* both of which his psychiatrist recommended. They met with the family therapist periodically to discuss how they were working together to prevent future episodes of illness.

Questions for Consideration

1. *Bipolar disorder is considered to be one of the most genetically determined and "biological" of all the psychiatric illnesses. Why was there so much involvement in David's care by the family therapist?* Bipolar disorder can be regarded as a disease of the brain, but if so it is a disease that is sensitive to emotional states, relationships, and health behaviors. Psychological and behavioral factors, such as excessive goal striving or sleep deprivation, can precipitate mania. Effective mood regulation requires psychoeducation about the natural course, treatments, vulnerability factors, and prevention strategies. Dr. Fred Goodwin, author of the bipolar disorder "bible," *Manic–Depressive Illness,* taught that bipolar patients should be seen together with couple partners, never alone (Griffith, 2005, personal communication). This was based upon his data showing that individuals during manic episodes lose their ability to self-observe, so that their self-reports to their doctors are often wildly at variance with reports from family members. Moreover, adherence to prophylactic mood-stabilizing medications is often challenging for bipolar patients without family support. Finally, family members often find it difficult to distinguish normal enthusiasm from early stages of mania without expert consultation.

2. *Why did the family therapist devote so much effort for David to learn a different story of his illness for family and workplace?* Stigma against those with mental illness and psychiatric treatment occurs in every culture. Stigma is a major reason why individuals prescribed psychiatric medications do not take them. There are different types of stigma, and an intervention must accurately target the specific type of stigma in order to be effective. In his workplace, David's employer was only concerned whether he was reliable with his work (disruption stigma). David's family, however, expressed moral stigma, viewing him as unworthy if he was in psychiatric treatment.

TREATMENT OF BIPOLAR DISORDER

Bipolar disorder can be challenging to treat and typically requires maintenance mood-stabilizer medications to prevent episodes; a different medication regimen to treat acute depressive, hypomanic, or manic episodes when they occur; psychotherapy; psychoeducation; and couple or family sessions that draw upon relational resources to strengthen the patient's mood stability (Miklowitz & Gitlin, 2014). Hypomanic or manic episodes are often accompanied by the patient's loss of awareness for how his or her conduct is affecting other people. Collateral information about family members' perceptions of patient's symptoms is often vital. Nonadherence to treatment is a frequent challenge, for which a strong alliance with couple partners or family members can be essential.

The importance of psychotherapy and family-centered care, in addition to medications, must be underscored (Miklowitz, 2008; Miklowitz et al., 2013; Moltz, 1993). When only psychopharmacology is utilized in bipolar disorder treatment, there is a 40% rate of relapse during a 1-year period, 60% rate of relapse over a 2-year period, and over 50% of patients have residual symptoms between episodes requiring psychosocial care (Miklowitz, 2008; Miklowitz et al., 2013). A number of psychosocial factors can contribute to relapse in bipolar disorder:

- High expressed emotion in family relationships
- Life events that disrupt daily routines, particularly sleep–wake cycle
- Excessive goal striving
- Factors contributing to poor adherence to medications (low education, lack of social support, lack of knowledge about the illness, or beliefs about its treatment)

Each of these can be targets for individual and family therapy. Family-focused treatment (FFT) is a manual-based psychoeducational intervention designed to reduce familial stress, conflict, and affective arousal by enhancing communication and problem solving among patients and caregivers (Miklowitz, 2008; Miklowitz et al., 2013).

During acute episodes, especially mania, hospitalization can be necessary. The turmoil and disruption resulting from mania, and its profound impact on judgment and behavior, may make it impossible to treat the patient on an outpatient basis. Furthermore, there are significant risks of aggravating existing medical illnesses, of physical injury to self or others, of dehydration, of physical exhaustion, and of suicide.

ACUTE MANIA/HYPOMANIA

Although presently only lithium, **valproic acid** (divalproex), and several atypical antipsychotics have been approved by the FDA as treatments for acute mania, clinicians prescribe a number of other medications as well for patients in the manic phase (Table 4.1). Carbamazepine is an anticonvulsant whose efficacy for bipolar disorder is supported by numerous research studies, although FDA approval for bipolar disorder was never added to its approval for epilepsy treatment.

Lithium carbonate is given orally. Sustained-release preparations of lithium can enable once- or twice-daily dosing. Within the human body, lithium is absorbed from the gastrointestinal track, enters the bloodstream, and is excreted unchanged through the kidneys, similarly in all aspects to how the body deals with sodium from table salt. Like sodium, lithium has a small margin of safety should blood levels rise too high. Doubling a therapeutic dose of lithium can be fatal. For this reason, dosing lithium relies upon adjustments of daily dose according to measured levels in the blood. Impaired kidney functioning can cause lithium levels to rise dangerously as excretion is slowed. For this reason, kidney function is checked at start of treatment and every 6 months thereafter. Lithium can produce inflammation within the thyroid gland that slows production of thyroid-stimulating hormone (TSH). For this reason TSH levels are checked at start of treatment and every 6 months thereafter.

Different patient populations respond best either to lithium or to anticonvulsant mood stabilizers, such as valproate or carbamazepine.

TABLE 4.1. Some Common Treatments for Acute Mania

Medication	Starting dose	Target dose/level
Lithium	600–1,200 mg/day	600–2,700 mg/day (0.6–1.3 mEq/L)
Olanzapine	5–10 mg/day	10–20 mg/day
Divalproex or valproate	500–1,000 mg/day	500–3,750 mg/day (20 ± 3 mg/kg/day)
Carbamazepine	300–500 mg/day	400–1,800 mg/day (6–16 µg/ml)
Aripiprazole	15 mg/day	10–30 mg/day
Quetiapine XR	300 mg/day	600 mg/day

Predictors of a poor response to lithium are listed in Table 4.2. Discontinuing lithium carries unique risks for patients who had been stably treated. Lithium is associated with a sixfold decrease in risk of suicide for bipolar patients compared to the normal population. However, subsequent cessation of lithium treatment is associated with a 20-fold increase in risk of suicide during the next year after stopping. Discontinuing lithium, then later restarting it, can be associated with a drop in efficacy for many patients.

Because of the potential effect it may have on other body systems and the risk of toxicity, a baseline medical workup is *de rigueur* in every patient who is a candidate for lithium therapy. This lithium workup includes laboratory tests aimed at evaluating kidney function, serum electrolytes, and functioning of the thyroid gland, at a minimum.

Lithium is effective within a certain range of concentration in the blood. Therefore, dosing must be tailored to the individual patient to reach levels that fall within the therapeutic range, usually between 0.6 and 1.3 mEq/L (milliequivalents per liter, the units used to express the concentration of lithium in the bloodstream). In general, levels for acute manic episodes fall in the higher end of the range, whereas for maintenance treatment the target level is lower. Exceeding the therapeutic level may result in severe and eventually lethal side effects. A properly managed patient receiving lithium must have periodic blood tests to ensure that the level is neither too low (ineffective) nor too high (potentially dangerous). Typically, blood levels are initially checked at least once a week until an appropriate blood level has been stably achieved. Once treatment is established and the individual dosing needs of the patient are better known, lithium level tests are done every 3 to 6 months. While lithium blood levels are valuable as guideline references, they are only meaningful in conjunction with an ongoing clinical assessment of the patient.

Lithium produces a number of side effects, even within the therapeutic range, and they will occur in a large majority of patients (Table

---

TABLE 4.2. Predictors of a Poor Response to Lithium

Predictors of a poor response to lithium, compared to mood-stabilizing anticonvulsants (valproate, carbamazepine, and others) include:

- Patients who show rapid cycling (four or more manic episodes per year).
- Mixed mania.
- Concurrent substance abuse.
- Secondary mania, due to steroids or other medication or right frontotemporal brain lesion.
- Previous poor response to lithium.

4.3). These effects may lead to treatment nonadherence and an increased risk of relapse. Sometimes, the side effects can be managed with blood-level adjustments and/or modifications in the daily dosage.

Lithium toxicity can become a life-threatening complication. The blood levels required for a therapeutic effect are close to those leading to toxicity. As mentioned above, doses of lithium typically are aimed at reaching blood levels of 0.6–1.2 mEq/L. Early signs of toxicity may appear at levels above 1.5 mEq/L and become quite serious above 2.0 mEq/L. If not recognized and treated on a timely basis, lithium toxicity can lead to serious CNS injury and even death. Older adults are particularly sensitive to even therapeutic levels of lithium, and their levels tend to fluctuate more unpredictably, thus requiring closer monitoring.

Lithium toxicity results from any situation that causes either excessive ingestion of the drug or insufficient clearance of it from the body (lithium is excreted via the kidneys). For example, patients who misunderstand the physician's directions or who otherwise take higher than prescribed doses can very quickly elevate their blood levels to a dangerous range. Dehydration, interactions with several other medications (e.g., nonsteroidal anti-inflammatory drugs, such as ibuprofen, which are commonly used and obtainable over the counter, and certain diuretics), certain medical illnesses, diarrhea, vomiting, anorexia, crash dieting, strenuous exercise, very hot climate, and pregnancy and delivery can all alter lithium levels and increase the risk of lithium toxicity.

Lithium toxicity constitutes a medical emergency. Because the need for early recognition and treatment are essential, its manifestations are included in Table 4.4 for reference.

TABLE 4.3. Lithium Side Effects

- Decreased renal ability to concentrate urine, leading to polyuria (increased urination) and polydipsia (increased thirst)
- Hand tremors
- Weight gain
- Sedation, lethargy
- Cognitive effects (slow thinking, dulling, impaired memory, confusion, decreased concentration)
- Motor coordination problems
- Gastrointestinal symptoms (nausea, vomiting, diarrhea)
- Hair loss
- Acne, psoriasis
- Water retention
- **Hypothyroidism** (may occur in up to 25%, more frequently in females)

Note. Data from Goodwin and Jamison (2007).

TABLE 4.4. Lithium Intoxication

Moderate
- Drowsiness, lassitude
- Dullness, disorientation, confusion
- Slurred or indistinct speech
- Blurred vision
- Unsteady gait
- Coarse hand tremor
- Restlessness
- Muscle twitches
- Lower jaw tremor
- Giddiness
- Vomiting

Severe
- Intensification of any of the above
- Marked apathy, impaired consciousness, may progress to coma
- Ataxia
- Irregular hand tremor
- Prominent generalized muscle twitches
- Choreiform/parkinsonian movements

Note. Data from Goodwin and Jamison (2007).

Since the observation made in Japan in the 1970s that carbamazepine, an anticonvulsant used for the treatment of epilepsy, was a promising antimanic agent, considerable research has been done on the use of this class of medications for the treatment of bipolar disorder. Carbamazepine and divalproex are anticonvulsants with substantial research support for their efficacy treating mania. **Lamotrigine** is ineffective for treating acute mania, but is effective as a prophylactic medication for reducing frequency of both mania and depressive episodes.

Divalproex is presently the drug most commonly used for the treatment of mania. It also requires doses to be adjusted to a blood-level range thought to be associated with optimal therapeutic benefit (50–100 µg/mL [micrograms per milliliter, the units used to express its concentration in the bloodstream]), but its therapeutic blood level is well below its toxicity level, making it, in this respect, an easier drug to use. Weight gain is the most common reason why patients discontinue valproate, with 50% of patients experiencing significant weight gain. Birth defects are a serious concern for women taking divalproex during pregnancy: 1.0–1.5% of pregnancies have **neural tube defects,** such as **spina bifida;** children born to mothers taking divalproex had persistent cognitive abnormalities, including lower average IQ compared to other groups of children (Velez-Ruiz & Meador, 2015).

Lamotrigine is an anticonvulsant agent approved for maintenance in bipolar disorder. Lamotrigine has limited evidence for effectiveness treating mania. However, it has been found to be useful in the adjunct treatment and in the prevention of the depressive phase of bipolar disorder. This is a particularly useful tool, considering the high prevalence of depression among bipolar patients. Lamotrigine use has been associated with skin rash in about 10% of patients. Rarely, this rash can be severe enough to require hospitalization and can be life-threatening. Gradual escalation in the dose over a period of several weeks is thought to significantly decrease the risk of a rash. In contrast to divalproex, lamotrigine appears to have the safest profile of anticonvulsants for use during pregnancy.

Atypical antipsychotic medications have also proved effective for treatment of mania. These medications, initially introduced for the treatment of schizophrenia and other psychoses, proved to have potent mood-stabilizing effects. Olanzapine was the first atypical antipsychotic approved for this purpose by the FDA, and others in this class soon followed. Use of atypical antipsychotic medications for treatment of bipolar disorder has been limited by their sedative side effects and risks for metabolic syndrome. All atypical antipsychotics carry an FDA black box warning for risk of metabolic syndrome (see Table 4.5). The **metabolic syndrome** consists of comorbid factors that speed progression of cardiovascular disease. These include **insulin resistance** that can progress into type 2 diabetes, hypertension, elevated serum triglycerides and cholesterol, and abdominal obesity. Risks for metabolic syndrome have taken on added significance during the COVID-19 pandemic. Mortality studies have shown that metabolic syndrome in COVID-19 infections increases the likelihood of death up to fivefold (Xie et al., 2020).

TABLE 4.5. Risks for Weight Gain and Metabolic Syndrome (Most to Least)

Clozapine (average weight gain = 9.8 pounds)

Olanzapine (average weight gain = 9.1 pounds)

Quetiapine (average weight gain = 8.0 pounds)

Risperidone (average weight gain = 4.6 pounds)

Haloperidol (average weight gain = 2.4 pounds)

Ziprasidone = Aripiprazole (average weight gain less than 1 pound)

Lurasidone (average weight gain less than 1 pound)

Atypical antipsychotics are most often utilized to initiate rapid control of manic symptoms, followed by a switch to lithium or an anticonvulsant as mood stabilizer for long-term mood stabilization.

Not infrequently, treatment (for maintenance or acute mania) with a single agent proves ineffective, and combinations are necessary. Some of the combinations physicians try are based on controlled studies, mostly of patients who suffered from persistent symptoms of hypomania or mania while receiving treatment with monotherapy. Some are based on case reports only. Common combinations include lithium + divalproex, lithium + atypical antipsychotics, and olanzapine + divalproex with or without lithium.

Also, ECT (see the discussion in Chapter 3) is an excellent antimanic treatment and, in fact, has been found to be more effective than the combination of lithium and haloperidol, a conventional antipsychotic.

BIPOLAR DEPRESSION

As mentioned earlier, bipolar depression is the phase of bipolar disorder that is most refractory to treatment and responsible for disability, primarily because antidepressant medications effective for unipolar depression are ineffective for bipolar depression and can even worsen its course. Bipolar depression is diagnosed with the same criteria as is MDD, except with an additional requirement that there must be a history of at least one episode of mania or hypomania. Bipolar disorder is mostly a disease of depression (Citrome, 2014).

Since bipolar disorder tends to manifest itself first with one or more depressive episodes before the first hypomania or mania occurs, an initial diagnosis of MDD, unipolar type, is often made in error—and later changed to bipolar only when the first episode of abnormally elevated mood and psychomotor function manifests itself. However, the more astute clinician will have inquired about family history and the presence of atypical depressive symptoms, which are more common in bipolar disorder than in unipolar depression. It has been suggested that certain clinical characteristics—for example, hypersomnia and profound **psychomotor retardation**—can help distinguish the two types of depression. However, there is considerable overlap of symptoms among unipolar and bipolar depression, making reliance on phenomenology alone an uncertain method.

Unlike unipolar depression, bipolar depression is among the psychiatric illnesses most difficult to treat. Three treatment regimens have received FDA approval for their effectiveness:

1. Quetiapine in high dose (trade name Seroquel)
2. Lurasidone (trade name Latuda)
3. Combination of fluoxetine and olanzapine (trade name Symbyax)

Unfortunately, all three of these regimens produce sedation that can be intolerable for some patients. Quetiapine and olanzapine introduce risks for metabolic syndrome, with weight gain, elevations in blood levels of cholesterol and triglycerides, type 2 diabetes, and cardiovascular diseases. Lurasidone appears not to produce weight gain or metabolic syndrome for most patients.

Antidepressants are the most commonly prescribed class of medications for bipolar disorder patients, despite lack of evidence for effectiveness. No tricyclic, MAOI, SSRI, or SNRI antidepressant has ever gained FDA approval for treatment of bipolar depression. Neither transient nor enduring improvement in depression has occurred when patients receiving adjunctive antidepressant medications, in addition to a mood stabilizer, were compared to patients receiving adjunctive placebo. Moreover, antidepressants introduce risks for switching from depression into mania or chronic rapid cycling. Rapid cycling occurs in approximately 25% of all bipolar disorder patients. In a randomized Systematic Treatment Enhancement Program for Bipolar Disorder (STEP-BD), patients continued on antidepressants experienced 268% more total mood episodes per year and 293% more depressive episodes per year, when compared to patients for whom antidepressants were discontinued (El-Mallakh et al., 2015).

ECT is the most effective treatment for bipolar depression. ECT is more effective than any of the available medication regimens. A multicenter, randomized controlled trial found that ECT was significantly more effective than algorithm-based pharmacological treatment for treatment-resistant bipolar disorder. Response rate was 74% in the ECT group and 35% in the pharmacological group (Schoeyen et al., 2015).

MAINTENANCE TREATMENT

Bipolar disorder is a lifetime condition, and accordingly, treatment usually must be given for the duration of the patient's life. The aims of maintenance treatment include relapse prevention, early detection and treatment of partial relapses, suicide prevention, mood stability, and improved daily life functioning. In particular, low-grade symptoms, like mild to moderate depressive symptoms and unpredictable mood fluctuations, can markedly impair daily life functioning. Improving treatment adherence is a good justification for couple or family sessions focused upon psychoeducation about the disorder, its treatments, and the need for long-term maintenance treatment (Miklowitz, 2008; Miklowitz et al., 2013).

PSYCHOTHERAPEUTIC INTERVENTIONS

Medications are the core feature in the treatment of bipolar disorder. Without their skillful application, there may be little hope for either symptom remission or a gratifying daily life. However, the illness and its course, coupled with the current limitations in medication effectiveness, make the use of psychotherapy and other psychosocial interventions essential. Bipolar patients are faced with myriad issues and obstacles that have a profound impact on how they perceive themselves and their future (Table 4.6).

The chronic, unpredictable, and recurrent nature of the illness creates fear and uncertainty in patients, their families, and their friends. Tremendous strain is put on marital relationships; frequent divorces and impulsive marriages are a common feature in the history of some of these patients. It can be difficult for couple partners and family members to distinguish a patient's normal expressions of enthusiasm or sadness from impending mania or depression, sometimes resulting in a hypervigilant "mania-watching" that is disabling for family life (Moltz, 1993).

Acceptance of the diagnosis, its implications, and its requirements for maintenance prophylactic treatment, even when asymptomatic, is a

TABLE 4.6. Issues for Psychotherapy in Bipolar Patients

- Patient education
- Family education
- Medication compliance
- Dealing with anger, denial, and ambivalence
- Dealing with reaction to partial treatment response
- Dealing with impact of side effects, including the "loss" of hypomanic mood
- Fears of recurrence
- Learning to discriminate normal from abnormal moods
- Concerns about spouse, family, other relationships
- Concerns about genetics
- Support groups

Note. Data from Goodwin and Jamison (2007).

difficult process for most patients. Treatment adherence is often an ongoing challenge, especially when the patient is doing well or during hypomanic states. The fear of transmitting the illness to one's children is ever present. All these issues form the core of the psychotherapeutic intervention, one that must be ongoing and long-term, with variable degrees of frequency, as the issues dictate. Regrettably, the major symptoms of hypomania and mania are basically immune to psychotherapy. During mania, the neurobiological processes involved in the illness disable a patient's self-observing capacities and capacities for reflective thought, hence making him or her unable to utilize most psychotherapeutic tools. Individual and family therapy can be effective in the depressive and maintenance phase of the illness but is usually used as an adjunct to medication.

The clinical management of bipolar disorder and its challenges make it a particularly appropriate condition for the collaborative model of care. There will be no successful medication treatment without psychotherapeutic intervention and no psychotherapeutic hope without medication. The prescribing physician—ideally a psychiatrist, given the need for specialized and often complex treatment—and the psychotherapist must work closely together to ensure the best possible results. The therapist must be knowledgeable about the natural course of the illness, its variability, the limitations and side effects of medication, and the need for different medication regimens imposed by the varying clinical manifestations. The therapist must be knowledgeable about common impacts of the illness upon the patient's sense of self and upon couple, family, and friendship relationships (Miklowitz, 2008; Miklowitz et al., 2013; Moltz, 1993). An excellent and detailed review of all these issues may be found in several texts specifically devoted to bipolar disorder, including the psychotherapy chapter in Goodwin and Jamison (2007).

In utilizing the collaborative care model in the management of bipolar disorder, as in unipolar depression, the therapist provides psychoeducation, supports the inherent coping skills of the patient, assesses progress and resistance, and tracks medication compliance. The psychotherapist and psychiatrist can inform each other of any changes that have occurred and/or are required, thereby resulting in a more comprehensive and quality-driven level of care.

ADDRESSING THE THREAT OF SUICIDE

Recognizing the inherent risk of suicide for patients with MDD or bipolar disorder is an obligation for every mental health professional (Adler, Slootsky, Griffith, & Khin Khin, 2016). Suicide is a behavior, not a mental illness. At least 10% of Americans who die by suicide do not have a mental illness. The motivating reason for suicide often matters more than the presence of mental illness. However, 60–70% of individuals who die by suicide have depression or mania, so it is appropriate to discuss suicide in the context of a chapter on mood disorders (Fazel & Runeson, 2020).

Reviewing a checklist of risk factors for suicide is an easy routine when gathering a clinical history. However, such factors alone predict suicide risk over a lifetime, not for the next 24 hours, which is the immediate concern of a therapist. Nevertheless, their presence in a clinical history serve as a signal that the therapist should conduct a more detailed inquiry to ascertain whether there are specific indicators for imminent risk.

Assessing imminent risk for suicide is best accomplished by an empathic interview that reveals the individual's existential predicament (feeling helpless, hopeless, isolated, desperate, trapped, guilty, or shame-ridden) while simultaneously building a therapeutic alliance. This enables assessment of warning signs for imminent risk, an assessment of level of lethality for the kind of attempt considered, and an evaluation of protective factors that could inhibit a suicidal impulse. An expanded inquiry about suicidal ideation or plan may then be necessary to maximize the accuracy of assessment. While several suicide assessment instruments have been produced, each has limited validity due to an excess of both false-positive and false-negative errors in detection, hence assessment instruments can supplement but not replace a clinician's systematic, multidimensional assessment (Lindh et al., 2019).

Most commonly, escape from despair is the driving motivation for suicide (Steeg et al., 2015). A compassionate interview begins with an effort to understand the patient's existential predicament and consequent experiences of pain, loss, and trauma. An empathic interview can discern motivations for suicide, while also engaging the patient in a shared effort to problem-solve the crisis and mobilize hope. Three sets of questions organize the interview (Bagge, Glenn, & Lee, 2013; Griffith, 2018):

1. Adversities—"What adversities are you facing? Which is the hardest?"
2. Impact—"How have these adversities affected you? What have they taken from you?"
3. Competencies for coping—"How have you responded to these adversities? How are you dealing with them? Do you feel trapped by them?"

The clinician listens for a perceived failure to attenuate stressors or to mobilize coping, which identifies a patient at potential risk for suicide. Suicide can seem to be the sole avenue of escape when a patient feels helpless, hopeless, isolated, and desperate. A clinician can ask a sequence of questions that gently open an expanding portal into a patient's experience of living (Adler et al., 2016):

- "When things are at their worst, does it ever feel that life isn't worth living?"
- [If answered, "Yes"] "Have you ever wished not to live?"
- [If answered, "Yes"] "Have you ever thought about ending your life through suicide?"
- [If answered, "Yes"] "Were these just vague thoughts, or did you think about specific methods of suicide?"
- [If answered, "Yes"] "How did you think through whether suicide would be the right thing to do? How did you think through what might be the best method for suicide?"
- [If answered, "Yes"] "Did you make a plan for suicide or implement any step of a plan for suicide?"

An estimated 17% of the U.S. population will have vague thoughts of suicide at some point. However, those who make a plan to die are likely to act upon the plan.

While listening, it can be important to keep in mind a list of less common motives for suicide. In each of these, the patient is protagonist in a drama that ends with death:

- Seeking reunion in death with a loved one
- Self-execution motivated by guilt over wrongs committed
- Self-erasure motivated by shame that one is unworthy of one's family, team, community, or religious faith
- Altruistic suicide as an act of self-sacrifice that spares suffering for others
- Ecstatic suicide that views death as only a portal to a beatific spiritual existence
- Suicide as a final act of revenge that also ruins the life of a hated person

Warning Signs for Imminent Risk for Suicide

Warning signs for suicide place a patient in a category of risk that warrants close monitoring, intensified treatment, or hospitalization. In clinical practice, four key areas should be routinely explored (Joiner, 2005):

1. Thwarted belongingness
   - "Has any close relationship ended or suffered a recent rupture?"
   - "Have you been feeling that you don't belong anywhere or to anyone?"
2. Perceived burdensomeness
   - "Have you felt that you are a burden to others?"
   - "Have you felt that others would be better off if you were no longer in their lives?"
3. Impaired emotion regulation
   - "Have you recently witnessed or suffered a traumatic or violent event?"
   - "How much alcohol or recreational drugs do you use? Has this use recently increased?"
   - "Are you having problems controlling your anger?"
   - "Have you recently engaged in risky or reckless activities?"
4. Lethal capability
   - "Do you own a firearm? Have you ever shot a firearm?"
   - "Have you ever committed an act of self-harm? How many times? Which was the most serious?"

The presence of alcoholism or substance abuse, or a psychotic, mood, anxiety, or dissociative disorder, can multiply risk (Inskip, Harris, & Barraclough, 1998). This is particularly so if there have been recent exacerbations of symptoms, due to neurobiological impairments in executive functions and emotion regulation that undermine problem solving and distress management. Joiner (2005) has shown that repeated acts of self-harm desensitize a person to natural fears of death.

Assessing the Risk of Lethality for Suicidal Ideation, Plan, or Behavior

Risk/rescue assessment provides a rough gauge for level of risk of lethality and intent for the kind of suicidal act imagined, planned, or attempted (Weissman & Worden, 1972). Risk/rescue assessment estimates the level of risk for the particular suicide method, together with the likelihood of rescue if the suicide attempt were to fail. For example, a patient was found comatose with a **benzodiazepine** overdose by accident because a maintenance worker came in his locked apartment to check the heating. The patient was assessed as having made a low-risk/low-rescue suicide attempt based upon method of suicide and likelihood of rescue if the attempt failed. Risk/rescue assessment must take into account the patient's factual understanding of the medical risks for the kind of attempt and whether that reflected accurately a desire to die.

Protective Factors for Inhibiting Suicidal Impulses

Protective factors are reasons for living that potentially can counter a desire for death. Many patients struggle with chronic physical or emotional pain. Chronically suicidal patients may feel on most days that life is not worth living, or they may even long for death. For such patients, reasons to live matter more than reasons to die. The critical question is "On a day when you sincerely wanted to die, what would lead you to choose to live instead?"

Fear, guilt, or shame can hold suicidal impulses in check for some patients. For example, J. M. was a 24-year-old graduate student admitted to the hospital after standing on a seventh-story ledge debating whether to jump. She stepped back to safety after imagining her friends finding her crushed, bloody body "and having to clean up the mess." Such avoidant coping provides little reassurance about long-term safety, since a patient can build the courage to act over time, or else use alcohol or substances to lessen binding anxiety.

Resilience factors expressed as assertive coping provide greater assurance of safety (Griffith, 2018). These factors most commonly are:

- Purpose for living—"What is important for you to accomplish in days to come?"
- Accountability to relationships—"Whom do you count on? Who counts on you?"
- Reliance upon a core identity—"In your heart, who do you know yourself to be? Who is the person that you would want to become?"
- Competent emotion regulation—"When life feels unfair and you feel really upset, what do you do to get through such hard times?"

Religion often provides hope—or a fear of hell—that can serve as a deterrent to suicide. However, religion also can motivate suicide due to yearnings to join God in an after-life, out of despair from feeling abandoned by God, as a just punishment for one's sins, or by sacrificing one's life in order to fulfill a perceived divine mission. It is essential to learn how religion actually informs moral reasoning about suicide (Griffith, 2010): *Is suicide the right thing to do? And why?*

Expanded Inquiry into Undisclosed Suicidal Ideation or Plan

Inquiry about suicidal ideation and plan is most accurate after an empathic relationship has been established, given that deception can be common with patients in distress. In a nationwide sample, 77% of inpatients who committed suicide while in the hospital had denied suicidal ideation in their final interview (Busch, Fawcett, & Jacobs, 2003). Collateral information from family members or close friends is thus critical, since patients may tell close relations about suicidal ideation or suicidal behaviors that are denied in clinical interviews.

The **Chronological Assessment of Suicide Events** (CASE) is a sophisticated interview strategy for eliciting suicidal ideation that has not appeared spontaneously (Shea, 2002). For example, normalization is used to diminish shame that prevents some patients from speaking openly about suicide: "Sometimes people who experience the loss of a loved one like you will have thoughts of killing themselves. Has this ever happened to you?" **Shame attenuation** reframes suicidal thoughts as part of the normal spectrum of responses to stressful situations: "Given the pain that you feel over the loss of your wife, have you been having any thoughts of killing yourself?" When a suicide attempt has been acknowledged, the CASE method reconstructs the behavioral incident—learning what happened just before the patient decided to take the pills, what the patient thought before they overdosed, how many pills the patient took, what kind of pills, how they decided which pills to take and how many, what thoughts the person was having after the attempt, what happened after they took the pills, and so on. By reconstructing the suicide attempt, the clinician can ensure that details that may indicate a lesser or greater intent to die during the suicide attempt are not omitted from the suicide assessment. Other techniques taught by the CASE method seek to prevent the patient from omitting important information, such as denial of the specific, by asking if the patient has ever thought about or attempted overdose, cutting, hanging, shooting, or jumping as different methods of suicide (Shea, 2002). Finally, the CASE method encourages use of symptom amplification to overcome possible minimization of symptoms: "How often do you have thoughts of killing yourself—40% of the day, 60% of the day, 90% of the day?" By symptom amplification and denial of the specific, as well as construction of behavioral incidents, the CASE method for suicide assessments can help clinicians circumvent the minimization of symptoms or omission of important information.

Effective suicide risk assessment must not only distinguish patients at risk for self-harm from others who are highly distressed. It must also be time-efficient and usable across a breadth of clinical conditions and in different clinical settings. It must be simple enough conceptually so as to leave a novice clinician's attentional focus, reflective thought, and emotional awareness unimpaired in their focus upon the patient. These aims are best met by first grasping a patient's human predicament as life's adversities are encountered (Adler et al., 2016). Such an empathic interview can create an alliance through which the patient willingly reveals thoughts and intentions for self-harm. A check of warning signs predictive for imminent risk and level of lethality for a suicidal act then completes the picture. Such an assessment can be brief enough to be usable and simple enough to be teachable.

CONCLUSION

Mood disorders are common in the general population. Depressive disorders are occasionally referred to as "the common cold" of psychiatry. In part this attribution speaks to the confusion between depression as the adjective for low moods from losses and disappointments and depression as a too-often malignant psychiatric illness. During the past half century, we have greatly enhanced our understanding of depression as a mood disorder, and now we know what was long suspected: Both genetics and the psychosocial environment play critical roles in the expression of major depression and manic–depressive illness.

We have also made headway in understanding the neurobiology of these illnesses and how this neurobiological understanding can guide treatment. We have medications that can substantially ameliorate their severity. These medications must be used skillfully by well-trained physicians in a constant effort to achieve the best cost–benefit ratio, that is, the most effectiveness with the least possible adverse effects—how best to initiate them, how long to use them, and with which patient populations. Failure to adhere to treatment and impacts of mood disorders upon couples and families are major problems for which contributions from the therapist are vital. When treatment collaboration between physician and therapist occurs regularly and is meaningful and goal-directed, treatment outcomes are optimal.

CHAPTER 5

Anxiety Disorders

Anxiety is a normal part of life. Our brains are "wired," as a result of thousands of years of evolution, to react to external threats or hazards with a protective and highly tuned set of psychological and physical alarm responses. We share this survival and escape reaction with most other species. In human beings, it includes rapid heartbeat and respiration, diversion of blood to the muscles, enlarged pupils, increased muscle tone, fear, and heightened alertness and awareness. It includes an urgently felt need to draw close with trustworthy others. This carefully modulated response occurs in a continuum and is generally proportional to the gravity of the threat. Within limits, it is quite beneficial. A little anxiety and alertness improves our performance when we take a test or give a speech. A reasonable fear that her children may be injured prompts a mother to insist that they wear helmets when biking. When this array of psychological and physical alarms exceeds the point where it helps us adapt and becomes an impediment to functioning in daily life, it becomes a disorder: The bright college student flunks out because he panics when faced with an exam, or a mother's pervasive fear of harm to her children prevents them from engaging in normal developmental activities. A person with an anxiety disorder either fails to make an adaptive response or fails to inhibit a maladaptive response when aroused by uncertainty or threat.

Unlike psychosis in which thoughts and emotions can be bizarrely inappropriate, the fear a person experiences with an anxiety disorder usually makes a certain amount of sense. The problem is that the fear comes on too quickly, becomes too intense, or lasts too long. Disabling anxiety is largely a problem of impaired **emotion regulation**. Some contributory factors that impair emotion regulation include genetic vulnerabilities, emotional neglect or abuse during the developmental years of childhood, or traumatic stress in childhood or adult life. Anxiety disorders can blend into normal fear responses that are adaptive because they are appropriate to uncertain or threatening life circumstances, sometimes making the diagnosis of anxiety disorder a difficult judgment call.

THE NEUROBIOLOGY OF ANXIETY

Neurobiologically, anxiety disorders are associated with abnormalities in brain systems that monitor threat, confer a sense of safety, or provide emotion regulation when adversities are encountered. As discussed in Chapter 1, the brain's salience network is tasked with screening incoming information from the external environment via the five senses and from the internal body organs via the **vagus nerve**. When an event is noticed in the environment or internally, salience network components, including the amygdala, insula, ventral striatum, and ventral anterior cingulate gyrus, generate an emotional response—surprise, fear, anger, sadness—appropriate to the type of event sensed. These initial steps of noticing a salient event and generating an emotional response are termed "bottom-up processing." It is then necessary to modulate the intensity and duration of this emotional response so that actions are aligned with overall priorities of the patient's life. This third task of dampening and adjusting emotional intensity is termed "top-down regulation." Top-down regulation is implemented by multiple neural pathways that descend from the prefrontal cortex and the **dorsal cingulate cortex** to inhibit arousal generated by the salience network. This top-down regulation is analogous to the cooling rods that when lowered into a nuclear reactor slow down the nuclear fission to a safe level and speed it up when they are lifted. The balance between bottom-up and top-down systems determines whether a person sustains a state of equanimity or experiences escalating fear. Grasping how this relationship between top-down and bottom-up processing constitutes emotion regulation is most important for a clinician. Both psychosocial interventions—psychotherapy, psychoeducation, family interventions, mindfulness meditation, aerobic exercise, spiritual practices—and medications exert their effects by adjusting the balance of top-down regulation and bottom-up processing of information.

Psychiatric medications generally strengthen a patient's capacities for top-down regulation, thereby attenuating intensity of fear-spectrum emotions, such as apprehension, dread, fright, or terror. The brain's major inhibitory neurotransmitter is **gamma-aminobutyric acid,** or **GABA.** Numerous local circuits that utilize GABA as a neurotransmitter are situated throughout the nervous system so that they can attenuate the salience network's capability for generating fear. The benzodiazepine class of drugs, which includes diazepam, chlordiazepoxide, alprazolam, and lorazepam among others, all augment the effects of GABA, thereby producing relaxation instead of anxiety, even when a potentially threatening event has been detected by the salience network. Alcohol works similarly. Some other medications, such as **pregabalin** and **gabapentin,** reduce anxiety by augmenting the efficiency of the brain's GABA systems (Mathew, Hoffman, & Charney, 2009).

The amygdala's role within the salience network centers upon detection of threats in the environment. Norepinephrine and serotonin receptors are placed within the amygdala so that activation of these two monoamine systems can modulate the level of arousal of the amygdala. Serotonin reuptake inhibitors, serotonin–norepinephrine (dual-action) antidepressants, tricyclic antidepressants, and MAOIs all have potent effects in diminishing anxiety systems by dampening the reactivity of the amygdala. While benzodiazepines and antidepressants are both effective in diminishing anxiety symptoms, they do so by these two different mechanisms.

TYPES OF ANXIETY DISORDERS

Anxiety disorders include a range of diagnoses in which fearfulness is a prominent feature. However, specific anxiety disorders, such as obsessive–compulsive disorder (OCD) or posttraumatic stress disorder (PTSD), have unique features other than exaggerated fear. Also, several other psychiatric disorders have anxiety as a prominent feature. For example, approximately two-thirds of depressed patients suffer from anxiety as a significant part of their symptomatology, raising diagnostic speculation as to whether major depression and generalized anxiety disorder may be different phases of a single illness (Liebowitz et al., 1990; Wittchen, Schuster, & Lieb, 2001; Cameron & Schatzberg, 2002).

Because there is considerable co-occurrence and overlap in symptoms, diagnosis can be tricky, but a correct diagnosis can make a big difference in whether a patient is referred for medication and which medication regimen a physician might choose. Consider, for example, a 27-year-old woman who has had panic attacks and is now unable to leave her house without considerable fear and anxiety. We would certainly think about panic disorder with agoraphobia, and we know medication can be very effective in blocking panic attacks. But as we probe further, we discover that her two panic attacks occurred in automobiles and she stays at home because she is afraid of cars that are ubiquitous in her urban environment, not because she fears an unprovoked panic attack. Now it begins to look as if she has developed a specific phobia. The distinction is important because there is no evidence that any currently available medication works for specific phobias. But if we inquire even further and find out that her fear of cars began when she was badly injured in a car accident, and she fears them because they prompt extremely distressing memories of the accident, we would be inclined to consider PTSD. Panic attacks are a frequent posttraumatic symptom, for which psychotherapy is usually the primary pillar of treatment, but for which antidepressant medications can serve an additional adjunctive role.

Making these distinctions may fall to the therapist, especially if he or she is planning to refer the patient to a primary care physician. In addition to the different diagnoses listed above, the physician will also explore many other causes of anxiety, including those induced by over-the-counter (OTC) medications and excessive caffeine from coffee, tea, and/or cola drinks. A number of medications prescribed for medical illnesses, such as asthma or decongestant medications, can produce anxiety symptoms as side effects. Anxiety symptoms and insomnia can represent withdrawal symptoms from hidden overuse of alcohol or sedative/hypnotic medications, which a patient may not yet have revealed to his therapist.

Anxiety disorders are the most common psychiatric disorders in the general population and appear commonly in primary and specialty care. Accurate detection and diagnosis carries added importance for physical health due to the high comorbidity of alcohol and substance abuse with most anxiety disorders. Anxiety disorders, particularly PTSD, panic disorder, and generalized anxiety disorder, largely account for patients who present medically unexplained physical symptoms. Poorly controlled anxiety symptoms, particularly panic attacks, are more ominous for suicide risk than is persistent depression (Hall & Platt, 1999; Fawcett et al., 1990).

CASE ILLUSTRATION: MR. MANSFIELD, GENERALIZED ANXIETY DISORDER

Mr. Mansfield, a 65-year-old engineer, arrived in an agitated state at his primary care physician's office. He paced around the office while waiting. When examined, he impatiently declared that he had been unable to sleep for three nights and was afraid of the effects of the stress on his heart. He had felt fatigued for over a month. He had been too keyed up to deeply relax for at least the past 6 months.

The physician learned that Mr. Mansfield had had similar episodes at intervals throughout his adult life, with the most recent one precipitated by worries about a crisis in his son's life. Despite his anxiety, he was still able to enjoy hobbies and denied experiencing a severely depressed mood. He did not have panic attacks, nor did he report obsessive thoughts, compulsive behaviors, or social anxiety. He ingested alcohol only as wine with dinner on social occasions. He had no history of alcohol or substance abuse.

The physician explained to Mr. Mansfield that he probably had had an anxiety disorder—generalized anxiety disorder—for most of his adult life, with improvements and recurrences happening in concert with life stressors. He told Mr. Mansfield to imagine this as a problem of his brain's threat detection systems—that they activated at too low a threshold. Both medications and cognitive-behavioral psychotherapy could reduce this vulnerability.

The physician prescribed a daily regimen of sertraline (trade name Zoloft), an antidepressant, which would expectably attenuate the anxiety in 2–3 weeks. In the meantime, Mr. Mansfield could take doses of alprazolam (trade name Xanax), a benzodiazepine, if he were to experience a severe episode. He also recommended that Mr. Mansfield meet regularly with a family therapist colleague who could provide psychoeducation on anxiety management, teach him cognitive-behavioral techniques, and give guidance on his efforts to help his son. Three months later, Mr. Mansfield's anxiety symptoms were in remission. He had discontinued the sertraline and only rarely needed to take alprazolam on stressful days.

Questions for Consideration

1. *What should the physician and therapist regard as a successful outcome of treatment?* The goal of anxiety disorder treatment is manageability, not cure. Generalized anxiety usually is a normal response to a stressor, but onset of anxiety comes too quickly, becomes too intense, or persists too long after the stressor remits. Treatment aims for anxiety responses to stressful life events to fall into a normal range. Symptoms should be reduced to a level that discomfort from anxiety is bearable and there is no constriction of daily life activities.

2. *Is alprazolam safe to use for generalized anxiety disorder, since it has a reputation for abuse?* Benzodiazepines, such as alprazolam, diazepam, lorazepam, clonazepam, and others, are among the most effective medications for generalized anxiety disorder and panic disorder. Unlike antidepressants that take 1–3 weeks to become effective, a benzodiazepine can relieve anxiety within an hour after ingestion. Benzodiazepines can be abused by patients with histories of alcohol or substance abuse in a pattern that parallels that of alcohol abuse. However, benzodiazepine misuse or addiction is almost never seen among in patients with well-diagnosed anxiety disorders who have no history of alcohol or substance abuse. Benzodiazepines have a high safety index; in the 60 years that benzodiazepines have been available, there have been almost no deaths reported worldwide from overdoses in suicide attempts, unless a benzodiazepine and alcohol were combined in overdose. Taking an accurate history for alcohol or substance abuse is thus critical when benzodiazepines are prescribed.

3. *Is it unusual for a patient to be able to decrease or discontinue medication for anxiety after psychoeducation and psychotherapy, as was the case Mr. Mansfield?* Many patients do require long-term maintenance medication in order for anxiety symptoms to be manageable. However, psychoeducation and psychotherapy are effective in attenuating severity and disability from anxiety disorders. Some patients can reduce or even discontinue medications provided that they continue the practices learned in psychotherapy in a disciplined manner.

GENERAL TREATMENT CONSIDERATIONS

Usually a patient with an anxiety disorder needs a treatment program with multiple modalities, not just one singular treatment. Patient and family psychoeducation about diagnosis and treatment serves an essential role in engaging patients and families in a successful treatment program (see Chapter 11). A comprehensive treatment program typically includes psychoeducation about the natural course of the disorder, including risk and resilience factors, psychotherapy or behavioral therapy, interventions to improve relationships, and life practices and lifestyle changes that strengthen emotion regulation (mindfulness meditation, exercise, spiritual practices, recreation, yoga), in addition to medication.

Some important principles that psychoeducation should communicate to a patient and his or her family include:

- While anxiety disorders occur commonly, coping strategies for usual stresses of daily life are often ineffective in controlling an anxiety disorder. Specific psychotherapeutic or pharmacological strategies may be required to control anxiety disorder symptoms.
- Most anxiety disorders emerge in early adult life and persist as conditions that relapse and remit over the course of a life, similar to migraine headaches, irritable bowel syndrome, herpes fever blisters, and other chronic relapsing medical illnesses. While a cure may be an unrealistic expectation, symptom control adequate for effective functioning and enjoyment of daily life can be achieved in nearly all cases.
- Psychiatric medications are often necessary for adequate treatment, but effectiveness of any medication can be overridden by an excess of stressors. Psychotherapy and lifestyle changes may be necessary to reduce stress to a manageable level.
- Symptoms of anxiety disorders diminish in nearly all cases when life practices are adopted that strengthen emotion regulation. There are dozens of activities and practices that can serve this role, enabling a plan to be tailored to a patient's unique preferences and resources. Thus, yoga, mindfulness meditation, spiritual and religious practices, aerobic and/or strengthening exercise, dance, music, knitting, or many other activities that promote equanimity and lowering of body arousal can serve this role.

The Role of Medications

As a general rule, all anxiety disorders respond to all SSRI antidepressants (see Table 5.1) (Schatzberg & DeBattista, 2015, p. 431). Most anxiety disorders respond as well to tricyclic and MAOI antidepressants. The major exception is OCD, which responds only to antidepressants that possess a robust serotonin reuptake mechanism, which includes all SSRIs but only **clomipramine** among the tricyclic antidepressants (Schatzberg & DeBattista, 2015, pp. 439–440).

Nearly all medications have one or more adverse side effects, in addition to beneficial treatment effects. Addressing potential medication side effects proactively can strengthen the therapeutic alliance by communicating implicitly the clinician's knowledge about and concern for any risks to the patient. As mentioned earlier, adverse side effects are a major reason for treatment refusal or poor adherence to treatment. If a physician prescribes a medication, their consultation should communicate to a patient:

TABLE 5.1. SSRIs, SNRIs, and Tricyclic Antidepressants Used in Treatment of Anxiety Disorders

SSRIs	All tricyclic antidepressants
• Citalopram	• Amitriptyline
• Escitalopram	• Clomipramine
• Fluoxetine	• Doxepin
• Fluvoxamine	• Imipramine
• Paroxetine	
• Sertraline	
SNRIs	
• Duloxetine	
• Levomilnacipran	
• Venlafaxine	

- "This is how we will assess effectiveness of the treatment."
- "This is how we will determine if negative side effects indicate a need to change the regimen."
- "If this treatment does not work, this is what we will do next."

The therapist typically meets with a patient more frequently than does the prescribing physician and has a wider window into the patient's quality of daily life. Thus, the therapist can play a vital role in monitoring treatment response to medication, side effects from the medication, and any comorbid medical or psychiatric conditions that appear during treatment.

Ms. T. was a 17-year-old woman who was a refugee from Central America. Her symptoms of depression and PTSD improved with her psychiatrist's treatment with a low dose of sertraline, an SSRI antidepressant. She also was referred for trauma-focused psychotherapy. During her psychotherapy sessions, however, the psychotherapist became concerned about Ms. T.'s recent poor school attendance and low grades. Further inquiry revealed that Ms. T.'s household was crowded with family members, such that Ms. T. was required to share her bedroom with her grandmother. With this added stressor, Ms. T. had developed obsessive fears and compulsive rituals about germs. As a consequence, she was spending evenings putting all her possessions in Ziploc bags and plastic containers, then checking and rechecking their security. The psychotherapist reported this to Ms. T.'s psychiatrist together with a *Yale–Brown Obsessive Compulsive Rating Scale* showing Ms. T.'s high score indicative of OCD. The psychiatrist, who had not suspected OCD as a possible diagnosis, added

OCD as a comorbid diagnosis and modified her medication regimen. Ms. T.'s obsessive–compulsive symptoms remitted.

PANIC DISORDER

A panic attack is a brief but intense experience of fear or distress accompanied by some of the symptoms listed in Table 5.2. Four or more symptoms are required to make this diagnosis but some patients can be severely anxious with fewer than four symptoms. A panic attack—or even several panic attacks—is not by itself a disorder. Many people have a panic attack at some point in their lives. However, about 4% of individuals develop recurrent panic attacks, and 3.5% actually meet DSM-5 criteria for panic disorder.

Panic disorder is diagnosed based on criteria listed in the DSM-5 or the ICD-11 diagnostic systems. If the attacks are always or frequently triggered by identifiable objects or situations, a specific phobia or social phobia may be a more likely diagnosis, although patients with panic disorder may also have some triggered panic attacks or may have both panic disorder and a phobia. Panic disorder may or may not be accompanied by agoraphobia (literally, "fear of the marketplace," once the most crowded public setting that people would typically encounter)—defined as anxiety about being in places where escape would be difficult or help might not be available if panic symptoms were to occur. In agoraphobia, which occurs in roughly one-third of patients with panic disorder, those situations are typically avoided, though a patient may be able to tolerate

---

TABLE 5.2. Symptoms of a Panic Attack

- Palpitations, racing or pounding heart
- Sweating
- Trembling or shaking
- Chest pain
- Nausea or abdominal pain
- Numbness or tingling sensations
- Chills or hot flushes
- Shortness of breath
- A feeling of choking
- Feeling dizzy, lightheaded, or faint
- Feelings of unreality (derealization) or of being detached from oneself (depersonalization)
- Fear of losing control, of "going crazy"
- Fear of dying

them with a companion or may suffer through them with considerable anxiety. Agoraphobia develops in panic disorder as a very crude kind of "self-help," that is, the patient's only perceived way of controlling what seem to be uncontrollable and intolerable symptoms. Typically, agoraphobia develops over time (most often during the first year after the onset of panic attacks) when initial efforts to seek help from medical or other resources don't produce a solution. As panic attacks recur, they provoke more and more anticipatory anxiety (worry about when the next one will happen). At the same time, patients give up on the sources of help they have tried and increasingly resort to avoiding any situation that might provoke an attack or be a frightening or embarrassing place to have an unexpected attack.

Panic disorder typically starts in the third decade of life, although it may start in childhood or late in life as well. It can become a recurrent, chronic, and disabling condition, in which relapses after remission are common. Panic disorder affects females twice as often as males, and after remission, women are more likely to relapse than men. The long duration of illness and the presence of agoraphobia portend a less favorable prognosis.

Panic disorder is a serious risk factor for ill physical health or premature death. Over a fourth of individuals with panic disorder misuse alcohol to self-medicate anxiety symptoms. Panic disorder increases odds of a suicide attempt 8-fold compared to the normal population, which is a greater risk than MDD alone (Weissman, Klerman, Markowitz, & Ouellette, 1989; Fawcett et al., 1990). When panic disorder, major depression, and substance abuse co-occur, the risks for suicide are additive (Weissman et al., 1989; Fawcett et al., 1990). Co-occurrence of panic disorder and depression should be routinely assessed.

Treatment

Treatment of panic disorder aims at stopping the panic attacks, treating any comorbid disorders (including agoraphobia and, if present, depression), and achieving and maintaining remission (see Table 5.3). In most cases, treatment options include two classes of medications—benzodiazepines and antidepressants—and CBT. Many patients see greater benefits from some combination of these treatments. As with other disorders, treatment here includes psychoeducational interventions and an invitation to the patient to become an active partner in the treatment effort. An example is the patient who, well informed of the mechanisms leading to the symptoms of a panic attack, learns to recognize and rate the intensity and frequency of panic attacks.

**TABLE 5.3. Goals of Pharmacotherapy
for Panic Disorder**

- Block panic attacks
- Treat comorbid conditions (e.g.,
  depression, substance abuse, or
  dependence)
- Achieve remission
- Maintain remission

Several different classes of medications have been used in the treatment of panic disorder; some are much more effective than others (Table 5.4). SSRI and SNRI antidepressants and benzodiazepines with slow absorption times after oral ingestion (i.e., lacking a "cocktail effect") are the medications of choice. Multiple studies have conclusively demonstrated the effectiveness of these medications. Antidepressants require 1–3 weeks before onset of effectiveness, while benzodiazepines, such as clonazepam (trade name Klonopin) can be effective within hours. Tricyclic and MAOI antidepressants also work, also following a several-week lag period, but their side effects generally make them the second choice. This period of waiting for the medication to begin working can be difficult for patients.

A significant disadvantage of most medications for panic disorder treatment is the appearance of side effects well before any benefit becomes apparent. Patients with panic disorder often are hypervigilant to body sensations and commonly stop antidepressants after a few doses due to early activating symptoms. Approximately 20% of patients treated with SSRI or tricyclic antidepressant medications experience "early adrenergic syndrome" side effects in which dysphoria ("feeling yucky") is combined with jitteriness, irritability, and insomnia, similar to an excess of caffeine. These side effects usually resolve after 2–3 weeks, but in the short term provide a reason to stop the medication for many patients. Some strategies for ameliorating their intensity include

**TABLE 5.4. Medications Used in the Treatment
of Panic Disorder**

- Selective serotonin reuptake inhibitors
- Tricyclic antidepressants
- High-potency benzodiazepines
- Monoamine oxidase inhibitors
- Other agents
- Combination treatments

a dramatic reduction in starting dose with slow increases over a number of days; addition of a beta-blocker medication, such as propranolol, that diminishes jitteriness; or addition of a benzodiazepine, such as clonazepam, to temper jitteriness and insomnia until the early adrenergic symptoms dissipate. Educating patients beforehand about anticipated side effects protects the therapeutic alliance.

Certain patients with panic disorder and substantial anticipatory anxiety have persistent free-floating anxiety, symptoms that have rendered them largely disabled in daily life. In these cases in which acute anxiety is so prominent, immediate or quick relief may be necessary. It then is useful to begin treatment not only with SSRIs but, concomitantly, with benzodiazapines (e.g., diazepam, clonazepam, alprazolam, and lorazepam). These medications have the advantage of producing antianxiety effects very quickly. Patients feel their effects shortly after taking them, and the drugs are very effective in blocking panic attacks and diminishing anticipatory anxiety. Sedation, heightened intoxication if ingested with alcohol, and possible risk of drug abuse usually make benzodiazepines a less attractive choice as a long-term treatment (see Table 5.5).

Used short term, a benzodiazepine provides immediate partial or complete relief and will "buy time" until the full effect of the SSRI becomes apparent several weeks later. Once the disorder is stabilized with the SSRI, the physician can then proceed with a gradual discontinuation of the benzodiazepine.

After daily use for more than a few weeks, sudden discontinuation of any benzodiazepine is very uncomfortable and can be potentially dangerous with a risk of withdrawal seizures. Patients should be strongly discouraged from ever discontinuing a benzodiazepine without proper medical supervision (Table 5.6). Benzodiazepines whose pharmacokinetic profile is that of rapid absorption, peak blood level, then rapid fall,

TABLE 5.5. Side Effects of Benzodiazepine Medications

- Drowsiness
- Dizziness
- Psychomotor dysfunction or incoordination
- Headaches
- Blurred vision
- Memory deficits
- Disinhibition and/or excitability (in children and the elderly)

TABLE 5.6. Manifestations of Benzodiazepine Withdrawal

Physical symptoms	Psychological symptoms
◦ Tremors	◦ Anxiety
◦ Headaches	◦ Difficulty concentrating
◦ Sweating	◦ Dysphoria
◦ Ataxia	◦ Insomnia
◦ Loss of appetite	◦ Irritability
◦ Nausea	◦ Depersonalization
◦ Vomiting	◦ Dizziness
◦ Seizures	◦ Visual misperceptions
	◦ Sensorial hypersensitivity

can produce "mini-withdrawals" between doses, characterized by anxiety symptoms often misinterpreted as a relapse of the primary anxiety disorder. This can result in an anxious waiting for the next dose, sometimes referred to as "clock-watching." Benzodiazepines that can encourage clock-watching include diazepam, lorazepam, and alprazolam. This does not occur with clonazepam or extended-release alprazolam.

For a limited number of patients, a benzodiazepine can be sufficient. For example, a patient who functions well between rare but unexpected panic attacks may prefer to have a diazepam or alprazolam handy for those infrequent occasions, rather than take a daily medication. Bear in mind that using benzodiazepines in this fashion will have no effect in blocking the panic attack itself, since the drug's action will not be apparent for 30–60 minutes, after the panic attack has reached its natural termination. However, the ingested medication may alleviate lingering generalized anxiety that often follows a panic attack. It can provide prophylactic protection, such as taking a dose an hour before a public presentation. Clinical experience suggests that for some patients, the simple awareness that a pill is available in their pocket or purse for immediate use if necessary can have a powerful placebo effect in preventing panic attacks or in assisting patients to better cope with them.

The third option for treatment of panic attacks is CBT. In some but not all cases CBT can be sufficient to prevent panic attacks, particularly if they occur only in response to specific stressors. Most often, especially when there is agoraphobia, a combination of medication and CBT is the preferred treatment (Barlow, 2002; Barlow & Craske, 2006). The medication will block the panic attacks but will not always treat the agoraphobia. In some patients, agoraphobia does resolve "spontaneously" (i.e., without the need for formal CBT) when the panic attacks are effectively being blocked and anticipatory anxiety is thus less intense. Usually, these patients are providing their own informal version of CBT. As the panic attacks lessen or stop, the patients cautiously venture out, try something previously avoided, and discover that no panic attack occurs (because of the medication). Then they try something else, perhaps more "daring." This exposure leads to success, and the agoraphobia gradually fades away. Other patients will need the structure and support of a more formal program of CBT.

In addition, patients with panic disorder may also have other disorders, although these may not be as apparent while the panic attacks are prominent. Specific phobias, social phobia, and depression are common problems comorbid with panic disorder that may need to be addressed directly. In fact, one of the advantages of using SSRIs over benzodiazepines is that the medication will not only block panic attacks but will also directly address the depressive symptoms.

Long-term follow-up of patients with panic disorder has shown that this condition tends to be chronic and recurrent in a significant number of cases. Medications have substantial benefits, but their effects are likely to be lost after discontinuation. Medication treatment should continue for at least 1 year. Then an attempt can be made to very slowly and gently taper off the medication over an extended period of time, perhaps several months. Should a relapse occur, treatment must be restarted. Some patients relapse quite quickly after discontinuation of medication, whereas others are asymptomatic for a year or longer before the panic attacks return. In this regard, CBT appears to be more effective in that its benefit is much longer lasting, possibly up to several years following discontinuation of formal CBT (van Dis et al., 2020).

SOCIAL PHOBIA

The hallmark of social phobia is an excessive and ongoing fear of being embarrassed or scrutinized in social or performance situations, including fear of being embarrassed by the physical symptoms of social phobia—trembling, blushing, or sweating. It can present in generalized form in which the fears are present in most social settings, including interactional and performance situations. Its symptoms can overlap with those of avoidant personality disorder.

Generalized social phobia is the most disabling of the social phobias. It tends to run in families and generally has a chronic course. In other cases, the phobia may be restricted to a single or to very few situations, usually of a performance nature. Fearful situations include those in which the patient must speak to or before others, as well as

TABLE 5.7. Typical Social Phobic Situations: Performance

- Speaking in public
- Performing in public (e.g., musical instrument)
- Eating in public
- Writing in public
- Urinating in a public bathroom
- Entering a room where people are already seated

Note. Data from Kessler et al. (1998); Stein et al. (1996, 2000).

other contexts in which the patient may be observed (urinating in public bathrooms, eating in public, or writing checks at the checkout line). See Tables 5.7 and 5.8.

Social phobia has a lifetime prevalence of about 13% and a 1-year prevalence of about 8% (Kessler et al., 1994), making it the third most common psychiatric disorder, after depression and alcoholism. It is estimated that approximately 30 million Americans suffer from social phobia, and it affects women twice as often as men. The disorder typically starts in the mid-teens, and some patients have a history of shyness or inhibited behavior dating back to childhood. Social phobia may start acutely—for example, following a particularly humiliating social experience—or it may develop insidiously, with no apparent precipitating event. Without treatment, symptoms tend to be continuous and become especially worse in certain particularly stressful situations. Once the individual reaches adulthood, some adaptation occurs, resulting in ameliorating manifestations or outright remission. Although it is more common among relatives, overall it appears to have low heritability. Further research is ongoing to clarify the possible contribution of genetic factors. Comorbidity in social phobia is quite common, as it may overlap with other anxiety disorders and with depression. Suicide risk is

TABLE 5.8. Typical Social Phobic Situations: Social Interactions

- Conversing on the telephone
- Meeting someone for the first time
- Attending social gatherings (e.g., parties)
- Asking someone for a date
- Dealing with people in authority (e.g., boss, teacher)
- Returning items to a store
- Making eye contact with unfamiliar people

Note. Data from Kessler et al. (1998); Stein et al. (1996, 2000).

increased, and substance abuse—interpreted by clinicians as an effort to self-medicate—is commonly seen among these patients.

Exposure to these social and performance situations consistently causes anxiety, which may or may not amount to a full-blown panic attack. Although patients recognize that the fear is out of proportion to the actual risk, their severe anxiety generally causes them to avoid the activities they fear or otherwise endure the situation at the cost of great discomfort and suffering (Table 5.9). It is easy to imagine the impact these symptoms can have on the social and occupational life of such an individual. For example, patients who are unable to use a public restroom may fear going to any place from which they could not immediately return home if necessary; as a result, they might be homebound to the extent that they appear (erroneously) to be suffering from agoraphobia.

Treatment

The goals of treatment for social phobia have been summarized by Davidson (2003), as seen in Table 5.10. A patient whose phobia is limited to relatively infrequent performance situations can sometimes be successfully treated with beta-blockers, such as propranolol. Beta-blockers are a class of medications normally used in the treatment of high blood pressure and other cardiovascular conditions. Beta-blockers work on a short-term basis by disconnecting emotional arousal from its physical manifestations. A patient on the verge of panic will find that propranolol blocks occurrence of tremor or shaky voice that would otherwise be witnessed by other people. Beta-blockers do not diminish the subjective experience of fear. However, they have great value in treating speech fright or performance anxiety.

TABLE 5.9. Concerns in Social Phobic Situations

- Doing or saying something embarrassing or humiliating in front of others
- Making a poor impression or being negatively evaluated by others
- Having hand tremble when writing in front of others
- Mind going blank when speaking to others
- Saying foolish things
- Blushing or showing other signs of anxiety that will be noticeable to others

Note. Data from Kessler et al. (1998); Stein et al. (1996, 2000).

TABLE 5.10. Treatment Goals for Social Phobia

- Eliminate anxiety/phobic avoidance
- Eliminate functional disability
- Remission of social anxiety and comorbidities
- Choose therapy that is tolerable for long-term

Note. Data from Davidson (2003).

Patients with generalized social phobia need ongoing treatment when the phobia interferes with their lives in many ways or on many occasions. Both CBT and certain antidepressants can treat social phobia effectively. As in other anxiety disorders, CBT can have a sustained effect over the long term. Among the antidepressants, SSRIs are the current medication of choice. Their characteristics have already been discussed in this chapter, and their use in social phobia is essentially quite similar to that in panic disorder (Schatzberg & DeBattista, 2015, pp. 411–462). Beta-blockers and the antianxiety drug buspirone have not been effective in the treatment of generalized social phobia. Some patients who are successfully treated with medication expand their social horizons on their own, but others may benefit from training in social skills they missed developing during childhood and adolescence.

POSTTRAUMATIC STRESS DISORDER

A traumatic event is a life experience that induces terror, horror, helplessness, or humiliation that is sustained too long or becomes too intense for recovery back to a baseline sense of safety and well-being. Since the appearance of PTSD is directly associated to the occurrence of specific traumatic events, its prevalence will vary significantly in different countries and even within countries. Exposure to war, torture, crime, natural disasters, traumatic social situations, motor vehicle accidents, and other traumatic events will all determine the rate of PTSD (van der Kolk, 2014).

PTSD is diagnosed based on criteria listed in the DSM-5 or the ICD-11 diagnostic systems. The core symptoms of PTSD include:

- Reexperiencing symptoms—recurrent dreams or intrusive daytime memories
- Avoidance behaviors—avoidance of any reminders or recollections of the event, sometimes even "forgetting" important elements of the event itself

- Negative alterations in cognition or mood—amnesia for the event; persistent fear, horror, anger, guilt, or shame; persistent exaggerated negative beliefs about oneself, others, or the world
- Hyperarousal symptoms—insomnia, irritability, sensitivity to lights and sounds, exaggerated startle response

Patients can experience a general blunting of feeling and detachment from others and from their normal interests. Positive emotions, such as joy or enthusiasm, disappear. Symptoms can be especially intense and long lasting when the trauma was intentionally inflicted by another person, such as in torture or rape.

Ninety percent of individuals experience a potentially traumatic event over the course of a lifetime. Most symptomatic individuals recover from PTSD without treatment by a professional. However, approximately 20% of traumatized individuals have persistent symptoms that characterize PTSD. Forty percent of traumatized individuals who are still symptomatic 2 years after a traumatic event will continue to experience posttraumatic symptoms throughout their lifetime. PTSD then becomes a chronic, relapsing illness (Kessler, Sonnega, Bromet, Hughes, & Nelson, 1995).

Both psychological and physiological risk factors influence whether symptoms of PTSD persist after a traumatic life event. Psychological risk factors include:

- Childhood physical, sexual, or emotional abuse
- Other prior traumatic life events
- Prior anxiety disorder, particularly panic disorder
- Female gender (women have fewer traumatic life events but twice the PTSD risk after a traumatic event)
- Severity of traumatic event
- Absence of protective and affirming social support after the traumatic event
- Additional life stressors, particularly if there is an ongoing absence of a safe environment
- Peritraumatic dissociation during or immediately following trauma (amnesia for the event, freeze response, emotional numbness, derealization, depersonalization)
- Depressive episode immediately following traumatic event

In the United States it is estimated that the lifetime prevalence for PTSD is about 8% (Kessler et al., 1995). PTSD is common among survivors of military combat and sexual assault, but it can also result from other events, such as being robbed or physically attacked; being kid-napped, tortured, or the victim of a terrorist attack; being diagnosed with a life-threatening illness; and experiencing natural disasters. Wit-nessing others being harmed or threatened in these ways and even hear-ing about them happening to people close to you can also lead to PTSD (see Table 5.11). Comorbidity is also common among patients with PTSD. Many suffer comorbid depression, panic disorder, alcohol or sub-stance abuse, and an increased risk of suicide comparable to that seen in major depression.

Treatment

Treatment outcome studies have generally shown psychotherapy to be the primary treatment modality for PTSD and the sole modality for post-traumatic dissociative symptoms. Psychopharmacology mainly serves an adjunctive role. However, pharmacological treatment is often essential for tempering severity of reexperiencing or hyperarousal symptoms so that psychotherapy can be conducted (Bajor, Ticlea, & Osser, 2011).

Most PTSD patients require a program of treatment, rather than one treatment modality. An effective treatment program integrates the following elements:

- Provide safety and security
- Provide psychoeducation about traumatic stress
- Attenuate risk factors
- Mobilize resilience factors
- (as indicated) Provide trauma-focused psychotherapy
- (as indicated) Prescribe medications

First-line treatment of PTSD utilizes an SSRI or SNRI antidepres-sant. Sertraline and paroxetine are FDA-approved for PTSD treatment,

TABLE 5.11. Common Traumatic Events

- Witnessing injury/death
- Sexual molestation/rape
- Natural disaster/fire
- Physical attack or abuse/threatened with a weapon
- Life-threatening accident
- Combat

Note. Data from Kessler et al. (1995).

while fluoxetine has substantial research support for its effectiveness. The U.S. Department of Veterans Affairs has added venlafaxine as a first-line treatment for combat PTSD (VA/DoD Working Group, 2010). Thirty-seven randomized placebo-controlled trials subjected to meta-analysis found only paroxetine, sertraline, and venlafaxine to have superiority over placebo (Baldwin, Anderson, & Nutt, 2014). Citalopram is an SSRI that has failed to show superiority over placebo. Venlafaxine has been found to be consistently efficacious across all trauma types in both men and women (Rothbaum et al., 2008).

When an initial antidepressant is ineffective, nefazodone and mirtazapine or a different SSRI or SNRI can be tried. Low doses of an atypical antipsychotic, such as olanzapine or quetiapine have been utilized to augment the initial antidepressant, particularly for sleep symptoms.

Prazosin and topiramate are medications that have been demonstrably effective specifically for treatment of posttraumatic nightmares. Due to greater side effects with topiramate, prazosin is regarded as first-line treatment for nightmares. As an example, an Afghan survivor of torture in a Russian prison during the 1980s had posttraumatic nightmares every night for a decade until treated with a combination of prazosin and topiramate. The patient described his experience: "Together, the prazosin and topiramate make me feel stronger like no worries. . . . My brain is not thinking about the past, no panic or anxiety, because of deep sleep."

Insomnia is a common complaint among PTSD patients. The Harvard South Shore Psychopharmacology Outcome Project has provided a well-reasoned treatment algorithm for PTSD treatment that first targets disturbed sleep with prazosin or trazodone before adding treatment with an SSRI antidepressant (Bajor et al., 2011). Many patients show broad attenuation of posttraumatic symptoms with restoration of normal sleep.

Patients with disabling hyperarousal symptoms, such as an exaggerated startle reflex, irritability, or intolerance of loud noises or bright lights, sometimes improve with clonidine or guanfacine, both alpha$_2$ agonists that tone down the sympathetic nervous system. Propranolol, a beta-blocker, can sometimes serve a similar role (Pitman et al., 2002). For example, a woman at midlife had been treated for chronic PTSD after multiple rapes 2 decades earlier. Nevertheless, she had such an exaggerated startle reflex if accidentally bumped that she avoided riding on elevators. Her startle reflex diminished dramatically after treatment with clonidine. As she put it, "There was a feeling of tranquility after the first couple of days with clonidine. The jumpiness stopped."

Although benzodiazepines can initiate sleep effectively, early studies found that benzodiazepines failed to ameliorate core PTSD symptoms. Some studies suggested that early use of benzodiazepines contributed to chronicity of PTSD. Use of benzodiazepines for PTSD treatment has been generally regarded as unwise.

GENERALIZED ANXIETY DISORDER

Generalized anxiety disorder is diagnosed based on criteria listed in the DSM-5 or the ICD-11 diagnostic systems. Worry is pervasive and is accompanied by physical symptoms, such as motor tension, autonomic hypersensitivity, or hyperarousal. Patients often present physical or psychological symptoms that have no medical explanation.

Despite its apparent benign character, generalized anxiety disorder is associated with a level of work and social disability similar to that of MDD. There is high comorbidity with other anxiety and mood disorders. Long-term remission rates are very low. Common symptoms include:

- Restlessness or feeling keyed up
- Being easily fatigued
- Difficulty concentrating
- Irritability
- Muscle tension
- Sleep disturbance

Generalized anxiety disorder typically appears in the mid-20s, with increasing rates at midlife and later. Its prevalence in the general population is 5%, but is 8% in primary care populations. It affects twice as many women as men and is associated with unemployment, divorce, loss of a spouse, and the role of a homemaker. It is the most common anxiety disorder in primary care populations but least common in psychiatric practices. Unlike social anxiety disorder, panic disorder, and PTSD, there is little evidence of self-medication using alcohol (Hans-Ulrich & Hoyer, 2001).

Treatment

Generalized anxiety disorder treatment is most effective with implementation of a multi-tiered treatment program, starting with psychoeducation. Patients may need to learn that they should:

- Avoid caffeine.
- Avoid excess alcohol and nicotine.

- Exercise moderately, preferably aerobic exercise. Exercise is more effective for physical anxiety symptoms, such as restlessness or "crawling out of my skin," than for psychic anxiety symptoms, such as worry or ruminations.
- Monitor OTC medications that can produce autonomic hyperarousal, such as nasal decongestants.

CBT that targets catastrophic thinking can serve as a primary treatment modality or can be implemented alongside pharmacological treatment. Couple, family, and interpersonal psychotherapy are valuable as they can resolve relational dissatisfaction, binds, and conflicts that exacerbate symptoms.

An SSRI or SNRI antidepressant is regarded as first-line pharmacological treatment for generalized anxiety disorder. There is little empirical evidence to argue the merits of one SSRI or SNRI over another, although some studies found venlafaxine to achieve early remission of symptoms. The major side effects of SSRIs and SNRIs are sexual side effects, particularly anorgasmia (Schatzberg & DeBattista, 2015, pp. 411–462).

Benzodiazepines with slow absorption from the GI tract (which minimizes abuse) and long duration of action (to minimize mini-withdrawal side effects) are an effective alternative treatment. Extended-release clonazepam and alprazolam fit well this profile. Benzodiazepines are extremely safe medications if overdosed, unless combined with alcohol. Their disadvantages are, in high doses, sedation, physical dependence, memory impairment, and incoordination.

Buspirone is a unique medication that can reduce general anxiety, although it is ineffective for preventing panic attacks. It is more effective for reducing psychic anxiety than for reducing somatic or autonomic symptoms. It can be combined with antidepressants. Buspirone has been found to be as efficacious as benzodiazepines in some studies. It does not have sedation, incoordination, or physical dependence side effects. It typically has a gradual onset of action over 5–10 days (Schatzberg & DeBattista, 2015, pp. 411–462).

OBSESSIVE–COMPULSIVE DISORDER

OCD is diagnosed based on criteria listed in the DSM-5 or the ICD-11 diagnostic systems. Obsessions are recurrent thoughts, impulses, or images that are intrusive and distressing. The person attempts to ignore or suppress the thoughts or to neutralize them with another thought or action. Compulsions are the repetitive behaviors or mental acts performed in response to an obsession or to accord with certain rules. Compulsions are intended to neutralize or prevent discomfort associated with an obsessive thought or impulse.

Obsessions are not simply worries about real-life problems. A person with OCD recognizes that the thoughts, or degree of worry, make no sense. Unlike psychotic delusions, the person recognizes that obsessions are a product of his or her mind, not imposed from without. Obsessions can be distinguished from delusions in that a person with an obsession has a dominant emotion of doubt; that is, he or she believes that there is only a slight possibility of validity to the thought. A person with a delusion has a dominant emotion of certainty about the validity of thoughts that other people would regard as bizarre or obviously false. With psychosis, there is no insight into the disorder.

A person with OCD often feels deep shame or self-hatred that he or she cannot control obsessive thoughts that he or she recognizes as irrational. For example, a middle-aged man was admitted to a psychiatric inpatient unit after he came to the hospital emergency room with suicidal impulses. When meeting with the inpatient psychiatrist, he revealed that he had persistent, intrusive thoughts of "Damn the Virgin Mary!" As a devout Catholic Christian, he felt that such thoughts were an unforgivable sin, and that he deserved to die as punishment.

There are many different types of obsessions, some of which bear little resemblance to other types. Different types of obsessions include:

- Contamination
- Fear of harm
- Need for symmetry
- Somatic concerns (preoccupations with bodily functions, such as defecation or urination)
- Religious
- Sexual impulses
- Hoarding

Likewise, there are different types of common compulsions, with perhaps the most common one being checking back:

- Checking back
- Cleaning/washing
- Repeating
- Mental rituals
- Ordering

- Hoarding/collecting
- Counting

The average age of onset is 20 years, with a 2% lifetime prevalence, and a roughly equal gender distribution. However, onset often occurs in 5- to 15-year-olds. OCD usually is unremitting over the course of adulthood with a gradual onset but continuous course through life (Eisen et al., 2013).

The existence of a personal ritual does not necessarily imply OCD as a diagnosis. For example, a professional baseball player may eat the identical meal before every game, line up his equipment in a specific order every day, wear the same (sometimes unwashed) socks or underwear as long as a hitting streak continues, and cross himself and tap his bat three times against his right shoe every time he enters the batter's box. He feels a strong need to do all this and would probably feel some distress if his lucky socks were accidentally washed. Although none of these behaviors are rationally connected to his ability to hit the baseball (and he would admit that, at least in the off-season), the ritual probably isn't OCD. The behaviors aren't distressing to him; he feels in control of them, and they are acceptable behaviors in the subculture of professional baseball. Thus, it can be important to consider cultural context in diagnosing OCD. Many cultural and religious groups prescribe rituals that may seem irrational or compulsive to outsiders but perfectly ego-syntonic and appropriate to members of the culture. On the other hand, people can develop obsessions and compulsions related to the content of their cultural rituals. A man whose religion forbids certain foods may develop an obsessive fear of accidentally ingesting a forbidden food and a compulsion to repeatedly check his kitchen for hidden traces of it. If a clinician does not know this man's culture, it might be helpful to find out whether his wife and his religious leader think his behavior is excessive to help the clinician distinguish between an unfamiliar ritual and a compulsive behavior of clinical significance.

Treatment

OCD treatment is most effective when a multimodality program can be implemented that emphasizes psychoeducation about the disorder and its treatment. This permits a collaborative relationship in which the patient and family can best work with clinicians in treating what is often the most challenging of anxiety disorders due to limited efficacy of currently available pharmacological and psychotherapeutic treatments.

As a general rule, medications are partially effective in diminishing severity of obsessions and compulsion, while behavioral therapy, utilizing exposure and response prevention strategies, most effectively diminishes compulsions and rituals that interfere with daily life (Foa & Yadin, 2012). Treatment responses to both are usually partial, and relapses occur when active treatment is stopped (Schatzberg & DeBattista, 2015, pp. 439–441).

The only consistently effective medications have been antidepressants that selectively inhibit serotonin reuptake, that is, clomipramine and the SSRIs. Generally, SSRI antidepressants are considered to be first-line treatments, particularly fluoxetine, fluvoxamine, sertraline, and paroxetine. Typical doses effective for OCD are two- to fourfold greater than for treatment of depression or panic disorder. Whereas depression or panic disorder often respond to antidepressant treatment in 1–3 weeks, OCD symptoms often require 6–12 weeks for a full response.

In the Collaborative Clomipramine Study Group Trial, the **Yale–Brown Obsessive Compulsive Scale (Y-BOCS)** score was reduced by about 40% in patients taking clomipramine as compared with 5% among patients taking placebo (Clomipramine Collaborative Study Group, 1991). In general, only 10–15% of OCD patients achieve full remission of symptoms with SSRI treatment, with 70% having a partial response. The average partial responder has a 40% decrease in symptoms. Chronic treatment is often needed, due to an 85% relapse rate within 1 or 2 months of stopping medications.

A typical program for OCD consists of:

- Psychoeducation.
- Adequate dosage with an SSRI for 10 weeks.
- Treatment with medication for 6–12 months before considering taper of medication.
- Couple, family, or interpersonal psychotherapy for family or interpersonal problems secondary to OCD compulsions or rituals, including family accommodation to compulsive rituals that is detrimental due to long-term effects upon family functioning.
- Behavior therapy. Exposure and response prevention can reduce severity of compulsions or rituals. Between 20 and 25% of patients with OCD refuse behavioral treatment out of fear of exposure to unacceptable levels of anxiety, so motivational enhancement is a key element of treatment. Basic principles of behavior therapy that all involved clinicians and family members can reinforce are:
  - "Confront the things you fear as often as possible."
  - "If you feel like you must avoid something, don't."
  - "If you feel like you must perform a ritual to feel better, don't."

CONCLUSION

Anxiety disorders are ubiquitous and, like affective disorders, are expressed clinically only when the combination of genetic vulnerability and psychosocial forces are critically combined in a given individual. Medications used for unrelated medical conditions and OCT drugs (even coffee) can induce anxiety disorders in susceptible individuals. This is also the case for recreational use of drugs.

Although anxiety disorders, when untreated, can be the cause of substantial personal suffering, disability, and marital and family disruption, progress has been made in treating panic disorder, OCD, and generalized anxiety disorder, and other anxiety disorders, making these conditions very gratifying to treat. Indeed, the skillful use of psychotherapies and medications can produce dramatic and lasting improvement in many patients.

Most medications used in the treatment of anxiety disorders are also those used in treating depressive disorders, and many comments made in Chapter 4 are applicable here, including the rational selection of medication, initiation, and duration of treatment, as well as the identification and management of side effects. It is important to note that patients with anxiety disorders have a tendency to relapse relatively quickly once medications are discontinued, whereas the impact of behavioral therapies appears to be longer lasting. Once again, a close collaborative effort between the therapist and the physician can guide the selection of the most appropriate form of treatment and/or combination of treatments, as well as their duration.

CHAPTER 6

Schizophrenia and Other Psychoses

Psychotic thinking can be loosely defined as an inability to distinguish accurately which perceptions are mostly, or entirely, a creation of one's inner thoughts and imagination and which reflect events in an outside, external world. Psychotic thinking can be hallucinatory, as when seeing, hearing, or touching people or physical objects when others present witness no one or no object present; delusional, as when holding a rigid belief at odds with accessible evidence to the contrary; or dissociative, as when perceptions of time, space, or self become distorted or there is a sense of leaving one's body. The distinction between an experience being psychotic or nonpsychotic largely turns on whether the experience would also be witnessed by observers other than the perceiver. As Simeon and Abugel (2006) have noted:

> If one person sees an angel hovering outside the window while no one else does, we think of them as either a religious visionary or, more likely, a person with schizophrenia. If 10 people see the angel, it may be a mass hallucination, and if everyone sees the angel, then we safely assume the angel is really there, whatever the explanation for her presence. (p. 17)

Distinctions between realities that are primarily imaginative and those properly regarded as objective events are often not clear-cut in everyday life.

Hypnotic processes with individuals or in groups can produce psychotic phenomena through suggestion. Hypnotists have been able to produce a variety of positive and negative hallucinations and dissociative phenomena through formal hypnotic inductions (Erickson, 1980; Erickson & Erickson, 1980; Kroger, 1977). Across the world's cultures, hallucinations and dissociative phenomena can be found within normative religious experiences. From hallucinations to delusional thinking to possession states, every form of psychopathology can be generated within some emotionally intense religious experience (Griffith, 2010).

Psychiatrists from Carl Jung to Karl Menninger have noted that some individuals have passed through episodes of psychotic mental illnesses to new lives of creative endeavors and mental health that they had never before achieved (Chadwick, 2009). Anton Boisen, for example, became a minister and established the discipline of pastoral counseling after enduring a psychotic episode (Boisen, 1936/1962). These experiences of psychosis produced transformational changes in people's lives that led to personal growth or insights that revitalized their cultures (Lukoff, 2007).

What these "normal" forms of psychotic thinking suggest is that a variety of interventions impacting brain physiology—drug intoxication, sensory deprivation, manipulation of brain attentional systems through hypnosis, controlled communications and relationships within closed ideological groups, or meditative Kundalini awakenings—may each interfere with routinized top-down regulation of sensory information entering the nervous system. The brain is then exposed to novel sensory patterns that can be interpreted as an awakening to a new world. The difference between a psychiatric disorder and "normal" psychoticism may rest primarily with the intactness of prefrontal cortex circuitry for working memory, executive functions, and emotion regulation as it responds to these novel patterns. During mindfulness meditation, these prefrontal cognitive systems are presumably operating at optimal efficiency, even as they are flooded by freshly unedited sensory input. This abrupt juxtaposition of reflective thought with raw sensory experience can become a formula for creativity. In schizophrenia, bipolar disorder, and dissociative disorders, however, there are diminished capacities for reflection, dialogue, and interpersonal relatedness due to impaired prefrontal regulation of other brain systems. In these illnesses, disorganized thought, rather than creativity, more often results if drugs or meditation flood the brain with raw sensory experience.

The schizophrenia family of disorders (schizophrenia, delusional disorder, schizoaffective disorder) are not the only psychiatric illnesses in which psychosis is a primary feature. In some, mood disorders, psychosis is present only during severe episodes. In others, like paranoid disorder, the main psychotic feature—the delusion—is an isolated feature,

TABLE 6.1. Disorders That Manifest Psychotic Symptoms

- Schizophrenia
- Schizophreniform disorder
- Schizoaffective disorder
- Delusional disorder
- Brief psychotic disorder
- Shared psychotic disorder
- Mood disorders (e.g., mania, psychotic depression)
- Brain tumors
- Stroke
- Head trauma
- Endocrine/metabolic abnormalities (e.g., severe hypothyroidism)
- Substance-induced psychoses
- Dementia (e.g., Alzheimer's disease)
- Delirium
- Neurological conditions (e.g., Huntington's chorea, Tourette's syndrome)
- Infections
- Other psychoses

and the rest of the patient's mental functioning is generally preserved (Table 6.1). The use of a number of substances, some prescribed for medical disorders and some used illegally for mind-altering purposes, can also result in psychotic symptoms (Table 6.2). It is estimated that about 5–6 million people in the United States suffer from psychotic symptoms at any given time.

SCHIZOPHRENIA

Schizophrenia is a frequently disabling, often chronic psychiatric illness that affects approximately 1% of the U.S. population. Florid symptoms most often begin in late adolescence or early adulthood, although onset

TABLE 6.2. Some Drugs Known to Induce Psychosis

Amphetamines	Indomethacin
Marijuana	Corticosteroids
Hallucinogens	Procainamide
Cocaine	Phenytoin
Beta-blockers	Carbamazepine
Bupropion	

can occur throughout the years of adulthood. Schizophrenia can be heralded by slow emotional and cognitive development during childhood, such as difficulties establishing a network of friends. There are five symptom clusters that can characterize episodes of illness. Variation can occur from one patient to the next as to which, or whether all, of these symptom clusters predominate. It is possible that different patterns of symptoms may be shown by researchers to constitute different illnesses in years to come (see Table 6.3).

One patient's symptoms may consist solely in "hearing voices," with a rich, full personality and an ability to interact socially that is fully intact. Such illness that is limited to **positive symptoms** can carry relatively little work disability or impairments in social roles. Severe **negative symptoms** and/or impaired social cognition can leave a patient socially excluded. Cognitive deficits, when severe, preclude many kinds of work that require judgment and complex problem solving.

Episodes of acute illness can occur frequently, often precipitated by heightened emotional arousal from life stress. Common stressors that precipitate acute psychotic episodes include (McFarlane, 2009, p. 646):

- Excessive sensory stimulation
- Prolonged emotional stress or heightened demands for cognitive performance

TABLE 6.3. Clinical Clusters of Schizophrenia

Cluster	Examples
Positive symptoms	Auditory hallucinations, delusional thinking, thought insertion or thought broadcasting (other people inserting thoughts into one's minds or listening to one's private thoughts)
Negative symptoms	Apathy, social withdrawal, paucity of thoughts (alogia), flatness in expression of emotions (flat affects), avolition, anhedonia
Cognitive deficits	Impaired executive functions, impaired immediate memory
Disorganized language	Loss of logical connections from one thought to the next or between words within a single sentence; use of newly created words that have only a privately understood meaning (neologism)
Social cognition	Misinterpretation of social cues; misjudgments in gauging appropriate social distance; inability to interpret accurately expressions of feelings, thoughts, or intentions of other people

- Rapid or frequent changes in environment, relationships, performance expectations
- Social disruptions
- Illicit drug and alcohol use
- Negative emotional experiences, particularly when involving blame, shame, or humiliation
- High expressed emotion (criticism, emotional overinvolvement) in the family environment

Remission of symptoms occurs to varying degrees between acute episodes. Acute positive symptoms, such as hallucinations or delusions, can largely remit in 5–15 days of treatment with antipsychotic medications. However, recovery from negative symptoms, such as apathy and social withdrawal, can take months even with treatment (McFarlane, 2009, p. 657). This slow recovery from negative symptoms is difficult for families to bear, since apathy as a symptom of illness can be difficult to distinguish between laziness or oppositional behavior. Our current antipsychotic medications unfortunately do not ameliorate disorganized thinking or cognitive impairments.

CASE ILLUSTRATION: MS. P., SCHIZOPHRENIA

Ms. P., a 53-year-old woman, visited her primary care physician, because she had been feeling pain in her arms, pressure around her eyes, and changes in her vision. The physician examined her, but found no medical cause for her complaints. He added them to the long list of symptoms she had reported over several recent visits that had found no clear medical etiology. She also told him that she had been feeling very "nervous and stressed out" over the past several weeks.

Ms. P. currently lived alone in a government-subsidized apartment complex. She had been married and divorced twice, maintained close contact with her mother, had an adult daughter who was refusing to speak to her, and had an adult son who was recently released from an inpatient substance-dependence treatment facility.

Beginning Collaboration

The physician referred Ms. P., a new patient, to an eye specialist. Concerned about her anxious demeanor, he also asked if she would like a referral to an in-house therapist for emotional support. She agreed, and the physician filled out a referral for one of the clinic therapists.

The therapist contacted Ms. P., who agreed to come in for an initial therapy session. She revealed several of her worries, including concerns about her health, her family, and her neighbors. She denied any symptoms of depression, mania, or psychosis and was given a diagnosis of anxiety disorder not otherwise specified. Over the next several sessions, the therapist began wonder if these anxieties were based in reality or were products of her imagination. Ms. P. had begun complaining about a discoloration of her skin that was not at all visible to the therapist. She later described an ability to smell food she watched cooking on television and an incident in which she saw her whole living room turn purple. In subsequent sessions, Ms. P. described several phone calls to the police and landlord about a neighbor stalking her, which were investigated and dismissed as unfounded. She also told the therapist about her special ability to know the thoughts of people she talks to on the phone, and to even hear special voices, as if she "has a satellite dish attached to her head." Throughout this time, Ms. P. held strong to her belief that she is "mentally sound" but that her problems were her doctor's failing to find diagnoses for her physical ailments, her bothersome neighbor, and her special abilities that most people don't have.

As the therapist gathered this information, she and the primary care physician conferred about the need for a psychiatric consultation. The therapist discussed with Ms. P. how she might benefit from "additional support of an extra doctor on her treatment team." As soon as Ms. P. heard the word "psychiatrist," however, she insisted that she was not mentally ill and had no need for "one of those kinds of doctors." One day, Ms. P. came to therapy particularly agitated. She described herself as feeling very stressed, unable to sleep, and unable to shut off her mind. The therapist again mentioned the idea of seeing a doctor who specializes in "dealing with stress," and this time Ms. P. agreed to the offer.

Ongoing Collaboration and Outcome

The therapist contacted Dr. M., a psychiatrist in her health care network. The therapist knew how important it would be for the psychiatrist to establish rapport with Ms. P. from the beginning due to Ms. P.'s ambivalence. She selected Dr. M. for his personal warmth and tactfulness with patients. She accompanied Ms. P. to the consultation so she and the psychiatrist, in a "warm handoff," could discuss the potential benefits of the consultation in Ms. P.'s presence.

In the psychiatric consultation, the psychiatrist avoided technical language in his explanation to Ms. P. for his treatment recommendations. He did not tell Ms. P. she was "psychotic" or possibly had "schizophrenia." Rather, he told Ms. P. that "too much stress for too long had worn down her nervous system," so that her thoughts "were becoming jumbled" and she was "having trouble discerning who to trust." He recommended a medication, risperidone, as an atypical antipsychotic that would improve her brain's effectiveness for thinking clearly. The risperidone would make it easier to determine who to trust and who not to trust so she could feel safe relaxing. Ms. P. accepted the prescription for medication, while her therapist asked the psychiatrist some questions so she could help Ms. P. take the medication correctly and monitor side effects. Ms. P. left the consultation expressing appreciation.

By her next therapy session, Ms. P. had read more information about her medication on the Internet and angrily told her therapist that it was for "people who are crazy," and she would not take it. The therapist assured her that taking medication did not mean she was "crazy" and reminded her that Dr. M. prescribed that medication in fact to help her think more clearly and to better shoulder stress without stress making her ill. The therapist encouraged Ms. P. to contact the psychiatrist to discuss her concerns. The therapist contacted both Ms. P.'s primary care physician and the psychiatrist so they were aware of Ms. P.'s hesitations.

Over the next several months, the primary care physician and therapist both worked closely with Ms. P. to take her medication as prescribed. Finally consenting to a 2-week initial trial, Ms. P. found that she liked how the risperidone helped her sleep and brought "a sense of peace" to her mind. Unfortunately, when she would feel better, she frequently discontinued her medication until she began feeling "stressed" again, despite her physician's and therapist's encouragement to take her medication as prescribed.

Questions for Consideration

1. Why did the therapist continue to see Ms. P. even though she clearly needed psychiatric care more than therapy? The therapist realized that therapy was not particularly helpful to Ms. P. while she was actively psychotic. She continued to see her so that she could serve as a bridge into the psychiatric care she saw as crucial to Ms. P.'s treatment. Because the therapist was located in the same office as the primary care physician, Ms. P. found it natural to come in to see her. Ms. P. often made medical appointments or had her blood pressure checked while she was at the clinic. This helped diminish a sense of stigma for seeking help from a mental health professional by keeping her symptoms in the category of "physical illness" rather than "mental illness," and it ultimately enabled her to trust the therapist enough to follow her advice to see a psychiatrist.

2. *Why did the therapist attend the psychiatry appointment with Ms. P.?* First, although the therapist knew and trusted the psychiatrist well enough to feel confident in his ability to establish a good rapport with Ms. P., she wanted to support Ms. P. overcoming her ambivalence about being stigmatized as "mentally ill." Second, she wanted to encourage Ms. P. to give information to Dr. M. that she might not disclose unless asked directly. Third, she knew that if Ms. P. disliked anything about the appointment, she would be quick to disregard everything Dr. M. said. Fourth, she knew that Ms. P.'s sense of trust in the process would be enhanced by having an open discussion about her problem with the psychiatrist in front of Ms. P. while she listened. Finally, she wanted to hear together with Ms. P. the psychiatrist's formulation and treatment recommendations so she could refer back to them in future meetings.

3. *How much should the therapist talk with Ms. P. about her psychotropic medications?* The therapist limited what she would say to Ms. P. about her medications. The therapist would often preface her statements about the medication by reminding Ms. P. that she was not the doctor, nor an expert on medication. However, she could help Ms. P. recall the doctor's recommendations about taking the medication and monitoring side effects. She then could help Ms. P. to organize questions she might want to ask her psychiatrist about the medication, such as possible side effects.

4. *Research suggests that many patients who are prescribed psychotropic medication fail to complete an adequate trial. They fail to take enough medication for enough time to see if it treats the symptoms. How did the therapist's presence influence the patient's adherence to the medication trial?* During the critical first weeks, the therapist was able to help Ms. P. address her worries and skepticism about the medication. She could address fears about stigma—whether taking medication meant that she was "crazy"—and she was able to help her get answers to the questions about the medication that emerged as she started taking it. Without the therapist's helpful encouragement, there was a good chance that Ms. P. would have simply stopped the medication and not returned to Dr. M.

The course of schizophrenia is often chronic and relentless, with periods of exacerbation marked by prominent psychotic symptoms interspersed between long periods with lesser psychotic symptoms but disabling cognitive, mood, interpersonal, and thought-process deficits.

Schizophrenia accounts for about 40% of mental health hospital beds and about 15% of all hospital beds. The costs to society are staggering: $150 billion per year in the United States for direct costs (hospitalization, physician and therapist services, and medications) plus indirect costs (disability, lost productivity, etc.). It accounts for 2.5% of all U.S. health costs and about 20% of the total days of Social Security benefits (McCutcheon, Marques, & Howes, 2020).

Patients with schizophrenia are also at a great disadvantage in other health concerns, reflected in a shortened life expectancy. Their mortality rates are between 1.6 and 2.6 times higher than those for the rest of the population, with a life expectancy about 20% shorter than the normal population (61 years vs. 76 years). While schizophrenia has a significantly elevated rate of suicide, this 15-year reduction in life expectancy is most related to poor physical health from poverty living conditions and homelessness. Patients with schizophrenia have smoking rates much higher than the general population and are therefore exposed to cardiovascular and pulmonary risks from long-term tobacco use. They are also more likely to be obese (some of this is medication-induced) and to suffer from diabetes, heart disease, and other conditions.

Patients with schizophrenia are at great risk for suicide. About half of patients with schizophrenia will attempt suicide sometime in their lives. Some suicide attempts are directly due to command hallucinations, delusions, or severe depression. However, other suicides occur due to the profound demoralization that can occur when a patient during a period of lucidity looks at his or her life circumstances and determines that this "is not a life worth living" (Shea, 2002, p. 77). Five to 10% of patients with schizophrenia will die as a result of suicide (McCutcheon et al., 2020).

OTHER PSYCHOTIC DISORDERS

Schizoaffective disorder can be regarded as either a "better prognosis" schizophrenia or a "worse prognosis" type of bipolar disorder. Schizoaffective disorder incorporates elements of thought disorder, hallucinations, and other psychotic symptoms typically observed in schizophrenia, with significant mood symptoms—depression, hypomania, and mania—classically associated with bipolar disorder.

Delusional disorder is characterized by the presence of a single unshakeable, nonbizarre delusion. Several subtypes of delusional disorder are recognized, emanating from the main delusional concern (erotomanic, grandiose, jealous, persecutory, somatic, and mixed).

Treatment for each of these psychotic conditions includes the use of antipsychotic medications similar to treatment of schizophrenia.

THE RECOVERY MOVEMENT

The **Recovery Movement** has challenged the historic nihilism about meaningful recovery from schizophrenia. It has refocused attention on significant numbers of individuals who, with the help of maintenance treatment, continue living fully functional lives. The Recovery Movement has disseminated and publicized long-term outcome studies showing that many individuals with chronic psychotic disorders were able to achieve significant degrees of life satisfaction and relational and work functioning over time, contrary to long-held expectations of mental health professionals. The Recovery Movement became a consumer-driven movement of social activism in which psychiatric patients sought to become partners in care and peer experts in counseling other patients (Myers, 2010; Peebles et al., 2007; Resnick, Fontana, Lehman, & Rosenhack, 2005).

The Recovery Movement regards a successful treatment outcome as about more than symptom reduction. Emphasis is placed upon:

- Increased life satisfaction
- Empowerment of the patient as a person
- Enhanced hope and commitment to recovery
- Improved ability to seek and maintain supportive relationships

The Recovery Movement is thus closely linked to the "common factors" of therapeutic change that include a highly collaborative treatment relationship, the fostering of self-efficacy, promotion of hope and expectancy that improvement will occur, and the social support of a treatment relationship (Griffith, 2018; Peebles et al., 2007).

In the Recovery Movement, patients assume a full partnership in treatment relationships with clinicians. Certified peer specialists are patients who are able to utilize their experiences coping with illness to advise and support other patients who are coping less well. Resnick and colleagues (2005) used data from the Schizophrenia Patient Outcomes Research Team (PORT) study to show that the different values forming the Recovery Movement coalesce into four key factors:

1. Gaining knowledge about the mental health system and how to acquire community assistance
2. Empowerment in which the self is experienced as an agent of change that is able to pursue needed services
3. Hope and optimism, including optimism about the future of one's mental health
4. Life satisfaction (family, social network, living situations, community concerns, sense of safety)

One consequence of such findings has been to place greater importance upon patient and family psychoeducation about the illness (natural course of illness, its symptoms, early detection of relapse, prevention of relapse) and its treatments (how medications work, side-effect management, guidelines for optimizing family environment). Effective psychoeducation enables patients and family members to collaborate with clinicians as partners. Such findings also have elevated the importance of **patient navigators** who help patients and families learn how systems of care operate and how to solicit system resources.

ANTIPSYCHOTIC MEDICATIONS

Antipsychotic medications constitute the backbone of pharmacological agents for psychotic illnesses. Antipsychotic medications primarily improve positive symptoms, with lesser improvement in negative symptoms. Their mechanism of action has been explained as compensating for dysregulation in brain circuits that utilize dopamine as a transmitter. These dopaminergic systems help regulate information processing within the prefrontal cortex and the salience network (amygdala, insula). All antipsychotic medications appear to exert their therapeutic effects by occupying (blocking) dopamine receptors in the limbic system and prefrontal cortex.

First-Generation or "Typical" Antipsychotics

The first generation of antipsychotics has been used in the United States since the 1950s. They have been largely replaced by newer agents that have fewer side effects, albeit without improved therapeutic potency. Examples of conventional antipsychotics appear in Table 6.4.

All typical antipsychotic medications share a common mechanism of action: They block the D_2 **dopamine receptor.** By blocking the dopamine

TABLE 6.4. Some Conventional Antipsychotics

- Chlorpromazine (Thorazine)
- Haloperidol (Haldol)[a]
- Thioridazine (Mellaril)
- Trifluoperazine (Stelazine)
- Fluphenazine (Prolixin)[a]
- Perphenazine (Trilafon)
- Thiothixene (Navane)
- Loxapine (Loxitane)
- Molindone (Moban)

Note. Trade names are in parentheses.
[a]Available in injectable depot (long-term) formulation.

receptor, they reduce activation of dopamine-activated circuits in the limbic system. The result is a noticeable reduction in positive symptoms, such as hallucinations and delusions. Unfortunately, the D_2 dopamine receptor that typical antipsychotics provide produces no improvement in the other four groups of psychotic symptoms that are more disabling.

The D_2 dopamine receptor blockade also produces two sets of side effects that characterize all typical antipsychotic medications: extrapyramidal symptoms (parkinsonian symptoms, akathisia, dystonia) and side effects from elevated blood levels of prolactin hormone (amenorrhea, gynecomastia). Extrapyramidal symptoms are produced due to the role that D_2 receptors serve in the motor systems that control posture and muscle tone.

Parkinsonian side effects include tremor, muscle rigidity, loss of balance, and stooped posture. These symptoms are identical to those of Parkinson's disease. Such symptoms can be relieved by anticholinergic medications, such as **benztropine** (trade name Cogentin) or **amantadine** (trade name Symmetrel).

Akathisia, a sense of intolerable restlessness and tension in leg muscles, responds poorly to anticholinergic medications, but can be relieved by propranolol or benzodiazepines. Table 6.5 lists the common side effects associated with conventional antipsychotic therapy.

Extrapyramidal motor side effects can occur as early as a few hours after administration of the first dose, such as acute dystonia in which frightening spasms of muscles can produce contorted body postures, or even eyeballs rotating back into the head. Acute dystonias most commonly occur during the first few doses of an antipsychotic medication ingested by a young patient (Schatzberg & DeBattista, 2015, p. 186). Acute dystonias resolve quickly with intramuscular administration of an

TABLE 6.5. Neurological Side Effects of Conventional Antipsychotics

Side effect	Clinical manifestations	Chronology of onset
Acute dystonia	Spasm of tongue, throat, face, jaw, eyes, neck, or back muscles (torticollis, facial grimacing, oculogyric crises)	24 hours to <1 week
Akathisia	Restlessness, inability to sit still, strong urge to move about	<1 week to 2 weeks
Pseudoparkinsonism	Bradykinesia, rigidity, sialorrhea, mask-like facies, resting tremor, "pill rolling," shuffling gait	~1 week
Tardive dyskinesia	Protrusion of tongue, puffing of cheeks, chewing movements, involuntary movements of extremities and trunk	3 months to years

anticholinergic medication, such as the antihistamine diphenhydramine (trade name Benadryl) (Schatzberg & DeBattista, 2015, p. 591).

After several months of treatment another extrapyramidal side effect, **tardive dyskinesia,** can appear. Elderly female patients are at greatest risk. The uncontrollable movements of facial muscles, and sometimes upper and lower extremities, are extremely distressing and bothersome to patients (Schatzberg & DeBattista, 2015, p. 186). Dread of extrapyramidal movement disorders contributes to the high rate of treatment nonadherence among patients with schizophrenia.

Approximately 50% of patients with schizophrenia will discontinue medications after 4–6 months of treatment, mostly because of side effects. It is important for therapists to develop some familiarity with this constellation of adverse effects, although their prevalence has diminished somewhat since the introduction of the atypical antipsychotics (see Table 6.6). Management of this class of side effects includes dose modifications and addition of agents specifically aimed at reducing or eliminating the movement disorder (see Table 6.7).

As a different type of side effect, dopamine D_2 blockade in the pituitary gland will increase the production and release of the hormone prolactin. Prolactin is normally elevated in pregnancy and is responsible for breast enlargement and milk production. Sometimes patients, including males, treated with these medications will develop breast enlargement

TABLE 6.6. Neurotransmitter Effects of Conventional Antipsychotics and Their Associated Side Effects

Neurotransmitter	Side effect
Histamine	Sedation, weight gain, hypotension
Acetylcholine (muscarinic)	Urinary retention, increased heart rate, memory deficits, confusion, dry mouth, blurred vision, constipation
Norepinephrine (alpha-adrenergic)	Low blood pressure, constricted pupils, increased heart rate
Dopamine	Parkinsonian symptoms, other motor symptoms, increased prolactin

(gynecomastia) and lactation (galactorrhea). In women, elevated prolactin can produce amenorrhea, polycystic ovary disease, or infertility (Table 6.8).

Neuroleptic malignant syndrome is a rare but potentially lethal side effect of antipsychotic medications. A patient may become confused and lethargic with a high body temperature (above 100 degrees Fahrenheit), and experience severe extrapyramidal symptoms, such as rigid muscles, drooling, grinding teeth, dystonic posture, or eyes rolling back (oculogyric crisis). Symptoms usually build over 1–3 days. Early recognition, discontinuation of all antipsychotic medications, and transfer to a medical intensive care unit is needed (Schatzberg & DeBattista, 2015, pp. 272–274).

TABLE 6.7. Drugs Used in the Treatment of Extrapyramidal Symptoms

Antimuscarinics
  Benztropine (Cogentin)
  Biperiden (Akineton)
  Ethopropazine (Parsidol)
  Orphenadrine
  Procyclidine (Kemadrin)
  Trihexyphenidyl (Artane)

Antihistaminic
  Diphenhydramine (Benadryl)

Dopamine agonist
  Amantadine (Symmetrel)

Note. Trade names are in parentheses.

TABLE 6.8. Clinical Effects of Hyperprolactinemia

Menstrual function	Sexual function
• Anovulation	• Decreased libido
• Shortened luteal phase	• Orgasmic dysfunction
• Oligomenorrhea	
• Amenorrhea	Bones
	• Decreased bone density mediated by estrogen deficiency
Breast	
• Engorgement	
• Nonpuerperal lactation	

Atypical Antipsychotics

An important leap in the treatment of schizophrenia occurred in the late 1980s with the introduction of the first of a number of medications that offered a wider spectrum of action and relatively improved tolerability. Some of these atypical antipsychotics, also called second-generation antipsychotics, are listed in Table 6.9. The first of the atypicals, clozapine [trade name Clozaril], produced results that raised expectations of antipsychotic therapy. For the first time, negative symptoms were amenable to treatment. This capability, along with the ability to block the dopamine receptor, has led some to call this new generation the "atypical" antipsychotics. Further clinical study showed that clozapine was able to induce noticeable improvement in patients hitherto unresponsive to other antipsychotics (efficacy in particularly refractory cases is not necessarily shared by the other atypicals, and it appears to be a particular advantage of Clozaril). Also, a worldwide study has

TABLE 6.9. Atypical (Second-Generation) Antipsychotics

- Clozapine (Clozaril)
- Risperidone (Risperdal)
- Olanzapine (Zyprexa)
- Quetiapine (Seroquel)
- Ziprasidone (Geodon)
- Aripiprazole (Abilify)[a]
- Paliperidone (Invega, Invega Sustenna)
- Iloperidone (Fanapt)
- Asenapine (Saphris)

Note. Trade names are in parentheses.
[a]Aripiprazole is sometimes called a third-generation antipsychotic because of its unique mechanism of action (see text).

shown that clozapine—in a distinct advantage over other antipsychotics, both conventional and atypical—has a specific effect to reduce suicide risk in patients with schizophrenia. Finally, clozapine and other atypical antipsychotics displayed a much lower incidence of extrapyramidal symptoms and tardive dyskinesia.

In spite of these advantages, clozapine use was accompanied by many side effects and dangerous adverse reactions, notably an increased risk of potentially fatal **agranulocytosis** (a severe drop in white blood cell count). This potential risk, which occurs in 1–1.5% of cases, requires patients to take weekly blood tests for the first 6 months of treatment, with a decreased frequency thereafter, for as long as they are on clozapine. Many patients have been unwilling to continue long-term treatment, in spite of the benefits obtained. Other side effects of clozapine that further limit its use are listed in Table 6.10.

In spite of its limitations, clozapine brought renewed impetus to the quest for improved antipsychotic medications. For the first time, negative symptoms, so disabling to patients in the interpersonal, social, and occupational spheres, were seen as amenable to treatment. This has been thought to result from a balanced effect on dopamine and serotonin receptors. Other antipsychotics also have a broader spectrum of action, leading to their proven use in the treatment of manic episodes and bipolar depression.

From the perspective of tolerability, these new atypicals are clearly superior to conventionals. The rates of extrapyramidal symptoms, tardive dyskinesia, and anticholinergic effects are much lower. However, as their use has become more commonplace, these drugs appear to have their own adverse effects, some of which have raised substantial concerns. They include increased rates of extrapyramidal symptoms at higher than usual doses, prolactin elevations, and electrocardiogram changes.

TABLE 6.10. Some Potential Side Effects of Clozapine (Clozaril)

- Risk of agranulocytosis
- Drowsiness and sedation
- Marked weight gain
- Orthostatic hypotension
- Hypersalivation
- Dizziness and vertigo
- Seizures
- Increased heart rate

Weight gain and metabolic side effects, in particular, merit special attention. Individuals with schizophrenia are at a higher risk for developing several chronic medical conditions, including heart disease and diabetes (Consensus Development Conference on Antipsychotic Drugs and Obesity and Diabetes, 2004). They tend to be more overweight and to have higher rates of obesity, and compared to the general population, they also have a shorter life expectancy. This is true also for bipolar patients, another diagnostic category in which atypical antipsychotics are being used with increased frequency (Kupfer, 2005).

Treatment with atypical antipsychotics—some more than others—has been associated with increased risks by promoting weight gain, **hyperglycemia** (elevated blood sugar), diabetes, and **hyperlipidemia** (elevated blood fats). The effect is significant enough to warrant recommendations for proper monitoring of patients in order to improve the chances of early detection (Consensus Development Conference on Antipsychotic Drugs and Obesity and Diabetes, 2004). All mental health providers should ensure that patients adhere to a program of monitoring as recommended by their primary care physician or psychiatrist (Marder et al., 2004). The program should include periodic monitoring of several parameters, including weight measurements and baseline and follow-up blood sugar and lipid levels. Furthermore, given that the evidence shows that not all atypical antipsychotics currently available are equal offenders in increasing the risk for metabolic syndrome (see Table 6.11), clinicians must give consideration to this, among other factors, when selecting antipsychotic medications.

Genetic risks for metabolic syndrome appear greater for certain ethnic groups, an ethnopharmacological concern. The long-term risk of diabetes and myocardial infarction on clozapine appears to be far higher

TABLE 6.11. Atypical Antipsychotics and Metabolic Abnormalities

Drug	Weight gain	Risk for diabetes	Worsening lipid profile
Clozapine	+++	+	+
Olanzapine	+++	+	+
Risperidone	++	D	D
Quetiapine	++	D	D
Aripiprazole[a]	+/–	–	–
Ziprasidone[a]	+/–	–	–

Note. D, discrepant results. Data from Consensus Development Conference on Antipsychotic Drugs and Obesity and Diabetes (2004).
[a]Newer drugs with limited long-term data.

for Blacks and Latinx in comparison to Whites. Blacks and Latinx taking atypical antipsychotics develop higher rates of metabolic syndrome, requiring attentive monitoring of body weights and blood glucose and lipid levels (Consensus Development Conference on Antipsychotic Drugs and Obesity and Diabetes, 2004).

CASE ILLUSTRATION: MR. F., DELUSIONAL DISORDER, SOMATIC TYPE

Mr. F., a 42-year-old man, visited his family physician with a myriad of health concerns, including aches, pains, rashes, numbness, fatigue, sadness, memory disturbance, and weight loss. He said that the symptoms began after an extramarital affair, which had occurred 2 weeks earlier. Mr. F. was particularly concerned that he might "have AIDS," since this was his only explanation for his health problems. He added he had already seen another physician near his mother's house in a neighboring community and reported similar complaints. This previous medical exam had included an HIV test that had been negative. Despite this reassuring news, Mr. F. still firmly believed he had AIDS, which was frightening him to the point of considering suicide.

Beginning Collaboration

The physician evaluated Mr. F. for suicidality and implemented a crisis intervention plan to ensure his safety. He met with Mr. F. for extended visits over the next 2 months, initiated treatment with an SSRI antidepressant, and referred Mr. F. to a therapist who worked in the same office. A general medical and cardiac evaluation was started as well. Over the course of 3 months, Mr. F. requested and received two more HIV tests, both of which were negative. Unfortunately, these negative results did little to weaken Mr. F.'s belief that he had AIDS. On a scale of 0–100, Mr. F. said he was 90% sure he had AIDS.

Ongoing Collaboration

Over the course of several months, Mr. F. had an extensive medical evaluation, including specialty evaluation by a neurologist, cardiac stress testing, podiatry evaluation, and laboratory testing including eight HIV tests. All evaluations were negative. At this point, the physician and therapist together recommended a psychiatric evaluation. Mr. F. reluctantly agreed to meet with a psychiatrist but found it unhelpful and refused to return after the first visit. The psychiatrist recommended an antipsychotic to be prescribed by Mr. F.'s primary care physician.

Outcome

Mr. F.'s certainty and worry about AIDS infection followed a predictable pattern: After a negative result, he felt relief and gratitude for the work of the health care team but would become increasingly anxious and irritable as time passed since his most recent HIV test. He began doubting the intent and honesty of his physician: "Maybe the AIDS test is positive but he's not telling me because he's afraid that I'll kill myself." He also questioned whether the therapist was doing enough to find the cause of his symptoms. His physician reassured Mr. F. that everyone was honest and attempting to provide the best possible care. In a joint meeting, the physician and therapist restated their commitment to helping Mr. F. and offered a referral to another primary care physician for a second opinion. Mr. F. declined this suggestion.

Questions for Consideration

1. *What role did collaboration play in Mr. F.'s treatment?* Success with Mr. F. would have been unlikely without close collaboration. Mr. F. demonstrated reluctance to follow through with referrals to a variety of specialists. When he did follow through with an initial appointment, rarely did he continue contact with these providers, such as the psychiatrist. The reason he attended the first and subsequent mental health appointments was due to the strong relationship between his physician and therapist, which was facilitated by the collocation of their practices.

Second, the medical clinic where Mr. F. received his medical care became a metaphoric "family" for Mr. F. This "family" included not only his medical providers but also front desk staff. When he arrived for his appointments, the staff greeted Mr. F. with familiar kindness and respect. His multiple needs could be met at one time and in one place. This "one-stop shopping" was convenient and secure.

Finally, his physician and therapist presented a united front, repeatedly reassuring Mr. F. When Mr. F.'s distortions convinced him that they were hiding information, such as a positive test result, they could provide consistent information because of their frequent communication and shared charting. Mr. F. was appreciative of this joint care, which communicated that he was an important patient and his doctors were working as a team devoted to giving him the best possible care.

2. *What are some risks and possible strengths of the close collaborative relationships that the physician and therapist had?* The close physical proximity, shared history, mutual respect, and frequent communications enable physician and therapist to create an emotional holding environment for Mr. F.

THE DOPAMINE PARTIAL AGONISTS

A new third generation of partial agonist antipsychotics has been introduced, with notable success for many patients. Partial dopamine agonist medications include aripiprazole, brexpiprazole, and cariprazine. The novel mechanism of action of these medications addresses several of the limitations of other atypical antipsychotics.

Dopamine partial agonists activate dopamine receptors to a mild degree, while physically attaching to the receptors in such a way as to block high levels of available dopamine from reaching the receptor. Aripiprazole thus will reduce dopamine drive where it is too high, while also increasing dopamine drive where it is too low, and it will have little effect where the drive is normal. In the case of schizophrenia, these drugs are expected to improve positive symptoms by *reducing* excessive dopamine drive in the mesolimbic pathway while improving negative symptoms by *increasing* reduced dopamine drive in the mesocortical pathway. They should also cause much fewer changes (or none at all) in the other two dopamine pathways, thus avoiding extrapyramidal symptom and prolactin elevations. In addition to its partial dopamine agonism, aripiprazole has serotonin receptor effects that have been associated with mood and cognitive improvements, both desirable features in treating schizophrenia. Aripiprazole does not alter serum prolactin levels and hence has none of the sexual and reproductive side effects of typical antipsychotics.

GENERAL TREATMENT CONSIDERATIONS
IN ANTIPSYCHOTIC THERAPY

Antipsychotic therapy is comparatively effective and at the same time disappointingly insufficient. Available medications best treat positive symptoms of the disorder but are less effective with negative symptoms and are ineffective with cognitive symptoms. The great majority of patients will have between 20 and 50% reduction in symptom severity. A small minority of patients will be entirely refractory to all forms of treatment currently available. While improvement in positive symptoms can be seen in 5–15 days, improvement in negative symptoms may take months. Robinson et al. (1999) showed that only 20% of patients responded after 4 weeks of treatment with conventional antipsychotics, whereas after 26 weeks the number of responders had grown to about 70%.

The most effective antipsychotic overall is clozapine, with response in 40% of subjects after 4 weeks and in 60% of subjects by week 17 (Kane et al., 2001). The time necessary for remission appears to be a function, among other factors, of the episode number being treated. It has been demonstrated that the average patient being treated for a first acute episode of schizophrenia reaches remission of symptoms in about 4–6 weeks, whereas the same average patient, now in the third episode, will take 4 months to reach the same benefit level. The duration of treatment is also a function of episode number. Experts recommend at least 1 year of treatment for the first episode, 5 years after a second episode, and lifetime after three episodes. The relapse rate would be cut in half if one could double the rate of adherence to maintenance treatment (Kissling, 1991).

The management of schizophrenia poses unique challenges, depending on the stage of the illness being treated. In an emergency room, where one may find psychotic patients with aggressive, hostile, and violent behavior, immediate symptom control is essential. During outpatient follow-up care, where the most severe symptoms are essentially controlled, adherence to treatment becomes a major issue, and simplicity of dosing and the ability to confirm compliance are preferable. In the interest of addressing the latter, pharmaceutical companies have developed different modes of administration for some of their products (Table 6.12).

It would seem plausible to speculate that a substantially better understanding of schizophrenia and other psychoses is perhaps not more than a decade or two away. Once the pathological processes leading to the clinical manifestations are elucidated, more specific treatments may then be possible. Given the protean nature of schizophrenia, it is likely that many different neural circuits are involved in multiple permutations, essentially moving us beyond the concept of one disorder with a few subtypes to the discovery of multiple conditions that will probably require medications or other interventions with more than just one mechanism of action, including interventions aimed at modifying genetic function.

TABLE 6.12. Routes of Administration for Antipsychotic Medications

Route	Examples	Comments
Intramuscular injection[a]	Haloperidol, ziprasidone, olanzapine	Maximum blood levels achieved in a short period of time
Dissolvable tablets	Olanzapine, risperidone, aripiprazole	Quicker absorption, provides alternative to injection
Liquid concentrate	Haloperidol, risperidone	Same as above
Tablets or capsules	All	Standard route
Injectable depot	Fluphenazine, haloperidol, risperidone, paliperidone	Slow release; allows for dosing every 2–4 weeks

[a]Intravenous route, which delivers quasi-instantaneous blood levels, is sometimes used. This constitutes an off-label use.

CONCLUSION

The most effective treatment for schizophrenia incorporates a multidisciplinary approach in which antipsychotic medications are a necessary but insufficient component. In order to achieve optimal outcomes, medication must be complemented by specific psychotherapy modalities. Skills training, psychoeducation, supportive intervention, vocational training, peer support groups, such as the Recovery Movement, and family psychoeducation are all important ingredients of treatment.

CHAPTER 7

Cognitive Disorders

An advertisement shows a picture of an elderly woman and a lovely child of about 6 years of age, and it reads: "70 years ago she learned to tie her shoes . . . yesterday she forgot how." The pain of dementia is shared by millions of families.

When evaluating a new patient, all therapists must be aware of disorders that often present with cognitive impairment or behavioral symptoms as their first sign of illness. A person may consult a therapist about relationship problems, stress at work, depression symptoms, or impulse control problems, and all of these could be symptoms of a dementing process at the early—and most treatable—stages. It is critical that therapists consider the differential diagnosis of cognitive impairment when deciding on a course of therapy and whether or not to recommend a medical evaluation specifically targeted to these symptoms.

DEFINITION OF DEMENTIA

Dementia is a **neurodegenerative** illness characterized by memory impairment, plus at least one additional cognitive deficit, which might include **aphasia** (a defect or loss of the power of communication by, or comprehension of, speech, writing, and signs), **apraxia** (inability to perform purposeful movements or to use objects correctly), **agnosia** (inability to recognize the nature of sensory input; e.g., not being able to tell the difference between a coin and a key placed in one's hand without looking is *tactile agnosia*), or a disturbance in executive functions (described above). The cognitive deficits must be severe enough to cause problems in occupational or social functioning, and they must represent a decline in function from the patient's previous level. The impairment must not occur exclusively during a delirium (American Psychiatric Association, 2013). Dementia is usually made as a clinical diagnosis. However, there are now definitive diagnostic tests that neurologists can conduct utilizing brain-imaging and cerebrospinal-fluid studies, in conjunction with neuropsychological testing.

In clinical practice, the **Mini-Mental State Examination** (MMSE; Table 7.1) is often used as a primary care screening tool for dementia. The MMSE has been widely used and standardized, but it does have limitations. A person who has had limited education may not do well, and a person who is very bright and well educated may have suffered a great deal of cognitive impairment and yet still score well; moreover, the MMSE is culture-bound. For example, when an elderly woman was asked what date it was, she answered, "Early in the season when the thunder sleeps." This was completely appropriate in her Navajo culture for a date in the middle of October. Many clinicians track serial MMSE scores, although some studies suggest that this is not a reliable tool for tracking dementia (Clark et al., 1999). The diagnosis and tracking of dementia is a clinical skill. There are many different types of dementia, sorted by differences that are known in their cause and/or in their symptomatic presentation.

A dementia is different from an **amnestic disorder,** in which there is impairment of memory but other functions are quite intact. Amnestic disorders may be due to brain injuries, such as head trauma or strokes, that damage the medial temporal lobe on both sides of the brain. Physiological brain impairment from alcohol intoxication or large doses of benzodiazepines can produce gaps in memory when brain memory systems were disrupted. These impairments in brain functioning can be mimicked by dissociative disorders in which memories cannot be accessed during spans of time associated with emotional trauma.

Dementia is also not *delirium,* which is a global impairment of cognitive processes due to metabolic derangements, such as blood glucose too low, blood sodium too high, inflammation from the tissue damage of surgery, or inflammation from bacterial infection in the body. The hallmarks of delirium are fluctuations hour to hour in conscious awareness and wakefulness, together with an impaired ability to maintain focus of attention. A person with delirium may have memory impairment as one symptom, but it is the difficulty in maintaining attention that is the hallmark symptom. Delirium can develop quickly, over minutes or hours, and it fluctuates over the course of minutes, hours, or

TABLE 7.1. The Mini-Mental State Examination

	Points
Orientation	
• "Name the season, day, date, month, year."	5 (1 for each correct)
• "Name our location (what building are we in, what floor of the building, what town, what state, what country?)."	5 (1 for each correct)
Registration of information	
• Identify three objects by name and ask the patient to repeat them immediately (e.g., cat, book, door).	3 (1 for each correct)
Attention and calculation	
• Serial 7s (subtract 7 from 100, then 7 from that) or spell "world" backward (D-L-R-O-W).	5 (1 for each correct)
Recall	
• "Tell me the three objects I named earlier."	3 (1 for each correct)
Language	
• "What is this?" (point to pencil, then watch).	2 (1 for each correct)
• "Repeat this phrase: 'No ifs, ands, or buts.'"	1
• "Do this exactly as I tell you: Take this paper, fold it in half, and place it on the table."	3 (1 for each step)
• "Do what I have written on this paper" (write CLOSE YOUR EYES on the paper and show it to the patient).	1
• Tell the patient to write a sentence on a paper (it does not matter what it says, but it must have at least a subject and a verb and make sense).	1
• Draw intersecting pentagons on a paper, and ask the patient to copy the drawing.	1
Total score	30

Note. Data from Folstein, Folstein, and McHugh (1975).

days. Slurred speech, language disturbance, or no speech at all can also occur. The person may become incoherent, see an electric cord on the floor and perceive it to be a snake, or see spots on a sheet or bedspread and perceive them to be insects; the person may be irritable and agitated in the night and hypoactive and apathetic in the daytime. Delirium is due to some physical cause, and time is critical in finding that cause and remedying it. Often the cause is the primary medical condition of the patient, such as head injury, insufficient oxygen delivery to the brain, heart failure, respiratory failure, kidney disease, liver disease, brain tumors, infections such as pneumonia, urinary tract infection, dehydration, and many other medical conditions. Delirium may also be due to the side effects of medications. This is such a common and readily treatable cause of delirium that the first question a physician asks when meeting a patient with delirium is this: "What are *we* giving to, or doing to, this person to cause this delirium?"

If a therapist thinks that the patient may have a delirium, the patient must be sent for medical evaluation for the specific symptoms of delirium that day, often in the emergency department of a hospital, since failure to treat the underlying cause may result in death. It is also important to recognize that delirium and dementia may coexist. If a patient who has dementia suffers an acute worsening of function, then a delirium may have developed in addition to the dementia, and the underlying cause may represent a potentially life-threatening emergency. Since possible causes of delirium are myriad, determining a specific etiology of delirium depends upon identifying what was time-linked with the first signs of confusion—Was there a new medication started? Was there a fever? Did the patient become dehydrated? Could the patient be withdrawing from alcohol?

Dementia is also not the mild decline in cognitive ability that is a normal process of aging, sometimes called *age-related cognitive decline* or *benign senescent forgetfulness*. People with age-related cognitive decline may have some trouble remembering names or may misplace objects, but they fully compensate by using notes, calendars, and other prompts. They take the small memory challenges in stride, and there is minimal or no impact on life functioning. Sometimes patients and their families worry about whether the mild symptoms that they observe are the precursor to dementia. Studies of those who suffer **mild cognitive impairment** (MCI), which is more significant than age-related cognitive decline, have shown that many of those with MCI, especially those who have significant impairment in executive function, will develop dementia (Petersen et al., 2001). Executive function refers to the ability to plan and think abstractly, to do things that require sequencing, such as gathering clothes for the laundry, starting the appropriate cycle on a washing machine, adding the soap, moving the clothes to the dryer, and removing and hanging them in the right closet. This is a simple task, yet it requires one to follow a sequence of planned actions. Other examples of executive functioning include making financial and other life decisions. Mild memory symptoms without difficulties in executive functioning may be just benign forgetfulness, but mild memory symptoms with significant disturbance in executive functioning could mean that the patient has MCI and may be a candidate for screening for dementia, with a particular focus on finding treatable, reversible causes.

A primary care clinician will typically consult a neurologist to confirm a dementia diagnosis and to determine which type of dementia, since different types produce different symptom profiles and rates of progression. This diagnostic evaluation may involve both a clinical neurological examination and also brain-imaging studies and blood and cerebrospinal fluid tests. A neuropsychologist can administer a battery of tests that provide guidance for treatment planning depending upon which specific aspects of cognition show impairment.

TYPES OF DEMENTIAS

While Alzheimer's disease is most common, other frequently occurring dementias are Lewy body dementia, vascular dementia, and frontotemporal dementia. These different dementias differ in their symptoms. Alzheimer's disease typically begins with impaired memory for recent events, word-finding difficulties, and getting lost easily, but with preservation of personality features and social graces. On the other hand, frontotemporal dementia can initially present with marked changes in personality and loss of impulse control. Lewy body dementia is often characterized by fluctuating levels of arousal and visual hallucinations. Vascular dementia usually shows loss of executive functions as a prominent feature, together with aphasia, apraxia, and agnosia (Health & Beller, 2019). These distinctions are best made by a neurologist working collaboratively with a neuropsychologist.

CASE ILLUSTRATION: SARA, COGNITIVE DISORDER

The M. family (Hector, 9-year-old son; Sara, mother; Maria, aunt/sister) arrived for counseling services at an urban free clinic complaining that Sara had significant problems with memory and was hitting Hector for no apparent reason. When Hector tried to take a piece of food from the table, Sara immediately reacted by slapping him in the face. Maria also reported that Sara had pulled Hector's hair when he sought food or water. Sara's behavior had been a concern for several months, following an incident of domestic violence involving her ex-husband that had resulted in her 2-week hospitalization for head injury and a coma. Prior to this incident, Sara had been hospitalized for overdosing on pills and alcohol. Sara stated that she arrived at the medical visit planning to apply for a job and did not think there was anything wrong with her or her family.

Beginning Collaboration

Because of Sara's previous cognitive impairment and current violent behavior toward her son, the therapist referred her to a physician at the free clinic for immediate attention. The therapist also reported the suspected child abuse to Child Protective Services (CPS).

A psychiatrist concluded that Sara had a history of hypoxic brain injury with consequent significant cognitive impairment, inability to perform activities of daily living, and impulse control problems (disinhibition because of her frontal lobe injury) in her role as a parent. Sara was prescribed a trial of trazodone to determine if it might attenuate her impulse-control problems. The therapist continued to work with Maria, Hector, and Sara to develop coping strategies for the family.

Questions for Consideration

1. *What are some of the legal issues inherent in this case? How can the collaborative team deal with them?* There are two key legal issues in this case: child protection and confidentiality. The therapist addressed the first issue by immediately reporting the situation to CPS. He set the tone for this referral by talking to the sisters about the need for outside support and help since Sara was a single mother with no health insurance. He framed the call to CPS as a call for help and resources and told CPS about this framing. The therapist also asked both Sara and Maria to sign releases so that he could talk with either of them at any time about clinical concerns. He did this to ensure that if he ever saw Sara alone and found out about dangerous or high-risk behaviors, he could immediately get Maria involved. At the same time, he talked to Maria about using the clinic and the team as a resource to help Sara be the best parent possible for Hector. The therapist reviewed these issues with the psychiatrist so they could plan together ways to help the family.

2. *The therapist has little knowledge about hypoxic brain injury. How can collaboration help him address his concerns about his unfamiliarity with the diagnosis?* While the therapist had never treated someone with hypoxic brain injury, he did feel confident in his abilities to help set boundaries, establish a safety net for Hector, encourage frequent communication between the clinic and the family, and help the family manage their lives despite uncertainty about the course and prognosis of

Sara's illness. He met with the psychiatrist to learn some basic information and to seek additional reference articles for study.

DEMENTIAS THAT ARE REVERSIBLE OR PARTIALLY REVERSIBLE

Persons can show apparent signs of cognitive impairment, but an undiagnosed medical or psychiatric problem is the cause, not a dementia. Often these causes are treatable. For example, a 47-year-old woman came to her therapist's office stating that she felt depressed, which she attributed to her excessive work schedule. The therapist elicited a history of fatigue, difficulty concentrating, and sleep problems, as well as a subjective sense of depression. She referred her patient to a physician for a medication evaluation, with a presumptive diagnosis of major depression. On the first visit with the physician, the patient gave the same history as she gave to the therapist, but the physician noted that the patient had no prior history of depression and most of her distress was related to her "memory problems." The patient owned her own business and took pride in filling her customers' orders "just exactly right—the right goods delivered to the right customer on the right day at the right time." But in recent weeks, she found herself making lots of mistakes, delivering goods to customers on the wrong day or delivering the wrong goods to a customer on the right day, and she was distraught: "I just can't think straight anymore!" The patient also complained of fatigue, crying about her deteriorating business, and feeling very grim about her future. An MMSE (Table 7.1) was administered to the patient. She scored 29 out of 30 points, missing the date by a few days, an incongruous error since she was very bright and well educated. MCI was suspected and laboratory tests were ordered. Her blood tests found that she had no detectable vitamin B_{12}. As is the case for a small number of other individuals, she absorbed vitamin B_{12} poorly from her diet. Life-long injections of vitamin B_{12} restored her memory, resolved her "depression," and restored health to both the patient and her business.

This clinical case involved cognitive impairment and mood changes due to vitamin B_{12} deficiency, sometimes called pernicious anemia. This is one of many illnesses that must be considered and tested for when a patient presents with cognitive symptoms. Other causes of cognitive impairment that are treatable are found in Table 7.2. It is critical that patients be examined and tested for these conditions as soon as symptoms are identified, since the passage of time may lessen the probability of cure or improvement in function.

TABLE 7.2. Causes of Dementias That Are Reversible or Treatable

Disorder	Management
Vitamin deficiencies, including B_{12}, nicotinic acid, thiamine	Therapeutic dose replacement
Endocrine disorders • Hypothyroidism • Parathyroid disorders • Adrenal disorders	Therapeutic dose replacement or adjustment
Infectious disorders • Chronic meningitis • Tuberculosis, fungal, parasitic • HIV disease • Tertiary syphilis • Slow virus (Creutzfeldt–Jakob disease)	Treatment of infection
Disorders with space-occupying effect • Primary brain tumor • Metastatic brain tumor • Subdural hematoma (posttrauma) • Normal-pressure hydrocephalus	Neurosurgical management
Toxic disorders • Drug, narcotic, heavy metals • Organic toxins • Medications (prescription) • Alcohol consumption • Dialysis dementia (aluminum)	Removal of offending toxin
Vascular dementia • Multi-infarct • Diffuse white matter disease (Binswanger's dementia)	Control of blood pressure
Miscellaneous • Vasculitis/inflammatory • Sarcoidosis/porphyria • Dementia pugilistica (recurrent head trauma) • Parkinson's disease/Huntington's disease • "Pseudodementia of depression"	Diagnosis and treatment varies

THE DEGENERATIVE DEMENTIAS

The most common types of degenerative dementias are listed in Table 7.3. Although Alzheimer's disease is the presumed diagnosis for the majority of patients who suffer from dementia, it is important for the therapist to be familiar with the clinical features of other types, because some of those discerning features are behavioral in nature. In the early stages of Alzheimer's disease, the symptoms may be subtle and attributed to forgetfulness. Alzheimer's disease is progressive, and as the symptoms

TABLE 7.3. Types and Features of the Most Common Dementias

Type	Selected features
Alzheimer's disease	Most common type; first symptoms often memory problems and word-finding difficulty, but behavior is socially correct in early stages. Progressive, with survival time 5–10 years after definitive symptoms. Diagnosis is presumptive in a living person and can only be certain at autopsy, with the finding of senile plaques, neurofibrillary tangles, gliosis, and amyloid angiopathy seen in neurons.
Pick's disease	Difficult to distinguish clinically from Alzheimer's disease at times; slowly progressive dementia; hyperoral behavior; disinhibition; irritability; persistent aimless wandering; memory loss; language difficulties; frontal lobe atrophy seen on brain imaging; diagnosed at autopsy by "Pick bodies" in neurons.
Frontotemporal dementia	Approximately 10% of dementias. Initial complaint is often personality changes. Disinhibition; withdrawal; apathy; hyperoral behavior (including weight gain); compulsions; memory problems; speech and language difficulty. Familial cases have approximately 40% autosomal dominant inheritance and may develop signs of Parkinson's disease.
Lewy body disease	Difficult to clinically distinguish from Alzheimer's disease at times and may coexist with Alzheimer's disease; frequent fluctuations in cognition and behavior (can look like delirium but persists); tremor and rigidity similar to Parkinson's disease; repeated unexplained falls; unusual sensitivity to neuroleptic medications (more side effects). Lewy bodies are found in neurons at autopsy.
Vascular dementia	Brain imaging (CT or MRI) reveals brain lesions, examination reveals neurological signs, usually there is a long history of hypertension

become more severe, they interfere with daily activities. Language skills deteriorate, as does comprehension and ability to perform the basic tasks of living and self-care. Hallucinations and delusions often develop, sleeping patterns deteriorate, and agitation puts tremendous stress on caregivers. At end-stage Alzheimer's disease, the patient is often bed-ridden, not eating or drinking, incontinent of stool and bladder, not recognizing family members, and showing primitive movements like sucking and snout reflex. Some patients have a continuously downhill course over 5–10 years, and others have plateau periods between times of deterioration, but the typical time course is similar. When there is an exacerbation in Alzheimer's disease symptoms, the patient should be examined to be sure that he or she has not developed an infection or other illness that is causing the acute change.

EPIDEMIOLOGY, COSTS, AND RISK FACTORS

Alois Alzheimer first described Alzheimer's disease in Germany in 1907. There are approximately 3–4 million people in the United States with Alzheimer's disease, about 10% of all those over 70 years of age. The health care cost of treatment is more than $80 billion per year, and the cost of caring for one patient with Alzheimer's disease is more than $50,000 per year when the disease is advanced. Alzheimer's disease is one of the most common reasons that a person is placed in a nursing home. Several genetic factors have been tied to Alzheimer's disease and other dementias, but very often there seems to be no family history, and the cause of Alzheimer's disease is unknown at this time.

BIOLOGY AND BIOCHEMISTRY OF COGNITIVE DISORDERS

A great deal of research is in progress to learn the cause of Alzheimer's disease and to understand its disease mechanisms and molecular biology. A full review of these exciting studies is beyond the scope of this book, but a few indicate the kinds of findings that may become clinically important in the future: Luukinen, Viramo, Koski, Laippala, and Kivela (1999) found that major head injuries caused in falls of those over 70 years of age were associated with increased risk of cognitive decline. And Petersen et al. (2001) found that MCI was associated with increased risk of developing dementia.

Current evidence suggests that an accumulation of beta-amyloid, a product of protein breakdown within neurons, produces gradual death of neurons. New brain-imaging techniques can quantify abnormal accumulation of amyloid in the brain, confirming a diagnosis of Alzheimer's disease and providing prognosis about its progression. High levels of tau protein in the cerebrospinal fluid characterize an early stage of Alzheimer's disease. These diagnostic tests are positive years before brain imaging shows atrophy of the brain (Turner, 2012).

TREATMENT PLAN FOR ALZHEIMER'S DISEASE

Medication Treatment

There is no cure for Alzheimer's disease. Historically, management has been aimed at enabling the patient to have the best life function for as long as possible, minimizing the distressing symptoms for the patient and family, and supporting family members and other caregivers through this very stressful time. In recent years, several medications have been developed that slow the progression of Alzheimer's disease, working best when they are started early. The comparative features of the most commonly used medications for cognitive impairment and dementia are listed in Table 7.4. None of these stop the progression of the dementia; all of them are expensive; and when they are stopped, the patient is in about the same stage of disease as controls who did not take medication. Nevertheless, any medication that can slow the progress of disease somewhat, and allow a person to remain in his or her own home longer because the symptoms are manageable, is definitely worth trying. The savings from avoiding a nursing home may more than compensate for the expense of the medication in many cases.

A new class of medication, an N-methyl-D-aspartate (NMDA)-receptor **antagonist** called memantine, was approved by the FDA and released in early 2004 under the brand name Namenda. It has been approved for the treatment of moderate to severe Alzheimer's disease and has been used in Germany for over 30 years. Clinical studies in the United States have shown modest effectiveness, with the main benefit being delayed deterioration of basic functions, such as the ability to go to the bathroom independently, feed oneself in a less messy fashion, be less easily distracted, and perhaps have less agitation. There is no evidence that it has any effect in the early stages of Alzheimer's disease or that it alters the ultimate course. Although these are modest benefits, they may allow a person to remain at home with family care and delay nursing-home placement for some period of time (Abramowicz, 2003).

Medications commonly used for the treatment of several target symptoms often seen in Alzheimer's disease are listed in Table 7.5. The

TABLE 7.4. Comparison of the Medications Most Commonly Used for Dementia in the United States

Tacrine (Cognex)

- The first medication demonstrated to have any effectiveness in slowing the progression of moderate Alzheimer's disease.
- 30–40% of patients who completed the drug trials showed modest improvement, compared to 10% of those receiving a placebo.
- Response is dose related (as is hepatocellular injury), and both response and increased liver function tests (LFTs) resolve with stopping the drug.
- Less commonly used now that several other medications are available that have fewer side effects.
- Side effects
  - 30% develop three times the upper limit of normal LFTs, and 5–10% must stop the drug because of increases of 10 times or more—this resolves with stopping the drug.
  - More common in women.
  - Tend to occur at about 6–8 weeks of treatment.
  - Spectrum of cholinergic side effects: nausea, vomiting, bradycardia, increased stomach acid.

Donepezil (Aricept)

- Improvement in cognitive function or no change (as compared to decline in controls) is seen in 80% of patients with Alzheimer's disease: improvement in 35–60%, stabilization in 20–45%.
- Benefits seen in up to 2 years of treatment.
- Return to controls 3–6 weeks after stopping the drug.
- Well tolerated, with no increased LFTs.
- Dosing/side effects
  - 5 mg/day to start: increase to 10 mg/day after 1 week, as tolerated.
  - Dose-related side effects: nausea, insomnia, diarrhea.
  - Incidence of treatment-emergent adverse events (68–78%) with both dosages was similar to incidence in group receiving a placebo (69%).

Rivastigmine (Exelon)

- Improvement in 25–30% of patients at 6–12 mg/day.
- Improvement maintained for about 40 weeks before declining.
- No liver toxicity.
- Fewer adverse drug interactions (not metabolized by CYP450).
- Dosing/side effects
  - 1.5 mg twice a day, which can be increased to 3, 4, 5, and up to 6 mg twice a day.
  - Should be taken with food.
  - Approximately 20% of patients were unable to tolerate because of side effects; most common were gastrointestinal in nature: nausea, vomiting, diarrhea, abdominal pain, loss of appetite.

(continued)

TABLE 7.4. *(continued)*

Galantamine (Razadyne)

- Superior to placebo at 16–32 mg/day.
- Improvement was sustained 6 months in some studies, 24 months in others.
- Liver metabolized by CYP2D6 and3A4, and high plasma levels may develop in the 7% of the population who lack CPY2D6 enzymes.
- Adverse drug interactions may occur if concurrent medications also metabolized by CYP2D6 and 3A4.
- Dosing/side effects
  - Start with 4 mg, twice a day; increased after 4 weeks to maintenance dose of 8 mg, twice a day.
  - Should be taken with food.
  - Avoid if liver or kidney impairment.
  - Most common side effects are nausea, vomiting, diarrhea, loss of appetite, weight loss, dizziness. Very slow heart rate may occur.

Memantine (Namenda)

- Approved for use in the United States in early 2004; used in Germany for more than 20 years.
- Main benefit is delayed deterioration of basic functions, such as self-feeding, toileting, decreased agitation.
- Only drug available that may work at more advanced stages of Alzheimer's disease.
- Dosing/side effects
  - Start with 5 mg/day; increase by 5 mg/day at weekly intervals to a maximum of 20 mg/day. Divide total daily amount into two doses per day when over 5 mg/day.
  - Most common side effects are headache, constipation, elevated blood pressure, confusion, and fatigue.

Note. All of these medications are used for the target symptom of cognitive impairment. Most are cholinesterase inhibitors, which result in an increase in ACH in the brain, and they are indicated for treatment of mild to moderate Alzheimer's disease. Data from Abramowicz (2000, 2001, 2003).

goal for the use of each medication is to assist the family and the patient by making the patient as comfortable and functional as possible, for as long as possible, with minimal side effects.

While agitation or insomnia can occur as severe and disabling symptoms late in the course of Alzheimer's disease, common remedies for such symptoms can be unsafe. All atypical antipsychotic medications carry FDA black box warnings about increase death rates in elderly patients treated for agitation. Benzodiazepines commonly used for insomnia or agitation can produce confusion and amnesia in cognitively impaired patients.

TABLE 7.5. Medications Used for Specific Target Symptoms in Alzheimer's Disease

Psychosis and agitation

- Assess why now—new medical problem, change in environment, depression, constipation—try all nondrug approaches first.
- When drugs are used, "start low–go slow" on the dose, and reevaluate need often.
- Antipsychotics, such as risperidone, haloperidol (0.5–2.0 mg/day), olanzapine.
- Non-FDA approved but commonly used: trazodone, buspirone, SSRIs.
- Anticonvulsants in treatment-resistant cases (carbamazepine, valproate).
- Avoid high-potency drugs (e.g., haloperidol) in Lewy body disease.

Benzodiazepines/sedation

- Save them for special needs (dental procedures, CT scans, etc.).
- Regular use results in habituation and ineffectiveness as a sedative; risks disinhibition and worsening cognitive impairment.
- Use only drugs with no active metabolites (lorazepam, oxazepam).
- Do not use flurazepam (too long a half-life) or triazolam (worsening dementia).

Depression

- First choice, SSRIs
  - Sertraline 25 mg/day to start (150 mg maximum)
  - Paroxetine 5–10 mg/day to start (40 mg maximum)
- Nortriptyline; low doses (often 10–50 mg/day) with drug level monitoring.
- Absolutely avoid amitriptyline as too anticholinergic.

Insomnia

- Sleep hygiene comes first—treat underlying problem (depression, agitation, etc.).
- Avoid benzodiazepines and others that exacerbate sleep apnea and cause rebound insomnia and worsening cognition.
- Avoid diphenhydramine (anticholinergic).
- Avoid amitriptyline (number one cause of anticholinergic delirium in the elderly).
- Trazodone 25–100 mg as needed for sleep.
- Zolpidem 5–10 mg nightly sleep.

Note. None of these medications have FDA indication for the treatment of Alzheimer's disease. The literature and practice guidelines support the use of these medications for specific target symptoms. The FDA has issued a "black box" warning regarding the use of certain antipsychotic medications in the elderly, especially haloperidol, olanzapine, and risperidone. The warning notes that the use of these drugs is associated with an increase in death rates when used by the elderly patients with dementia.

There are no FDA-approved drugs for the treatment of these symptoms in persons with dementia. All antipsychotics, when used in patients with dementia, carry a small but measurable increased risk of death.

Side Effects

The most common side effects of the Alzheimer's disease drugs are listed with each drug in Table 7.4. The most common side effects of the other drugs are listed when they are discussed in detail (e.g., the SSRIs). The point here is that any drug can cause anything, and the therapist can encourage the patient and family to tolerate minor reactions and talk to their physician about the important side effects. A comprehensive list is beyond the scope of this text.

The Therapist's Role in Treatment

A patient may come to a therapist with many complaints that are early symptoms of Alzheimer's disease or other types of cognitive impairment, and the therapist's first responsibility is to recognize the importance of prompt medical evaluation and treatment. The therapist may also be assisting a patient with MCI and depression, a common co-occurrence. Because medications are likely to be indicated for major depression in Alzheimer's disease, the patient may benefit from the therapist's assistance in learning to cope with mild symptoms. Most likely, the therapist will work with the family members and caregivers of those who suffer from Alzheimer's disease and other dementias.

Assisting Families and Caregivers

When a patient and family have learned that the diagnosis is presumptive or probably Alzheimer's disease, there is often widespread dismay, and all the stages of grief may be expressed at one time or another. Because they need time to process this dismaying news, the family may have difficulty planning such necessary items as wills, trusts, durable power of attorney for health care, and the patient's wishes for end-of-life care. The therapist should encourage early planning of these matters because once the patient's dementia has progressed to the point that he or she is not considered legally competent, the patient can no longer have input into these critical decisions. For example, helping the family by mentioning the need to attend to matters of safety, such as driving and wandering, as well as the patient's type of residence may be necessary. If a move to a different residence will be needed eventually, it is best to help the patient to settle into the new living situation early in the course of the disease to maintain stability as long as possible. Moves at a later stage in illness will be poorly tolerated. The therapist can be of tremendous help to the family in setting realistic goals and plans and supporting the family through what might be a guilt-provoking time when it becomes necessary to transfer the patient to a nursing facility.

The therapist can also help the family by advising them of educational sources and available support groups, such as the local chapter of the Alzheimer's Association, social service and home health agencies, assistance with home behavioral management, Meals on Wheels, transportation and recreational programs, and respite care. A helpful website is the Alzheimer's and Disease Education and Referral Center (ADEAR), a service of the National Institute on Aging of the National Institutes of Health at *www.nia.nih.gov*. The website of the Alzheimer's Association, *www.alz.org*, also provides resources and information for patients, families, and caregivers. Alzheimer's disease and other dementias rob patients and families of what is arguably their most precious belonging—their very identity and personhood. The therapist can play a key role in helping the patient and family cope with this trying and long illness.

CONCLUSION

While the focus of this chapter has been on the patient with cognitive disorders and providing resources to family members, attending to the needs of caregivers is essential. Depression is very common among caregivers of patients with Alzheimer's disease. With the typical course of illness being 10 years—beginning with gradual onset, then progressive memory loss, cognitive decline, and, on average, institutionalization for the last 3 years of life—caregivers are vulnerable to mental illness exacerbations (or illness *de novo*) because of the hard work of care. Prevention of caregiver burnout treats two patients and benefits the extended family indirectly. The therapist should be vigilant for signs that the caregivers are overwhelmed; at that point the patient will be institutionalized. The most common symptoms that acutely precipitate institutionalization of patients with Alzheimer's disease are insomnia with night-time wandering, urinary or fecal incontinence, or agitation with aggressive behaviors.

CHAPTER 8

Alcoholism and Substance Abuse

Alcoholism is a mental health problem that has persisted due in part to societal ambivalence about use of alcohol. For example, Mississippi was the last state to legalize sales of alcoholic beverages. Prohibition finally ended in 1966, although there had long been a "black market tax" that required purchasers of illegal alcohol to pay a tax to the state. This ambivalence about the benefits and ills from alcohol were captured colorfully by Mississippi legislator Noah S. "Soggy" Sweat who gave a speech to fellow legislators still known as "If By Whiskey" (Safire, 1997):

> My friends, I had not intended to discuss this controversial subject at this particular time. However, I want you to know that I do not shun controversy. On the contrary, I will take a stand on any issue at any time, regardless of how fraught with controversy it might be. You have asked me how I feel about whiskey. All right, here is how I feel about whiskey: If when you say whiskey you mean the devil's brew, the poison scourge, the bloody monster, that defiles innocence, dethrones reason, destroys the home, creates misery and poverty, yea, literally takes the bread from the mouths of little children; if you mean the evil drink that topples the Christian man and woman from the pinnacle of righteous, gracious living into the bottomless pit of degradation, and despair, and shame and helplessness, and hopelessness, then certainly I am against it. But, if when you say whiskey you mean the oil of conversation, the philosophic wine, the ale that is consumed when good fellows get together, that puts a song in their hearts and laughter on their lips, and the warm glow of contentment in their eyes; if you mean Christmas cheer; if you mean the stimulating drink

that puts the spring in the old gentleman's step on a frosty, crispy morning; if you mean the drink which enables a man to magnify his joy, and his happiness, and to forget, if only for a little while, life's great tragedies, and heartaches, and sorrows; if you mean that drink, the sale of which pours into our treasuries untold millions of dollars, which are used to provide tender care for our little crippled children, our blind, our deaf, our dumb, our pitiful aged and infirm; to build highways and hospitals and schools, then certainly I am for it. This is my stand. I will not retreat from it. I will not compromise. (p. 876)

Throughout history, such ambivalence about alcohol and other substances has stood as a moral dilemma between a choice to seek the pleasures of substances in the moment or to refuse them due to long-term pain and destruction. However, the advent of "alcohol" and "substance use disorders" in the language of mental health professionals recasts this dilemma as a problem of functional brain circuitry and not primarily a problem of moral choices. The neurobiological investigations of Volkow, Koob, and McLellan (2016) and others have framed craving for alcohol or drugs as a loss of top-down regulation by prefrontal cortex over the bottom-up processing of the ventral striatum with its dopamine circuitry. In simple terms, circuitry required for top-down regulation no longer works within the brains of addicted individuals.

Substance use disorders (SUDs) are collectively the most common coexisting condition that therapists will see in their patients who present with relationship problems, depression, or anxiety disorders. SUDs are common and often unrecognized, at least in the initial evaluation of the patient and family. This has changed with the recent spike in opioid abuse since 2011. The fivefold increase in overdose deaths has captured national attention as a public health crisis.

ALCOHOLISM

Definition

Alcoholism is the most common SUD and the prototype for discussion of other SUDs. A person is diagnosed with alcoholism, or **alcohol use disorder,** if he or she continues to drink alcohol despite awareness that this continued use will lead to adverse consequences in health, school, employment, relationships, or the law. A person with alcoholism may know that alcohol use can cost a person the loss of career, family, friends, liberty, or health, and yet the person shows no control over the use of alcohol and continues to drink in spite of the consequences.

It is the behavioral evidence of loss of regulation that primarily defines alcoholism, rather than the amount or kind of alcohol ingested (Nisavic & Nejad, 2018a, 2018b).

Several terms require definition:

- **Tolerance** refers to the need to consume progressively larger quantities of the substance (e.g., alcohol, benzodiazepines, or opiates) to achieve intoxication or the desired effect, or the state of needing a progressively increasing dose in order to maintain a sense of normality.
- **Withdrawal** is a syndrome of very unpleasant cognitive, psychological, and physical symptoms that occurs when the amount of the substance declines in the bloodstream. The onset of withdrawal symptoms generally brings an intense craving for the substance, and use of the substance results in resolution of the withdrawal syndrome.
- **Dependence** refers to any one or the combination of cognitive, behavioral, and physical symptoms that indicate that the individual continues to use the substance in spite of significant harm or life problems. Typically a person who has substance dependence also experiences tolerance and withdrawal, as well as compulsive use and drug-seeking behavior.
- **Abuse** is the maladaptive pattern over at least a 12-month period of substance use, leading to impairment or distress, but this does not include substance dependence, tolerance, or withdrawal.
- **Blood alcohol level (BAL)** refers to serum levels of alcohol that correlate with typical behavioral effects (see Table 8.1).

TABLE 8.1. BALs and Cognitive and Behavioral Impairment

BAL	Cognitive and behavioral effects
20–30 mg/dL	Slowed motor performance and thinking ability (i.e., after one or two drinks).
30–80 mg/dL	Mild incoordination and slowed thinking (80 mg/dL is the legal intoxication limit in California).
80–100 mg/dL	Overt incoordination and impaired judgment (legal intoxication in most states).
200–300 mg/dL	Nystagmus, marked slurring of speech, and blackouts.
>300 mg/dL	Respiratory arrest, impaired vital signs, and death.

Note. Data from Schuckit (1995).

Tolerance may occur to the point that patients can appear to be alert and talking coherently with BALs in excess of 400 mg/dL, but these individuals are still at risk of respiratory arrest and death at that level of intoxication. Later, they will not remember what occurred during this time (they are in a blackout), and they may experience alcohol withdrawal symptoms when their BAL drops from 400 to 200, a level that is still indicative of intoxication for most people.

CASE ILLUSTRATION: MS. A., ALCOHOL USE DISORDER

Ms. A., a 25-year-old woman, presented to her primary care physician, Dr. D., with myriad health concerns, including skin rashes, symptoms of "panic attack" (described by the patient as periods of dizziness, increased heart rate, tingling sensations and extremity numbness, shortness of breath, and feeling trapped), headache, hopelessness, and weight gain. Dr. D. assessed Ms. A. for depression and anxiety and referred her to an in-clinic therapist for regular individual therapy. She met with the therapist weekly over the next 2 months. During these sessions, she stated concerns about her drinking, as well as her concurrent symptoms of depression and anxiety.

Beginning Collaboration

Ms. A. reported that her symptoms began after a traumatic experience—her mother's near-fatal car accident that had occurred 3 years earlier. Ms. A. was particularly concerned because she since then had become more and more dependent on alcohol as a way to "get through the stress." She drank four or more glasses of wine daily. Ms. A. noted that her mother had been an active alcoholic for 20 years. Even though she was drunk at the time of her accident and was almost killed, she continued to drink heavily. Ms. A. had moved back home since her mother's accident in order to provide her mother with care. She wondered if she had inherited an "addictive personality trait" from her mother. She had become increasingly concerned that she was losing control over her own drinking. Over the course of the last year, she had begun drinking more regularly and more heavily, to the point of intoxication on most occasions. She feared that she had the potential to be an alcoholic. Now she felt she was "losing ground" in battling her drinking.

Over the course of 2 months, Ms. A. had an extensive medical evaluation with Dr. D. The therapist met weekly with Ms. A. in order to address her alcohol abuse and concurrent anxiety. Ms. A. acknowledged that she needed to drink to alleviate stress and feelings of guilt, hopelessness, and feeling trapped in her situation. She was aware of the emotions connected to her urge to drink. Familiar feelings of rising tension, worry, and restlessness subsided as soon as she began drinking alcohol.

The therapist and Ms. A. identified links among her past life events that were connected to her drinking. These included her mother's alcoholism; the trauma of her mother's accident and 3-month coma; Ms. A.'s return from college to become full-time caretaker; Ms. A.'s anger at giving up her own life to care for her mother; and the guilt she felt when angry at her mother for "trapping her" with the accident, recovery, and her care needs. Ms. A.'s drinking followed a predictable pattern.

The therapist worked collaboratively with Dr. D. to address Ms. A.'s many health concerns: a skin disorder, her symptoms of anxiety and depression, her weight gain, and her continued alcohol abuse. Physician, therapist, and patient made explicit their awareness of the connection among the various problems she experienced. Months passed with no improvements in her physical or emotional health, as she continued to turn to drink as the only way to combat the anger and frustration she felt about her life.

The therapist continued to identify, normalize, and encourage Ms. A.'s expression of her frustration and resentment. Finally, the therapist recommended that Ms. A. attend Alcoholics Anonymous (AA) meetings in order to gain the support of a group with whom she could meet regularly.

Question for Consideration

1. *What role did collaboration play in Ms. A.'s treatment?* A favorable therapeutic outcome would have been difficult to achieve without close collaboration. Ms. A. initially presented physical symptoms of illness to her physician. Emotional components to her symptomatology would have been difficult to identify had Ms. A.'s only contact been with her primary care physician. Successful treatment in this case required a number of lengthy, regular, "nonrushed" sessions with Ms. A. to allow her the time and space to reflect on her past, to begin investigating and identifying possible maladaptive behavioral patterns, and to build the therapeutic trust required to finally express the intense anger and frustration underlying her physical presentation.

The medical clinic where Ms. A. received her medical care and attended regular therapy sessions provided a safe haven for her. It was essential for her to find a place physically apart from her family and home, where she could begin to express her anger and frustration.

As she herself reported, having trust that her therapist and physician would work together to care for her, not let her "slip through" when she lacked the motivation and energy, aided her continued treatment and eventual improvement.

    2. How was time an important variable in treating Ms. A.? By "time" we refer to both having enough time to talk to the patient, often 30–45 minutes weekly, and the passing of weeks and even months when Ms. A. felt connected to the clinic team. Her physician usually had 10–15 minutes set aside for his appointment with Ms. A. He often felt frustrated by the lack of time, because they often had only enough time to go through their mutual problem list.

    A resource the therapist could offer was the added time that she could spend with Ms. A.—45 minutes every week for several months. That time, in turn, gave them the chance to explore the connections among Ms. A.'s early life, her current life, her physical symptoms, and her alcohol use.

EPIDEMIOLOGY AND RISK FACTORS

Over 90% of adults in the United States drink alcohol, and nearly half of men and 3–10% of women develop significant alcohol-related problems at some point in their lives (Schuckit, 2001). Many drinkers of alcohol will have an occasional problem involving excess drinking, and this does not mean they are alcoholics. However, the National Institute on Alcohol Abuse and Alcoholism (NIAAA) identifies "at-risk" drinkers as four or more drinks on any day during the past year for men, and three drinks on any day for women (NIAAA, 2019).

    Up to 40% of men in their late teens and early 20s have experienced at least one blackout (drinking to the point of amnesia concerning all or part of the time during which they were drinking and awake), but most of them do not develop alcoholism (Schuckit, 2001). Only 5% of alcoholics are homeless; most alcoholics have a job, marriage, and family and are living in mainstream America. Many studies demonstrate the genetics of alcoholism. There is a fourfold increased risk for children of alcoholics to develop alcoholism themselves, even if adopted at birth and raised without knowledge of the alcoholism in their biological parents (Schuckit, 2001). A 15-year follow-up of 453 men originally studied at age 20 has shown that sons of alcoholic fathers showed a lower level of response to alcohol: They felt less intoxicated, less impaired on cognitive and psychomotor tests, and more willing to drive even though they were more intoxicated than their peers who did not have alcoholic fathers (Schuckit, 1994, 2001; Schuckit & Smith, 1996). This low level of perception and response to intoxication at age 20, when they were alcohol-naïve, was a powerful predictor of the development of alcoholism later in life. In short, they seemed genetically vulnerable in that they could not tell when "enough is enough."

Genetic factors can protect against alcoholism. Approximately half of Asian populations have a gene that interferes with the metabolism of alcohol, and a toxic metabolite of alcohol accumulates in their body. When they drink alcohol, acetaldehyde accumulates, and they experience the very unpleasant symptoms of rapid heartbeat, flushing, heat, and dropping blood pressure, and they feel intoxicated with very low levels of alcohol in their blood. These individuals rarely, if ever, abuse alcohol. All the genetic factors combined explain about 60% of the risk of alcoholism, with environmental factors contributing about 40% (Schuckit, 2003).

Approximately 20% of the patients entering a primary care medical office are alcoholic, and alcoholism is a significant factor in at least 25% of all hospitalizations. If the drug "alcohol" was just discovered today, most likely it would not be released by the FDA because it would be regarded as too toxic to bodily organs and too dangerous to release to the public. The prohibition of alcohol in the United States in the 1920s did not work, as alcohol has been around a long time and is an integral part of many cultural celebrations.

TREATMENT PLAN

Establishing the Diagnosis

Most patients who say they are alcoholic are already in recovery. Those with an active disease most often deny that their alcohol use is causing problems in their lives, and collateral historians play an essential role in understanding alcohol's true impact. Very often, the patient will stress that he or she consumes "only a few [usually two] beers a day" and therefore could not possibly have alcoholism. That patient, and possibly the family as well, will need education and support to understand that the amount and the type of alcohol consumed do not by themselves define alcoholism. Rather, it is the impact of the alcohol on the person and the inability to stop its use that define the problem.

Alcoholism is ubiquitous and often occult. All physicians are instructed to screen for SUDs, and this is also an essential component of every mental health assessment. There are many tools to accomplish this, and one of the simplest was advocated by the American Medical Association (AMA). The AMA has suggested the **CAGE questions** about alcohol use as a routine screening test for every adult and adolescent (see Table 8.2; Kinney, 1989).

Whether a therapist or physician uses the CAGE questions or any other questionnaire or style of inquiry, it is important to have a regular method for screening every single patient. One should ask adolescents and most adults the alcohol-screening questions when interviewing them alone, and then ask collateral historians the questions again later. Some adolescents, for example, will be more honest when asked alone; others will deny the importance of their substance use, and it will be the family's history that brings it to light.

Sometimes the patient denies alcoholism, yet there are physical signs and symptoms that make the therapist suspect it. The person who suffers from alcoholism for an extended period of time may have any of many physical findings: redness of the palms; disproportionately large abdomen ("beer belly"); elevated blood pressure; frequent trouble with the stomach (gastritis or ulcer disease); hemorrhoids; problems with recurrent abdominal pain (due to pancreatitis); male impotence (due to shrinkage of the testicles and liver dysfunction, leading to the accumulation of estrogen); liver cirrhosis, leading to bleeding problems; and heart problems. In advanced stages of alcoholism, there may be cognitive difficulties and neurologic complications, some of which may improve greatly if the person abstains from alcohol.

Alcohol Dependence and Withdrawal

A person who is addicted to alcohol may begin to show signs and symptoms of physical withdrawal within hours of abstinence. These may include tremors, insomnia, anxiety, craving for alcohol, loss of appetite,

---

TABLE 8.2. CAGE Questionnaire for Screening Risk of Alcoholism

Have you ever . . .

- Thought about Cutting down?
- Felt Annoyed when others criticize your drinking?
- Felt Guilty about your drinking?
- Used alcohol as an Eye opener?

Score 1 point for each positive answer. A score of 2–3 is suggestive of alcohol problems

---

Note. Data from Kinney (1989).

nausea, vomiting, sweating, high blood pressure, rapid heartbeat, agitation, and irritability (see Table 8.3). Withdrawal symptoms may start within hours of a decreased intake of alcohol, usually peak at 48 hours abstinence, and often resolve within 4 or 5 days. As mentioned, a person who has very severe alcohol tolerance and dependence may start to have withdrawal symptoms even when his or her BAL is still quite elevated. During alcohol withdrawal, one or two generalized seizures historically termed "rum fits" may occur, usually within 24–48 hours after decreased alcohol intake, and some patients may develop a more severe withdrawal syndrome, including hallucinations, with or without **delirium tremens** (DTs). Those who are dependent on other central nervous system (CNS) depressants, such as benzodiazepines, meprobamate, or barbiturates, may have a similar withdrawal syndrome. It is critical for the therapist to quickly recognize the patient with a withdrawal syndrome from alcohol or other CNS depressants in order to determine whether he or she can be managed as an outpatient (low risk and mild symptoms) or whether hospitalization will be necessary. If the withdrawal syndrome progresses to full DTs, there can be up to a 15% mortality rate, even when well managed, so hospitalization is essential when there is a history or probability of DTs.

Many alcohol-dependent patients manage their withdrawal outside of the hospital when they have only mild symptoms and are in generally good health. Very often these patients will visit their primary care physician, seeking a short course of benzodiazepines (such as diazepam or chlordiazepoxide) for a few days, as well as some prescription-strength vitamins and thiamine to assist in their withdrawal and recovery. It is critical that a responsible adult monitors these patients around the clock

---

TABLE 8.3. Signs and Symptoms of Physical Withdrawal from Alcohol

- Tremor
- Insomnia
- Anxiety
- Craving for alcohol
- Loss of appetite
- Nausea
- Vomiting
- Sweating
- High blood pressure
- Rapid heartbeat
- Agitation
- Irritability

to be sure that they are not developing confusion, unstable blood pressure, or other abnormal vital signs and to provide essential support for the detoxification process.

Treatment Approach to Alcoholism and SUDs

A comprehensive review of the therapist's role in the treatment of patients with SUDs is an entire text in itself and beyond the scope of this book. Here we consider the therapist's role as a collaborator with physicians and others in the health care system in the management of a patient with SUDs. This can generally be organized into six areas of collaboration:

1. Accurately identifying the alcoholism or SUD.
2. Empathically confronting the patient so that he or she can acknowledge the illness; this often involves a specific intervention session with the patient and family.
3. Ensuring that the patient is referred for management of the detoxification process; this may be a "social detox" or a "medical detox" program, depending on the severity of the dependence and the probability of life-threatening withdrawal.
4. Ensuring that the patient is referred for a comprehensive medical history and physical examination in order to obtain treatment for the medical and psychiatric complications of the alcoholism or other SUD.
5. Referring the patient to alcohol and substance abuse rehabilitation programs that will help him or her to:
   a. Maintain the essential motivation for abstinence.
   b. Learn to adjust to life and friends without alcohol.
   c. Prevent relapse.
   AA is one readily available resource that every recovering alcoholic should know about.
6. Providing counseling or therapy to the patient in the inpatient or outpatient setting, as appropriate, with the same long-term goals as listed in number 5. Cognitive therapy may be particularly beneficial to the recovering person, who is learning to reframe many events that have, in the past, been triggers for alcohol use and abuse.

After successful completion of an alcoholic rehabilitation program, at least 60% of middle-class alcoholics will maintain abstinence for at least 1 year, and many for a lifetime (Schuckit, 2001). There is no evidence to support the claims that any one specific recovery approach is any better than others, so it is best to keep the treatment approach simple, to ensure that it is something that the patient can do and that it is something the patient is willing to work with. There is no place for dogmatism in the treatment of SUDs since it is harmful to the patient to be forced into a treatment paradigm that may be the only one in the therapist's belief system but a poor fit for the patient. Twelve-step programs, such as AA, have a strong track record of success, and most patients should be encouraged to incorporate AA into their recovery plan. But some patients cannot work with AA, and they can do well with other approaches. The therapist must help the patient find a good fit that will maximize the probability of successful treatment, regardless of the therapist's own biases.

Medications in Alcoholism Recovery

During acute withdrawal from alcohol, benzodiazepines (e.g., lorazepam, diazepam, clonazepam, or chlordiazepoxide) are administered in a slow detoxification schedule. Benzodiazepines are cross-tolerant with alcohol and can prevent progress of withdrawal into DTs. Detoxification usually occurs in a hospital setting or within an outpatient program that has adequate medical consultation. Detoxification first replaces the alcohol with an equivalent daily dose of a benzodiazepine, then progressively decreases the benzodiazepine doses until the patient is medication-free. Failure to detoxify in a controlled manner can result in alcohol withdrawal seizures, hypertension, or a full-blown DTs with confusion, hallucinations, and agitation. Beyond that acute phase, however, benzodiazepines should not be used.

Naltrexone was approved by the FDA for the treatment of alcohol dependence. This opioid-antagonist drug was proposed for the treatment of alcoholism after several small studies suggested that it is useful in decreasing alcohol craving, decreasing the probability of relapse, and shortening the time of relapse should it occur (Schuckit, 2003).

Acamprosate is a medication that produces similar results to naltrexone. Acamprosate increases abstinence from alcohol by mimicking the action of alcohol in reducing activity of the excitatory neurotransmitter glutamate and augmenting activity of the inhibitory neurotransmitter GABA. Acamprosate has been found effective in treatment trials between 13 and 52 weeks. When effectiveness is partial, acamprosate can be combined with naltrexone in group or individual psychotherapy.

Disulfiram, also known by the brand name of **Antabuse,** is the old-est available medication for the treatment of alcoholism. Disulfiram interferes with the metabolism of alcohol, resulting in the accumulation of its first metabolite, acetaldehyde. Acetaldehyde causes very unpleas-ant symptoms, some of which are potentially life-threatening cardiac and neurologic symptoms, including a risk of stroke or heart attack. The use of disulfiram can be dangerous for patients with heart disease, blood pressure problems, neurological problems, diabetes, and many other medical conditions. Currently, disulfiram is rarely used. Most physicians prescribe disulfiram only to patients who have a clear history of success-ful use of it in the past, and often these patients have used disulfiram successfully to get through holidays or other specific times that are high risk for relapse.

No medication is widely recommended for the treatment of alco-holism per se; each individual patient should be assessed to see if there are other physical and mental conditions that need treatment in order to maximize the probability of sustained recovery from alcoholism. In addition, all patients recovering from alcohol should receive a vitamin supplement that is rich in the B-vitamins, especially thiamine at 50–100 mg per day for the first month of recovery.

OPIOID ABUSE AND OVERDOSES

Patients with opioid abuse and dependence may have needle marks ("tracks") at the site of injections (the marks are often hidden in tat-toos) and constricted pupils. They may complain of chronic constipa-tion. Patients in opiate withdrawal may experience nausea, diarrhea, coughing, teary eyes, runny nose, sweating, muscle twitching, goose-bumps, elevated body temperature and blood pressure, diffuse body pain, insomnia, frequent yawning, and craving for the drug of abuse. Opiate withdrawal is very uncomfortable and the discomfort puts the patients at a high risk of returning to abuse and dependence, but opiate withdrawal does not have the fatal potential of withdrawal from alcohol or benzodiazepines.

Between 2011 and 2017, deaths from drug overdoses in the United States went from less than 20,000 in 2011 to more than 72,000 in 2017, with the largest factor related to opioid overdoses (Parthvi, Agrawal, Khanijo, Tsegare, & Talwar, 2019). While opioid abuse and addiction have long existed, widespread opioid addiction and overdoses as a pub-lic health crisis burst unexpectedly into national consciousness due to unethical and illegal marketing of opioids by major pharmaceutical corporations. As reported in national media, Purdue Pharma developed **Oxycontin** as a slow-release form of the opioid oxycodone. Pharmaceutical company representatives and other marketing campaigns conveyed to prescribing physicians that Oxycontin was safe with little risk for addiction due to its slow-release mechanism (Horwitz, Higham, Bennett, & Kornfield, 2019). Despite substantial evidence of abuse and diversion of the medication to illegal prescribers, Purdue Pharma and other pharmaceutical companies collected massive profits by continuing aggressive marketing campaigns that fostered addiction among chronic pain patients. When these pharmaceutical companies eventually were made accountable, they were punished with massive legal penalties for damage to communities. However, the damage was done. As prescribers' access to legally prescribed opioids diminished, patients turned to heroin purchased on the street. Organized crime opportunistically then began supplying increasing supplies of heroin, followed by illegal supplies of fentanyl, another opioid far more potent than heroin. The advent of fentanyl resulted in high rates of overdose deaths when users failed to appreciate the potency of fentanyl.

This opioid crisis has expanded addiction medicine to include educating medical professionals and first responders, such as police and firemen, on distinctions between opioid intoxication and overdose from other medications. **Naloxone,** a rapidly acting opioid antagonist, is now widely distributed for use by both opioid users and first responders to rescue individuals found overdosed from opioids. A new emphasis is now placed upon **medication-assisted treatment** as a component of addiction treatment.

MEDICATION-ASSISTED TREATMENT

Historically, Narcotics Anonymous (NA) has avoided introducing medications as a component of recovery from opioid addiction. However, large empirical studies have found medication-assisted treatment (MAT) to reduce opioid use, lower risk of relapse, improve adherence to treatment, and improve patients' functioning and quality of life.

Three medications—naltrexone, buprenorphine, and **methadone**— are available for use in MAT (Kampman & Jarvis, 2015). Naltrexone, similar to its use in alcohol withdrawal, blocks effects of opioids by blocking opiate receptors in the nervous system. It can be used in outpatient programs with administration either as a pill or a monthly injection.

Methadone is an opioid with a long duration in the body. It prevents withdrawal symptoms from occurring that would otherwise prompt drug craving. Methadone can only be administered by a licensed outpatient clinic and must be administered daily as a liquid for oral ingestion.

Buprenorphine is an opioid-agonist that both stimulates opioid receptors and also blocks their activation by other opioids, such as prescription drugs or heroin. It can be used in an office-based practice and is administered as either a dissolving tablet, a cheek film, or a 6-month implant under the skin. Because buprenorphine itself is an opioid more potent than morphine, it can be abused by individuals who crush the tablets to ingest larger quantities at once. For this reason, a combination of buprenorphine/naloxone has been produced to dampen the experience of a "high" when taking buprenorphine.

MAT should always provide only one component of a recovery program. A psychosocial needs assessment, supportive counseling, involvement of family supports, and referrals to community services should also be elements of every program (Kampman & Jarvis, 2015).

ABUSE OF OTHER SUBSTANCES

Selected Features of Other Commonly Abused Substances

Substance abuse should be suspected whenever there are inconsistencies in the person's presentation from time to time. Patients who abuse amphetamines may present with wide mood swings, including euphoria, mood elevation, irritability, and a high sense of energy one day; another day they may be exhausted, paranoid, delusional, and psychotic. They may have rapid heart rate, elevated blood pressure, large pupils, weight loss, and complications such as stroke and heart failure or abnormal heart rhythm. Acute amphetamine intoxication can be indistinguishable from schizophrenia at times, and a urine drug screen at the time of the psychotic presentation is essential.

Patients who abuse cocaine may appear similar to those using amphetamines. Cocaine is actually an anesthetic that is used on the surface of the membranes inside of the nose, sinuses, and throat so that the surgeon can operate there. Cocaine is considered much too dangerous and toxic to use in the body as a whole due to risks for heart attacks or stroke, and it is limited to topical application to these small areas. Cocaine abusers may use it orally, sniffing it into the nose; inhale it into the lungs; and inject it intravenously, sometimes combined with heroin ("speedballing"). Patients may thus have irritation of the inside of the nose, problems with their lungs, or tracks where they injected the drug.

Smoking freebase cocaine, which is very potent, leads to the onset of the euphoria in 8–10 seconds, but this rapid increase in drug level in the blood also increases the risk of complications, such as irregular heart rhythm, heart failure, and stroke. Often the abuser will try to modulate the effects of cocaine by drinking alcohol at the same time. The use of alcohol and cocaine together results in a compound called ethylcocaine, which has heart and stroke risks similar to cocaine alone, and the toxic consequences to heart and brain can be additive when ethylcocaine and cocaine are present together. Acute cocaine intoxication or overdose is a true medical emergency, and patients should be referred to the emergency department of a hospital. If they have also been drinking alcohol, they will probably be managed in the intensive care unit.

Patients who use marijuana may have red eyes, a rapid heartbeat, and apathy and memory problems. Many daily users of marijuana develop tolerance for the rapid heartbeat, and they may also develop lung disease and chronic bronchial irritation.

A more sinister drug of abuse is known as **K-2**, "spice," or synthetic cannabinoids. Although sold legally as a synthetic marijuana-like drug, K-2 sold on the street often contains other substances, such as methamphetamine. K-2 intoxication can produce agitated, psychotic states that resemble schizophrenia. K-2 is unfortunately not detectable by current urine drug screens, so diagnosis often must be presumptive.

Patients who use lysergic acid diethylamide (LSD) will have a rapid heartbeat, large pupils, elevated blood pressure, tremors, and elevated body temperature, along with hallucinations. Patients who consume phencyclidine (PCP), a veterinary anesthetic, will appear to be excited and agitated. PCP intoxication can produce a high-energy state of agitation combined with psychotic thinking and a dissociative anesthetized-like state. PCP intoxication produces difficulty talking, motor incoordination, abnormal eye movements, flushing, sweating, and sensitivity to sounds. Drooling, vomiting, muscle twitching, fever, delirium, and coma can occur. Both LSD and PCP can lead to stroke. Patients who are intoxicated with PCP lack normal pain sensation, and they may be very seriously injured when they fight those who are trying to bring their dangerous behavior under control. Patients can appear unable to feel the pain of self-inflicted injuries. There are occasional reports of those under the influence of PCP threatening police officers with weapons; the officers respond with nonlethal force (bean bag guns, electric shock [Taser], or even a nonlethal bullet wound), but the abusers do not stop their aggression because they do not feel the pain of these interventions. Those under the influence of PCP can be dangerous to manage in the hospital.

Patients with **polydrug** use commonly present for care, so that even if the therapist or physician is aware of one drug of abuse, there may be others that need attention in the acute management of very ill patients. A urine drug screen may be essential in establishing that diagnosis. These signs and symptoms are summarized in Table 8.4.

INTERVENTION AND MANAGEMENT OF THE SUDs

Smoking Cessation

Patients who are addicted to nicotine in the form of cigarette smoking have a common but expensive and deadly addiction. Nicotine addiction is the most common cause of preventable death in the United States. Most smokers started in their teen years, and it is very hard for them to quit—possibly the hardest of all of the addictions. Patients with nicotine addiction are at a much increased risk of a long list of cancers, heart disease, and stroke, but they will definitely develop chronic lung disease if they do not die of one of the other risk factors first.

A smoker may need one or more intervention sessions in which education about the impact of smoking on his or her life is presented, just

TABLE 8.4. Signs and Symptoms of Substance Abuse

Drug	Signs and symptoms of use
Opioids	Needle marks, small pupils, constipation.
Amphetamines	Wide mood swings: euphoria, mood elevation, and high energy to exhaustion, paranoid, delusional, and psychotic; rapid heart rate, elevated blood pressure, large pupils, weight loss, stroke, heart failure or arrhythmia.
Cocaine	Nose irritation, lung problems, injection marks, heart failure or arrhythmia, stroke.
Marijuana	Red eyes, rapid heartbeat, apathy, memory problems, lung disease, bronchial irritation.
LSD	Rapid heartbeat, large pupils, elevated blood pressure, tremors, elevated body temperature, mental status changes.
PCP	Excited, agitated, difficulty talking, poor motor coordination, abnormal eye movements, flushing, sweating, exaggerated hearing, mental status changes, drooling, vomiting, muscle twitching, fever, delirium, coma, abnormal pain sensation.

as the person with alcoholism needs an intervention to demonstrate the impact of the alcohol use on his or her life. Physicians will often use a visit for a sinus complaint, sore throat, or even fatigue as an opportunity to talk about the impact of smoking—for example, "Unless you quit smoking, this is the first of many, many visits you will have for bronchitis; it will become a permanent problem, and we're going to be seeing a lot of you . . . until you need the oxygen tank every day and then you *have* to quit."

More than 90% of former smokers quit without formal intervention, and about 80% of those who quit do so cold turkey. For those who utilize the support of others, there are national quit days, 1-800-NO-BUTTS telephone support, and group therapy meetings. Nicotine gum and patches are available without prescription in the drug store; however, the best results will be achieved if patients use them only in conjunction with a support group. If used alone, the risk is that patients will use the nicotine replacement patch or gum and will also keep smoking, thus greatly increasing the risk they face from nicotine. For those who are motivated to stop, the nicotine replacement patches and gum can be a very helpful adjunct to their resolve. If in the course of a medical visit, a physician simply says, "You should stop smoking because of your health," that will double the spontaneous stop-smoking rate. We often utilize a transitional object to reinforce the message to stop smoking by telling the patient that we almost never "guarantee" anything in medicine, but we will give the patient a note written on a prescription, such as the one in Figure 8.1. Patients have taken this home and placed it on the

---

Margaret McCahill, MD
123 Any Street
Some Town, CA 90000

Name: *Mr. John Q. Patient*   Date: *Today*

Rx:

I guarantee you emphysema and a life of gasping for breath attached to an oxygen tank. You may also get lung cancer, but you will definitely get COPD, emphysema, and heart problems, if the cancer doesn't get you first. This guarantee is only good if you continue to smoke—you could stop smoking NOW and void this guarantee. I hope you will stop smoking.

Signature: *M. McCahill, MD*   Refills:

FIGURE 8.1. Sample "prescription" for smoking cessation.

bathroom mirror or the refrigerator as a way to repeatedly deliver the message and the feeling of the intervention. They have come in weeks to years later to say they have now gotten this message and that they really intend to quit smoking.

Patient and Family Education

Families are often significantly affected by a family member's SUD. There are few areas in mental health care where patient and family education are as important as they are in the treatment of SUDs. The initial management and intervention described above is focused on educating the patient and family about the nature of SUDs and the need for abstinence. The process of intervention is rarely effective in a single visit, and typically the therapist must conclude the effort with a mutual agreement to keep the door open for future discussion. Referral to AA, Alanon, and Alateen may provide the patient and family with excellent information and educational materials.

As we follow patients who continue to abuse substances, it is important to present the evidence of the illness and need for treatment in a nonjudgmental way with each therapeutic opportunity. We have all heard trainees and colleagues say, and we may have ourselves said, "Why should I waste my time talking to him about alcoholism *again* today? He knows and he continues to drink anyway—why bother?" It would be a mistake to give up on a person with an SUD when it may be that for this patient to really hear the problem and enter recovery, he or she needs to hear it repeatedly over an extended period of time.

Whereas mental health professionals are most accustomed to supporting the morale of distressed persons, the path to recovery may be most aided by questions that undermine morale by challenging denial:

- "What are some of the things that alcohol has taken from your life since you started drinking heavily?"
- "Which losses have you most regretted?"
- "What is likely to be the next loss?"
- "At the current rate, how long before you have nothing left?"

CONCLUSION

Considering the far-reaching and damaging effects of drug and alcohol abuse, one might wonder what the mental health professional can do to assist individuals and families in preventing them. We cannot change genetics, but we can educate our patients about genetic influences and encourage them to use the knowledge of these disorders to make healthy choices. We can point out that most of the SUDs begin in childhood, adolescence, or young adulthood and that peer group choice plays an important role for many young people. Parents should be advised to be vigilant about the peer group their children associate with, and youth should be encouraged to "hang out" with academic teams, supervised team sports, scouts, church groups, and family groups, all of which are likely to discourage or clearly forbid substance use. Families should teach their children and adolescents about the norms and appropriateness of alcohol use. Medical personnel usually advise teens and young adults about their family history for diabetes, hypertension, and cancer, and they should also tell them about the possible consequences of any family history of SUDs. Physicians should advise adolescents and young adults that if they have a parent with alcoholism, they have a fourfold increased risk of developing it themselves, and they need to consider that fact in their own decision of whether or not to drink and how to monitor how much they drink. When we see that young man who "holds his liquor well"—that is, he seems to be able to drink more than his friends and not show it or not realize it—we should advise him that research shows that this trait may indicate that he is more vulnerable to developing alcoholism later, and he will need to be extra cautious in his relationship with alcohol. There is no pill to cure alcoholism and other SUDs, but we can help those who are the most vulnerable shape their behavior toward alcohol and other substances in a healthy manner.

CHAPTER 9

Physical Health and Illness

Symptoms of anxiety, mood, or thought disorder are common reasons why psychotherapy is recommended. However, such symptoms can represent secondary effects of either a medical illness or medical treatment. The term *due to another medical condition* is used in the DSM-5 to refer to depressive, manic, anxiety, or psychotic symptoms that are a direct pathophysiological consequence of another medical condition. This use of language is unfortunate in that it can suggest that there exists some commonly shared mechanism through which physical illnesses engender depression, mania, anxiety, or psychosis. Rather, medical diseases producing psychiatric symptoms do so through processes unique and highly specific to that disease. For example, the high rate of depression in Parkinson's disease appears due to degeneration of dopamine and norepinephrine mood-regulating systems within the brain, not just the emotional stress of a physically disabling illness. An extraordinarily high rate of depression and suicide in Cushing's disease is related to the high blood levels of cortisol, which has a role in emotion regulation but bears no resemblance to the pathophysiology of depression in Parkinson's disease. On the other hand, high rates of depression in **chronic pain** syndromes are due to interminable suffering and physical disability that robs life of pleasurable and joyful experiences for a person whose brain is presumably normal.

Most commonly, psychiatric symptoms associated with medical conditions are side effects of the medical treatments, not the diseases themselves. For example, depression occurs commonly, and mania less commonly, when patients are treated with corticosteroids, such as prednisone. Many commonly used medications have anticholinergic side effects that can impair concentration and memory in older people. In this chapter we will review the "usual suspects" that are medications commonly producing adverse effects upon mood and cognition. Then we will look at the important roles therapists may play in helping patients manage chronic physical illnesses through psychoeducation, resilience-building interventions, family-centered care that organizes family and community support, and interventions that strengthen adherence to medical treatment programs.

PATIENTS TAKING MEDICATIONS FOR GENERAL MEDICAL CONDITIONS

Detailed knowledge about medications with psychiatric symptoms as side effects is the responsibility of the prescribing physician, but it is important for therapists to be familiar with some of the most common culprits so that they can help provide surveillance for adverse effects. In addition, therapists may wish to use reference tables, which are published periodically. One table is published as a single issue approximately every 2 years from *The Medical Letter on Drugs and Therapeutics*. It is available online at *www.medicalletter.org*, where single issues may be purchased. *Medscape, MDEdge,* and *Mayo Clinic Health Letter* are reliable sources of information. One reference that is usually *not* very helpful for the nonphysician inquiring about side effects is the *Physicians' Desk Reference* (PDR), which is published annually. This widely distributed text contains the pharmaceutical manufacturers' list of everything imaginable for which they wish to have legal documentation for warning patients of risks for harm. It provides a degree of legal protection for the pharmaceutical industry by warning patients about every possible side effect. However, it also can unnecessarily heighten patients' fears about obscure side effects that undermine needed adherence to treatment. Likewise, the Internet is filled with misinformation about medication side effects in personal anecdotes and blog postings by patients.

COMMON PHYSICAL DISEASES THAT CAN PRODUCE PSYCHIATRIC SYMPTOMS

As a general rule, any disease affecting the endocrine system will have high rates of psychiatric symptoms, most commonly mood symptoms, but sometimes cognitive impairment with confusion. Thus, hyper- or hypothyroidism, hyperparathyroidism, diabetes, Cushing's disease (excess of steroid hormone), and Addison's disease (insufficiency of steroid hormone) are associated with secondary mood symptoms, usually depression. Fifty to 80% of patients with Cushing's disease have depression and anxiety due to high levels of the steroid hormone cortisol in the bloodstream (Goebel-Fabbri, Musen, & Levenson, 2010).

Diseases that damage mood-regulating systems of the brain also can have direct effects that produce depression or, less often, mania. Brain circuits that constitute the salience network, discussed in Chapter 1, lie in the medial temporal lobe of the brain. Neurological diseases specifically affecting the temporal lobe, such as complex-partial seizure disorders, also carry high rates of depression. In general, injury to the left, dominant-for-language hemisphere of the brain with strokes or head injury is more often associated with depression, while similar injuries to the right, nondominant-for-language hemisphere can be associated with mania.

Inflammatory gastrointestinal diseases, such as Crohn's disease, celiac disease, and gluten intolerance have high rates of depression for a different reason. Inflammation in the gastrointestinal tract produces cytokines, small molecules that are part of the body's immune response. When cytokines are carried by the bloodstream to the brain, they produce all the familiar symptoms associated with influenza: malaise, lethargy, and mood changes difficult to distinguish from depression.

While pathophysiological processes of different diseases can produce mood, anxiety, or psychotic symptoms, disturbances affecting mood or thinking are far more common as side effects of prescribed medications. Medications that dysregulate mood, generate anxiety, or produce confusion are most often medications that impact functioning of the body's endocrine system (steroids), or monoamine system that regulates mood (some antihypertensive medications), or cognitive system that supports executive functions, attention, and memory (anticholinergic medications and benzodiazepines). Medications at greatest risk for producing confusion or agitation are listed in Table 9.1.

Most published literature on drug-induced mood disorders has consisted of isolated case reports with few randomized studies involving large samples of patients. A systematic review of drug-induced depression concluded that some medications can produce low moods or fatigue, but no medication has been demonstrated to produce a typical major depressive episode (Patten & Barbui, 2004). Medications most at risk for contributing to depressive symptoms are listed in Table 9.2.

TABLE 9.1. Medications at Highest Risk for Contributing to Confusion or Agitation

Type of medication	Use
Anticholinergic (including antihistamines)	Treatment of allergies, gastrointestinal symptoms, Parkinson's disease, or extrapyramidal side effects of antipsychotic medications
Dopaminergic (L-dopa, amantadine, pramipexole, ropinirole)	Treatment of Parkinson's disease or restless legs syndrome
Interferon alpha	Treatment of hepatitis C
Psychostimulants (methylphenidate, dextroamphetamine)	Treatment of attention-deficit/hyperactivity disorder, or excessive daytime sleepiness
Anti-inflammatory hormones— corticosteroids (prednisone)	Treatment of allergic, rheumatological, or autoimmune disorders

Note. Data from Caplan (2018).

TABLE 9.2. Medications at Highest Risk for Contributing to Depression Symptoms

Type of medication	Use
Anti-inflammatory hormones— corticosteroids (prednisone)	Treatment of allergic, rheumatological, or autoimmune disorders
Interferon alpha	Treatment of hepatitis C
Interleukin-2	Treatment of metastatic melanoma and other cancers
Gonadotropin-releasing hormone agonist	Treatment of endometriosis and infertility
Mefloquine	Treatment and prevention of malaria
Progestin-releasing implanted contraceptive	Birth control

Note. Data from Patten and Barbui (2004).

Among other medications, a few commonly used antibiotics have been reported to cause psychiatric symptoms. For example, clarithromycin (trade name Biaxin)—which is frequently used to treat respiratory illnesses, ear infections, and skin infections—has been reported to cause mania in some patients. Metronidazole (trade name Flagyl), which is used to treat many types of infections—from parasites to vaginal infections and abscesses—has been reported to cause depression, agitation, confusion, hallucinations, and mania. Trimethoprim and sulfamethoxazole in combination (trade names Bactrim and Septra)—which is used for urinary tract and sinus and ear infections—has been reported to cause delirium, psychosis, depression, and hallucinations in rare cases. The fluoroquinolone antibiotics—such as ciprofloxacin (trade name Cipro), levofloxacin (trade name Levaquin), ofloxacin (trade name Floxin), trovafloxacin (trade name Trovan), and others of this class—can cause psychiatric symptoms in vulnerable patients, including confusion, agitation, depression, insomnia, mania, paranoia, and psychosis.

Among antihypertensive medications, beta-blockers, such as propranolol, have acquired reputations for producing depression. However, some investigators may have misinterpreted fatigue as depression. Most randomized studies using validated depression measures have failed to demonstrate an association between beta-blockers and depression. Angiotensin-converting enzyme inhibitors (ACE inhibitors), calcium channel blockers, clonidine, and methyldopa are other antihypertensive medications reported to be associated with depression in case series. However, no causal relationships have been verified in controlled studies using validated measures of depression (Patten & Barbui, 2004).

Similarly, depression has been attributed to use of histamine-2 receptor blockers (H-2 blockers) for hyperacidity in the stomach and gastric reflux. H-2 blockers are available over the counter without a physician's prescription. Cimetidine (brand name Tagamet), has been associated with confusion and aggression in the elderly—especially at night. However, methodologically sound studies have failed to establish a relationship between other H-2 blockers, such as ranitidine, and depression (Patten & Barbui, 2004). Cimetidine should be avoided in the elderly and those with serious medical illnesses at risk for encephalopathy and confusion.

SLEEP DISORDERS

More than one-half of adults in the United States have sleep disturbances, some of them transient and some of them persistent. If a person consults a physician about insomnia, it will be attributed to a "psychiatric disorder." While accurate for some patients, it is not always the case that sleep problems are due to a mental disorder.

A useful role that a therapist can serve in assessment of sleep problems is to help a patient to collect 1 or 2 weeks of **sleep logs** that can be provided to the patient's physician. A sample sleep log can be downloaded from the website of the National Sleep Foundation at *www. SleepFoundation.org*. A patient can use sleep logs to record systematically bedtime, time falling asleep, number of awakenings during the night, awakening time, and number of naps during the day. Two weeks of daily sleep logs provide the patient's physician far more information at a glance than an impressionistic account of "not sleeping well." Such use of sleep logs clarify the differences between sleep-onset insomnia, awakenings during the night, awakening too early in the morning, and excessive daytime sleepiness. A sleep problem often can be the heralding sign of another physical illness. Some of the more common causes of poor sleep *not* primarily due to a psychiatric disorder are listed in Table 9.3. It is also valuable to obtain a sleep history from the bed partner or other appropriate family member since the patient may be unaware of sleep problems such as apneic episodes (obstructed breathing), periodic limb movements (leg jerks during sleep), or other symptoms.

TABLE 9.3. Common Causes of Sleep Disturbance That Are Not Primarily Due to a Psychiatric Disorder

- Transient situational insomnia—sleep difficulty that is acute in onset and directly related to a stressor.
- Inadequate sleep hygiene (good sleep hygiene is discussed in the text).
- Psychophysiological insomnia—may have started with transient situational insomnia but persisted after the stressor was resolved.
- Sleep apnea syndrome—a serious structural, medical problem.
- Periodic limb movement disorder—previously called nocturnal myoclonus.
- Restless legs syndrome.
- Altitude insomnia.
- Drug- or alcohol-dependent insomnia.
- Sleep disorders associated with neurological disorders.
- Sleep disorders associated with other chronic medical conditions, for example, asthma, chronic lung disease, cystic fibrosis, chronic pain, kidney and liver failure, congestive heart failure, gastroesophageal reflux, thyroid disorders, and menopause.
- Shift work sleep disorder.
- Sleep disturbance due to parasomnias, such as sleepwalking, sleep terrors, bruxism (teeth grinding), and enuresis (bedwetting). Note that family members may need to provide history about these behaviors, which are probably unknown to the patient.

Regardless of the type of insomnia, proper sleep hygiene is always a good initial step in its management. The therapist may often be the first to provide education to the patient and make some recommendations for lifestyle change. For example, patients should be advised to avoid all drugs of abuse, and they should limit, and preferably stop, the use of alcohol, nicotine, and caffeine. As few as three to five cups of coffee early in the day can result in insomnia in some patients. Although most patients realize that coffee is a significant source of caffeine, they often do not realize that caffeine is also found in various forms of cola, chocolate, and tea. Additional sleep hygiene instructions are shown in Table 9.4.

When sleep hygiene is insufficient management for insomnia, a therapist can incorporate cognitive-behavioral interventions for insomnia into the psychotherapy. Medications can be employed for persistent insomnia. There are OTC sleep aids (including herbals) that although popular, frequently are unreliable and sometimes present more risk than prescription medications. There are five classes of medication utilized for sleep-onset insomnia or to improve maintenance of sleep (Bianchi, Smallwood, Quinn, & Stern, 2018):

1. *Antihistamines.* The histaminic brain system utilizes histamine as a neurotransmitter to help sustain wakefulness. Antihistamine medications that block histamine receptors, such as diphenhydramine (trade name Benadryl) are sedating. Several psychiatric medications are also potent antihistamines, such as quetiapine (trade name Seroquel), doxepin

TABLE 9.4. Useful Sleep Hygiene Instructions

- Have a regular schedule for retiring to bed and getting up in the morning.
- Avoid large meals or vigorous exercise for several hours before sleep.
- Do not watch television or read in bed—the bed is used only for sleep and sexual activity.
- Go to bed only when sleepy, and if unable to get to sleep in approximately 20 minutes, get up and do some very routine, boring activity. Do not read or do anything that requires intellectual activity—folding laundry is an example given by many people as a fairly nonstimulating task. Go back to bed when feeling sleepy, and if sleep does not come in another short period, get up again and repeat this sequence.
- Get up at the same time each day, even if not much sleep was obtained during the night—it is important to establish a regular schedule.
- Do not take naps during the day.
- Avoid the use of caffeine in any form (coffee, tea, chocolate, or cola).
- Avoid the use of alcohol, nicotine, and recreational drugs.

(trade name Silenor), or mirtazapine (trade name Remeron). They each produce drowsiness and can be used for insomnia. Most OTC sleep aids, such as Nyquil, contain an antihistamine as their active ingredient. The main drawback for use of antihistamine for insomnia is tolerance to their sedating effects that occurs after 1 to 2 weeks of continuous use.

2. *Benzodiazepines.* The major "standbys" for insomnia treatment are the benzodiazepine medications, such as diazepam (trade name Valium) and lorazepam (trade name Ativan), and others, together with nonbenzodiazepine medications that nevertheless activate the benzodiazepine receptor in the brain, such as zolpidem (trade name Ambien) and eszopiclone (trade name Lunesta). Development of benzodiazepines in the 1950s revolutionized use of sleep medications. The barbiturate class of sleeping pills of the 1930s and 1940s were lethal in overdose, quickly addicting, and resulted in dangerous withdrawal syndromes when discontinued. By contrast, benzodiazepines had few side effects in prescribed doses other than sedation. Deaths from overdoses were nonexistent when only benzodiazepines were involved. Benzodiazepines and benzodiazepine agonists, such as zolpidem, eventually proved to show tolerance with high-dose, continuous use and have acquired notoriety for contributing to overdose deaths when combined with either alcohol or opioids. Nevertheless, benzodiazepines remain the most effective, safest, and least side-effect class of medications available to facilitate sleep induction and maintenance when medications are required.

3. *Serotonin receptor blockers.* Medications that block type 2A serotonin receptors in the brain, such as trazodone, induce emotional quietude that can facilitate falling asleep. A benefit of trazodone is its lack of risk for addiction or abuse. While highly effective with some patients, however, trazodone has had an erratic record of effectiveness as a sleep aid.

4. *Melatonin.* Melatonin is a hormone released within the brain at sleep onset. Used for sleep induction, melatonin has had a mixed history, effective for some individuals but not others. Some sleep studies have suggested chronic use of melatonin may contribute to disorganization of sleep architecture.

5. *Prazosin and topiramate.* Prazosin, an antihypertensive medication, and topiramate, an anticonvulsant, can facilitate sleep for patients with posttraumatic stress disorder and secondary light, fragmented sleep due to heightened vigilance for threats. They are particularly helpful for patients with posttraumatic nightmares that disrupt sleep (Taylor & Raskind, 2002; Berlant, 2006).

Pharmacological sleep aids, herbal or prescribed, optimally should only be used for 3 or 4 consecutive days. Some patients do function best with chronic use of medications for sleep maintenance, but this should be the judgment of a physician who has conducted an adequate diagnostic evaluation. For persistent insomnia, sleep disorder centers are broadly available in most urban settings. A sleep disorder specialist can conduct a sophisticated diagnostic evaluation that may include a **polysomnogram** study of the patient's sleep.

The greatest health risks from sleep problems come with excessive daytime sleepiness, rather than insomnia. Obstructive sleep apnea occurs when a person's airway closes during sleep, producing choking or cessation of respirations. Undiagnosed sleep apnea accounts for motor vehicle accidents and other injuries due to daytime sleepiness. Left untreated, sleep apnea produces secondary hypertension that contributes to cardiovascular disease. A bed partner may describe a history of snoring, choking, or cessation of breathing. Patients with apnea are not refreshed by a long night of sleep. They often awaken with a headache and feel it necessary to take multiple naps during the day. A therapist can play an important role in recognizing these symptoms and ensuring that they are reported to a patient's physician.

OBESITY

According to the Centers for Disease Control and Prevention (CDC), it is estimated that more than two-thirds of adults in the United States are overweight, an epidemic that has been increasing steadily over the last 50 years. **Obesity,** which is a state of excess fat tissue in the body, is best defined through the body mass index (BMI), which is equal to weight in kilograms divided by height in meters squared. A BMI of 30 or more is generally considered obesity, and a BMI of 25–30 is usually considered medically significant. Children and adolescents are classified as normal weight, overweight, or obese depending upon age and sex-specific growth charts developed by the CDC. Children in the 85th–95th BMI percentile for age and gender are classed as overweight, while those above the 95th percentile are obese. Almost 9% of children and adolescents are greater than 120% of the 95th percentile, an alarming statistic (Cook & Evans, 2018).

The consequences of obesity are legion and include high blood pressure, arthritis (especially in weight-bearing joints), diabetes, lung disorders, gallstones, certain cancers, and premature death due to heart attack and stroke. In addition to these well-known physical consequences, the

United States is a society in which obese people have faced stigmatization and discrimination in the workplace and other social settings. We live in a society that generally regards thinness as the only acceptable standard. Therapists can help their patients by providing commonsense, accurate information in a setting of psychological support.

Obesity is a consequence of interplay between genetic, environmental, and psychosocial factors. We know that if people consume more calories than they utilize in energy, they will gain weight. If a person takes in an average of 3,400 kilocalories above their energy expenditure, they will gain 1 pound of weight. Population studies suggest that the current prevalence of obesity is related more to increased caloric intake in U.S. culture, rather than a decreased energy expenditure from physical activity (Cook & Evans, 2018).

How many calories a person needs varies from person to person. Suppose two women, each 5 feet, 6 inches tall and both weighing 140 pounds, have similar job activities that they do daily with no other exercise. Yet, one may require many *fewer* calories than the other even with the same activities. When she eats the same as her peer, she will gain weight. The genetic factors contributing to obesity are complex and not fully known, but it is believed that there is a subset of obese individuals who are predisposed to obesity and have the capacity to become obese initially, without an absolute increase in caloric consumption (Flier, 2001; see Table 9.5).

Currently available drugs for weight loss are all aimed at reducing appetite. None address the issue of the varying utilization of energy from one person to another, and the appetite suppressants all have risks, especially to the cardiovascular system. Sometimes the risk is worthwhile because the obesity itself is causing a more life-threatening risk than the drugs, but for most patients who consult a therapist about their weight, the risk of weight-loss drugs is not worth taking. The fundamental issue of how the cells of the body use energy will remain, and the patient

TABLE 9.5. *Just* an Apple a Day . . .

We have all heard the saying "An apple a day keeps the doctor away." However, if you are genetically vulnerable to obesity, and you eat just one apple a day (80–85 calories) more than your (lower than most people's) caloric need, you will be consuming enough extra calories in a year to gain about 9 pounds. It does not take much to gain steadily, and for those with obesity genes, that weight gain over the years stays with them. Their best strategy is to understand what is going on and to work rigorously and continuously to develop a lifestyle of vigorous diet and exercise that is much more intense than their genetically thin peers.

would be better off learning how to balance diet and exercise. In cases of extreme obesity and failed weight-loss programs, gastric surgical procedures can be considered. Such procedures can be safely conducted and have produced sustained weight loss for refractory morbid obesity when conducted with a comprehensive, long-term weight-loss program after the surgery. Psychiatric consultation is obligatory prior to any consideration of the surgical management of morbid obesity.

For typical obese patients, therapists can help patients reduce self-shaming through education about the complex nature of obesity—the fact that it *really is true* that they did not eat more than their peers in a day but still gained weight. The patient did not create the problem yet must take charge of the solution with diet and exercise and a very long-term perspective. The therapist also can help their patients understand that drugs do not work on a long-term basis for most obese people, and the most effective tools are a diet that leads to gradual weight loss and sustains that loss for a lifetime, and sensible, aerobic exercise. The therapist can be a very effective educator and supporter of an obese person who is resolving to lose weight by teaching the genetic components of obesity, relieving guilt when appropriate, addressing the stigma that obese persons face, and teaching behavioral strategies for sustained weight loss.

EATING DISORDERS

Anorexia Nervosa

Patients who suffer with anorexia nervosa fail to maintain at least 85% of their expected weight; they have great fear of gaining weight, and they resist any treatment that urges them to return to a goal of approximately 90% of predicted weight. The patient appears unduly thin and may have soft, longer than normal, downy hair growth, especially on the back and the arms. The patient may have prominent cheeks from enlarged salivary glands and a slow pulse. She may report that her menstrual periods have stopped. There are many physiological signs and symptoms of starvation the physician will look for in a medical evaluation, but they will not be apparent in the therapist's office.

A question that may raise the suspicion of anorexia nervosa is asking an unusually thin patient how she feels about her current weight. The patient who is thin because of some other illness will usually reply that she feels she is too thin; however, the patient with anorexia nervosa typically responds that she feels that she is "too fat" or obese, even though she is extraordinarily thin. When anorexia nervosa is suspected, it is important that the patient (and her family) be served by a multi-disciplinary team. Anorexia nervosa has the highest death rate of any psychiatric illness with an estimated mortality rate of 10% (Insel, 2012). Patients often require inpatient treatment in order to stabilize them when they are in a life-threatening phase of the illness. No medication has been proven to be of superior efficacy for anorexia nervosa, and a long-term treatment program for the individual and the family is indicated. This is a specialty area for both psychiatry and psychotherapy, and the therapist who will be working with anorectic patients and their families is encouraged to obtain specialty training in this area.

Bulimia Nervosa

Although a minority of patients with anorexia nervosa engage in binge eating, it is universal in bulimia nervosa, and this is one of the diagnostic criteria. Binge eating is often followed by some activity to eliminate (or purge) its consequences, such as self-induced vomiting and misuse of laxatives. Others do not purge but engage in fasting or excessive exercise to compensate for the binge eating. Patients are often ashamed of their behavior; they may not easily volunteer information about it, and they may appear to be of normal or even above normal weight. Very few physical signs suggest bulimia, and they occur only in those who induce vomiting. There may be a reddish roughening of the skin around the knuckles of the hand; there may be large cheeks from enlarged salivary glands, and the front teeth may appear discolored or damaged from the stomach acid injury to the dental enamel. The primary way in which a therapist will learn about the existence of bulimia is the development of enough rapport with a patient so that a very candid history can be obtained.

Neither anorexia nor bulimia have specific indications for pharmacological treatment, but improvement in either can occur when medication can be used to treat depression or an anxiety disorder that is comorbid with the eating disorder.

CASE ILLUSTRATION: LAURA, ANOREXIA

Laura, a 17-year-old dancer and honors student, made an appointment to see Dr. P. because her dance teacher suggested it. Actually, Laura's mother called to make the appointment because Laura was so reluctant to do so. Laura had been diagnosed with anorexia 4 years earlier and was barely able to maintain her minimal weight. She had never had a menstrual period and currently reported numerous symptoms of starvation. Laura was being treated for the medical aspects of anorexia by a pediatrician who had expertise in treating eating disorders.

During the initial sessions, Dr. P. spent a great deal of time asking about Laura's life apart from the anorexia. Dr. P. felt comfortable taking time for this inquiry because she knew Laura's condition was being monitored by her pediatrician. Dr. P. learned that Laura was an honors student applying to Harvard College. She loved modern dance and was concerned about social justice. Laura and Dr. P. looked at a BMI scale together, and Laura chose a target weight gain that would move her into the (barely) normal range.

Dr. P. also met with Laura's parents, who were very concerned about Laura's eating disorder. They also worried about what Laura might do if she were not to be accepted into Harvard. They were concerned about her ritualized, private eating; the fact that she had never menstruated; that she didn't want to see a nutritionist; and that she was unwilling to give up her exercise and dance routine, even for a day.

Beginning Collaboration

After several sessions, Laura and Dr. P. began to establish rapport. At this time, Laura told Dr. P. that she had been "cheating" when she was weighed, in both unscheduled weigh-ins by her mother at home and at her regularly scheduled appointments at her pediatrician's office. She did this by adding weights inside her clothes. Laura said that she hated deceiving her parents and her physician but forbid Dr. P. from telling anyone.

Dr. P. decided to go over several treatment options with Laura: setting weekly eating and weight goals; being hospitalized; seeing a nutritionist; bringing her dance instructor, Eren, into a few sessions to get her perspective; meeting with Dr. S., a psychiatrist colleague of Dr. P.; and other options. Laura declined medication but liked the ideas of bringing Eren into therapy, setting weekly goals, and possibly seeing a nutritionist. Over the next month, many of these treatment options took place, and Dr. P.'s relationship with Laura continued to grow stronger. Laura dismissed the nutritionist as naïve after their first meeting but in time agreed for Eren to join a therapy session. She also agreed on some weight-gain goals.

After much prodding from Dr. P., Laura agreed to tell her parents that she had been cheating on her weigh-ins. This led to a dramatic family session, but afterward Laura felt free for the first time from the guilt of deceiving her supportive family.

Laura slowly began to gain weight. She told Dr. P. about an important success: She allowed her friends at school to observe her eating some sugar. Laura's family, Eren, Dr. P., and a caring English teacher become her cheerleaders as they watched her make tentative, small gains. However, several months into the treatment, Laura's progress stalled. She still had not had a menstrual period—the goal she had set.

Ongoing Collaboration and Outcome

Again, Dr. P. brought up the idea of trying a psychotropic medication: "I'm not asking you to agree to *take* medication. I'm asking you to agree to find out if it might help *us* in achieving our goals. I have a colleague that I respect a great deal. She knows a lot about eating disorders, and I'd like to get her opinion. In fact, I'll go with you to see her in her office." Reluctantly, and perhaps to please Dr. P., Laura agreed. Dr. P. consulted her colleague, Dr. S., because Dr. S. was a woman, and Laura felt more comfortable with female physicians. Dr. S. was knowledgeable about eating disorders but was conservative in recommending treatment with medications.

When Dr. S. met with Laura, she obtained all the needed medical information, occasionally asking for Dr. P.'s thoughts or observations on an issue. She acknowledged the gains Laura had made and validated the fact that Laura was in charge of her own body. Toward the end of the session, Dr. S. suggested that an antidepressant medication could help Laura achieve her goals. Laura and her parents questioned how the medication would be helpful. Dr. S. discussed how Laura often struggled with anxiety and that an antidepressant medication might help diminish this anxiety, which was as an added burden for her to cope with. At the end of the session, Laura agreed to take a "trial dose" of the medication.

Although the medication effects of the next few months were not dramatic, Laura did start slowly achieving her target goals again. She eventually had a menstrual period. Her body changed color, her skin became less wrinkled, and she had to buy new clothes. The following September Laura moved to the Northeast to start attending Harvard College. Before she started, she visited its counseling center, found a new therapist that she liked, and reluctantly agreed to stay on her medication during her first semester.

Questions for Consideration

1. Dr. P. involved Laura's parents in her treatment, coordinated with her pediatrician, and referred her to a psychiatrist. She even

included her supportive dance instructor in her care. Laura declined the services of the "naïve" nutritionist that she met but accepted the support of her English teacher. Why is a "team approach" so important in treating anorexia? What are the challenges that a private therapist faces when trying to develop "a team"?

2. Laura was 17 years old when she started treatment with Dr. P. Dr. P. spent a lot of time establishing rapport with Laura and obtained her consent on treatment goals. She supported Laura's decision to decline the nutritionist's help but encouraged her to be honest with her family about using weights during the weekly weigh-ins. Anorexia is a dangerous illness and patients can die. How and when would Dr. P. need to step-up her care to an in-patient setting regardless of whether Laura agreed?

3. Medication is not a primary treatment for eating disorders. But medication can help treat other symptoms such as anxiety and depression. How and why should a therapist decide when to initiate a medication referral?

CHRONIC PAIN

Chronic pain is defined as a pain state that is persistent and for which the cause cannot be removed or otherwise treated and, in the generally accepted course of medical practice, no relief or cure is possible or none has been found after reasonable efforts. Approximately one out of three Americans suffer from a chronic pain condition, most commonly chronic back pain or headaches but also including arthritis, diabetic neuropathy, and chronic pain from falls and physical injuries (Kohrt, Griffith, & Patel, 2018).

A decade of research on the mechanisms of pain transmission to the brain has led to improved understanding and improved methods of pain control. The Joint Commission on Accreditation of Healthcare Organizations (JCAHO) now requires all accredited health care organizations to fully assess pain in all patients, teach patients pain management options, provide appropriate pain management, and record the results of that strategy (Curtiss, 2001). Some states have enacted legislation that requires physicians to take courses in pain management before they can renew their medical license. Patients can now file a legal complaint against their physicians for inadequate pain management. The care of the chronic pain patient is now legally more important than it was in the past, and the therapist will be asked to be a part of the treatment team for patients who suffer from chronic pain. See the various treatments listed in Figure 9.1, which is organized through a multidisciplinary approach for patients with chronic pain.

Patient care for chronic pain should aim at tailoring treatment to each person's unique experience, with self-management of pain by the patient an objective (Institute of Medicine, 2012). Since there is no singular "magic bullet" for most patients with chronic pain, this requires creation of complex, individualized treatment plans that integrate in a rational matter evidence-based interventions of different types. Rarely does an effective pain management program consist solely of pain medications. More often, management of chronic pain requires an integrated program of medications, psychotherapy, physical therapy, and complementary and alternative therapies. Therapists serve an important role in helping patients communicate more effectively with their physicians and in organizing a comprehensive personal program of pain management.

Biology and Biochemistry of Chronic Pain

At a biological level, pain is a signal that body tissues are threatened with injury. The role of pain is to ensure safety. However, not all signals to the brain accurately reflect danger. If the brain's first information-processing task is to organize flight from sources of pain, then the second task is to detect false warnings, when incoming nociceptive signals are benign.

In human beings, a "pain matrix" has evolved to accomplish this dual mission. The pain matrix receives sensory inputs through each of the five senses as well as from internal body organs. The pain matrix

Medical	Physical Therapy	Psychological
Medication trials:	Active mobilization	Support
Lidocaine	Desensitization	Motivation
Gabapentin	Myofascial release	Stress management
Mexilitine	Aerobic conditioning	Treatment for depression
Opioid		Hypnosis
Nerve block		Imagery
neurostimulation		Biofeedback
	Functional improvement	

FIGURE 9.1. Multidisciplinary treatment of complex regional pain syndrome.

enables interplay between bottom-up processing of tissue nociceptive sensations as danger signals and top-down regulation of the nociceptive information to temper behavioral reactions to the sensations. **Nociception** refers to the body's system of sensory organs in body tissues that detects potential tissue damage, such as from heat or pressure. Nociceptive organs throughout our tissues send signals over peripheral nerves to the spinal cord, which in turn relays this information to the brain, alerting the person to danger. If nociception refers to the physical transmission of danger signals from sensory organs in body tissues, then pain refers to a person's interpretation of those nociceptive signals as a valid warning of danger. Bottom-up processing refers to the brain's analysis and interpretation of incoming nociceptive information.

Top-down processing refers to a set of mechanisms through which the brain can dampen or suppress incoming nociceptive information, tempering any behavioral responses to it. Top-down regulation of nociception is essential for effective living. As anyone who has had a migraine headache during a workday knows, it can be essential to shift attention away from the pain and onto the work of the day, rather than spending the day distraught. Patients with chronic back pain must learn ways to manage the pain so that they can work, engage in relationships, and enjoy pleasurable activities—without the ever-present back pain becoming a constant preoccupation. Different systems for top-down regulation of nociception make this possible.

This interplay between bottom-up and top-down processing of nociception can be regarded as the brain's summary "opinion" as to the state of bodily safety. The complexity of the pain matrix provides multiple points of entry where an intervention can reduce overall suffering from pain by either attenuating the bottom-up transmission of nociceptive information or by amplifying effectiveness of top-down regulation of the information.

The Brain's Analgesia Systems: Multiple Systems for Providing Top-Down Regulation of Nociception

At multiple levels of the pain matrix, different control systems are in place that can limit transmission of nociceptive signals. These top-down control systems provide the underpinnings for our different pain management interventions:

1. *Gate control.* Large-caliber nerve fibers carry non-nociceptive information from sensory receptors regarding touch, temperature, or movement (see Figure 9.2). As these fibers enter the spinal cord, they

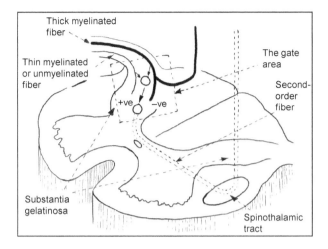

FIGURE 9.2. Cross section of the spinal cord: The gate area connections.

inhibit transmission of pain sensations upward to the brainstem and cortex. This inhibition is the basis for pain relief through rubbing or scratching the skin. Medically, it is the basis for use of **transcutaneous nerve stimulator** or **dorsal column stimulators** that neurosurgeons can implant on the surface of the spinal cord in selected chronic pain patients.

2. *Endogenous opiate system for analgesia.* An enkephalin is a neurotransmitter involved in regulating nociception in the body. Enkephalins activate opiate receptors in the brainstem, which in turn activate descending **serotonergic pathways** and **noradrenergic pathways,** both of which descend to inhibit pain transmission within the spinal cord (see Figure 9.3). Activating the endogenous opiate system

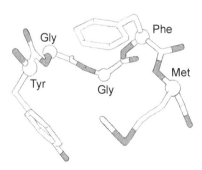

FIGURE 9.3. Three-dimensional structure of enkephalin.

is the neurophysiological basis for opioid medications, as well as for acupuncture and the placebo response. "Dual-action" SNRI antidepressants, such as amitriptyline (trade name Elavil), venlafaxine (trade name Effexor), or duloxetine (trade name Cymbalta) enhance the effectiveness of this **endogenous opiate system.**

3. *Placebo response.* Placebo responses also activate the endogenous enkephalin system, utilizing the same neural circuitry as opioid medications, such as morphine. Placebo responses are blocked by administration of naloxone, an opiate-receptor blocker.

4. *Attention allocation.* Within the brain, "attention trumps emotion." By shifting focus of attention, no emotional distress may be experienced in response to pain sensations. This is the neurophysiological basis for hypnosis and other strategies that utilize absorption and distraction to manage pain. These effects operate by attenuating activation of the amygdala and insula by nociceptive stimuli. However, this reallocation of attention does not utilize the endogenous opiate circuitry that opioid medications, acupuncture, and the placebo response utilize.

5. *Perspective taking (cognitive appraisal).* Beliefs, values, and expectations shape how the prefrontal cortex regulates level of alarm responses of the amygdala and insula in response to nociceptive information. Through these mechanisms, beliefs, values, and expectations can suppress activation of the amygdala and insula by nociceptive stimuli.

6. *Secure attachment and confiding relationships.* In mammals, the **mirror neuron system** and associated neural circuitry link person-to-person relationships to the pain matrix so that relational pain evokes the same responses as does pain from tissue injury. The intimacy of a securely attached relationship can dampen pain-evoked responses of the amygdala and insula to nociceptive stimuli, similarly to physical comfort measures and provision of a safe environment (see Figures 9.4 and 9.5).

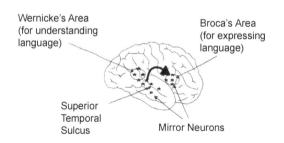

FIGURE 9.4. Mirror neuron and language systems.

"I feel your pain."

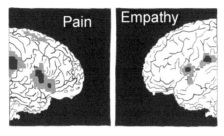

FIGURE 9.5. Mirror neurons with pain and empathy.

Linking information streams from mirror neurons to the pain matrix provides the neural infrastructure for empathy. Over the course of evolution, the original function of the pain matrix for managing physical pain was doubly co-opted, first by adapting it to respond to emotional as well as to physical pain, then by adapting it further to perceive and respond to pain in other people.

Vicarious experiencing of another person's pain activates the same structures within the brain as does pain in one's physical body. Relieving pain of the other also becomes a method through which one's own pain is relieved. Empathy enables acts of compassion to become vehicles for regulating pain that is vicariously experienced.

The Role of Medications in Treating Chronic Pain

The key to successful chronic pain treatment is a multimodality program that integrates different kinds of evidence-based interventions. Usually medications have a role but rarely are medications sufficient as a sole intervention. It is almost never the case that chronic pain treatment should consist only of an opioid prescription.

It is helpful to appreciate how different classes of medications best treat different kinds of pain. Each of the following classes of medications have different roles in treatment of different kinds of chronic pain.

- *Nonsteroidal analgesics (ibuprofen, naproxen):* Block activation of C-fibers in injured peripheral tissues.
- *Dual-action antidepressants (amitriptyline and other tricyclic antidepressants, venlafaxine, duloxetine):* Amplify effectiveness of endogenous opiate system by augmenting activation of

descending serotonergic and noradrenergic pathways that block nociceptive transmission within spinal cord.

- *Anticonvulsants (gabapentin, pregabalin):* Stabilize membrane potentials of injured nerves.
- *Opioids:* Activate the brain's endogenous opiate system.

In general, the type of medication prescribed should be determined by the type of pain syndrome. Each of the above medication classes tends to fit best in treatment for different types of pain:

- *Active tissue damage:* nonsteroidal analgesics, opioids
- *Neuropathic pain (damaged peripheral nerves):* anticonvulsants, such as gabapentin (trade name Neurontin), pregabalin (trade name Lyrica)
- *Pain from central sensitization (fibromyalgia, irritable bowel syndrome, migraine):* "dual-action" SNRI antidepressants, such as amitriptyline (trade name Elavil), duloxetine (trade name Cymbalta), venlafaxine (trade name Effexor)

CASE ILLUSTRATIONS: TREATMENT OF CHRONIC PAIN

A 45-year-old woman presented to the orthopedic clinic unable to raise her right arm above shoulder. She had been noticing increasing pain in her right shoulder when working out with a particular machine at the gym prior to the day it suddenly worsened. The orthopedic surgeon ordered a magnetic resonance imaging (MRI) scan that showed a mild rotator cuff tear. She did not wish to have surgery on her shoulder, so the surgeon prescribed physical therapy with naproxen (nonsteroidal anti-inflammatory analgesic) for pain. He also prescribed a limited supply of hydroxycodone (opioid) for awakenings during the night when pain disrupted her sleep. While this anti-inflammatory/analgesic medication regimen relieved her acute distress, her orthopedic surgeon emphasized that her recovery most depended upon a several-month regular program of physical therapy to restore strength to the injured muscle.

A 60-year-old man with diabetes developed symmetrical numbness and intolerable burning pain over both feet up to the ankles. His internist explained that he suffered from diabetic neuropathy. While no medication could restore feeling where there was numbness, gabapentin (anticonvulsant) was a medication that sometimes could help such burning pain. After titrating upward the dosage from 100 mg daily to 800 mg daily, the patient reported the pain to be 75% improved. Treatment of neuropathy pain is one of the few types of pain for which treatment consists almost exclusively of a daily regimen of anticonvulsant medications.

A 40-year-old woman presented with chronic fatigue, headaches, and multiple areas of tenderness over her back and shoulders. She often experienced a detached "brain fog" that made concentrating at work difficult. Treatment with Percocet (opioid) and ibuprofen (nonsteroidal analgesic) for pain had been ineffective in relieving either her pain or associated symptoms. Her new internist diagnosed her symptoms as fibromyalgia and instituted a multimodality treatment program consisting of yoga, physical therapy consultation for additional at-home exercises, mirtazapine at bedtime (sedating dual-action antidepressant), and duloxetine in the morning (nonsedating dual-action antidepressant). After 6 weeks, her pain symptoms diminished and energy level had improved.

Central sensitization is a condition of the nervous system that is associated with the development and maintenance of chronic pain. When central sensitization occurs, the nervous system goes through a process called "wind-up" in which circuits for bottom-up nociceptive transmission within the pain matrix stay in a persistent state of high reactivity. Central sensitization has two main characteristics, both of which involve heightened sensitivity:

1. **Allodynia**—experiencing pain with things that are normally not painful; for example, light touch to skin feels painful.
2. **Hyperalgesia**—a painful stimulus feels more painful than it should; for example, light pressure feels too painful to tolerate.

Central sensitization appears to play an etiological role in fibromyalgia, irritable bowel syndrome, migraine headaches, and other chronic pain conditions. Dual-action antidepressants and anticonvulsant medications often contribute to recovery, as with the patient in the above illustration.

Use of Opioids in Chronic Pain Treatment

Opioids have been a mainstay of pain control throughout the history of civilization. However, opioid abuse and deaths from opioid accidental overdoses or suicide have recently become the most pressing public health concern facing the United States. Deaths from suicides or accidental overdoses increased by 250% from 2000 to the present, with 40%

of these involving opioids. Opioid dosage per person per year increased 600% between 1997 and 2007. This dramatic increase has appeared due to three factors:

1. Concerns over untreated pain in the 1990s led to promoting the practice of viewing "pain as the fifth vital sign" and increased prescription of opioids.
2. "Diseases of despair" (alcohol abuse, alcoholic liver disease, opioid and methamphetamine abuse, suicide) escalated in prevalence in working-class communities with high unemployment, social deterioration, and economic insecurity following the 2008 recession.
3. Pharmaceutical companies, particularly Purdue Pharma, Insys Therapeutics, and Johnson & Johnson, began aggressively promoting high-potency opioids for chronic pain treatment without monitoring illegal diversion of medications. In some cases, pharmaceutical company executives were convicted and imprisoned for bribing doctors to prescribed highly addictive opioids (*Washington Post*, 2020).

A recent patient presentation illustrates these issues. A 28-year-old man was diagnosed with opioid use disorder as he faced a 2-year sentence for illegal possession of heroin. He had been sniffing 8–10 bags of heroin a day for the past 6 months after using 120–150 mg of oxycodone (opioid) daily for the past 5 years. Initially, he had used oxycodone recreationally and only on weekends drinking with friends. Over a few years the drug became a daily habit that he needed to get through the day as a construction worker. He has never been in drug treatment. He says that every time he has tried to stop, he became irritable with coworkers, suffered intolerable anxiety and insomnia, and had withdrawal symptoms of nausea, diarrhea, and muscle aches.

Due to alarm over opioid addiction, measures to dramatically curtail chronic pain patients' access to opioids produced a secondary public health crisis when rapid tapering of opioids led to patients seeking street heroin for pain control (sometimes with accidental overdoses) and suicides by patients unable to tolerate pain without opioids. While current recommendations are to avoid both long-term use and doses of opioids for pain above 40 morphine milligram equivalents (MME), it has been increasingly recognized that some "legacy" pain patients who have been taking 100 MME of opioids for years may never be able to taper off opioids. It is now recommended that any tapering be done slowly (10% or less per month) and in collaboration with the patient.

A casualty of the opioid crisis have been those chronic pain patients who do need an opioid medication as one component of a well-designed treatment regimen. In the aftermath of the opioid crisis, some physicians have become reticent to prescribe opioids for any reason.

CONCLUSION

Successful chronic pain treatment has the triple aim of reducing pain symptoms, improving functioning in daily life (including recreational activities), and strengthening resilience as a whole person who lives richly and fully despite the ongoing presence of chronic pain.

The therapist's role in the first aim of reducing pain includes helping patients and families to understand, at a basic level, how nociceptive systems operate and how each element of the patient's treatment program—medications, physical therapy, exercise, mindfulness practices, sleep, and diet—makes its contributions to pain management. Perhaps the greatest challenge for chronic pain patients is demoralization when despair makes daily adherence to physical therapy exercises and mindfulness practices seem pointless and too tedious to sustain. The therapist's most important role is to help a patient to sustain hope as a practice, to cope assertively despite whatever obstacles present themselves, to sustain an attitude that "there is never a time when nothing can be done" (de Figueiredo & Griffith, 2016; Griffith & Gaby, 2005).

The therapist has a critical role in improving functioning by helping a patient to stay focused on achieving a steady functional improvement in activities and work roles, rather than a preoccupation with whether or not pain persists. Useful reading for patients is Jerome Groopman's (2004) landmark text, *The Anatomy of Hope,* in which he described his personal struggle with disabling back pain and how he learned to revise the meaning of his pain. Patients must learn to plot accruing progress in terms of "what I can do now" versus "what I could do at start of treatment."

For the third aim, the therapist works with the patient to build resilience by "putting the illness in its place." This entails accepting residual pain that cannot be eradicated while working to reduce space that the pain takes up in one's life (Gonzalez, Steinglass, & Reiss, 1989).

CHAPTER 10

Special Populations

This chapter presents selected background information and clinical guidance to help therapists with specific populations. We present a brief overview of collaborative issues in the treatment of problems in childhood and special considerations essential to the care of women and older adults. We provide not an exhaustive discussion of these issues, but rather a general discussion of common challenges.

CHILDREN AND ADOLESCENTS

Use of psychiatric medications in children and adolescents is still at an early stage of development. Ethical concerns about conducting clinical research trials of medications have limited the evidence base for guiding use of medications in children. Clinicians cannot assume that the immature brain of a child will show the same therapeutic effects and side effects from a medication that an adult would show. Most use of medications in children is off-label, lacking formal approval by the FDA.

Mood and anxiety problems in children are nearly always addressed first with a combination of CBT and family interventions. When a medication appears necessary, fluoxetine has had the largest registry monitoring side effects and so has usually been the medication of choice. Children may be treated with a range of medications on an off-label basis, depending upon the experience and expertise of the specialist. Most general psychiatrists and primary care clinicians will either avoid treating children with medications or limit treatment of mood and anxiety problems to fluoxetine.

The one exception to this limited scope of pediatric psychopharmacology is treatment of attention-deficit/hyperactivity disorder (ADHD). ADHD is relatively common, with prevalence estimated at 3–7% of school-age children (American Psychiatric Association, 2013). The therapist can assist in making an accurate diagnosis when ADHD is considered, and if the diagnosis is confirmed, the therapist can provide essential education to the parents and, in many cases, to the child.

ADHD is both overdiagnosed and underdiagnosed in our society. It is critical that parents, teachers, therapists, and physicians work together to ensure that the correct diagnosis is established. The **Conners Comprehensive Behavior Rating Scales** are commonly used, and there are questionnaires for parents, teachers, adolescents, and adults who might have ADHD themselves. The Conners scales are "B-level products," which require documentation of professional licenses and qualifications before ordering them. Most school counselors' offices have the Conners scales for screening children for ADHD. Table 10.1 lists other conditions that should be considered in the differential diagnosis of ADHD symptoms.

If the diagnosis of ADHD appears likely, the therapist may consult with the child's family physician or pediatrician for possible medication management. A child psychiatrist may be needed when there is an inadequate response to treatment or if the diagnosis is not clear.

The impact of untreated ADHD on a child can be large and enduring. Some of the consequences of untreated ADHD are listed in Table 10.2.

In spite of these factors, parents often worry about giving their child a "mind-altering drug." They understandably look for other explanations and interventions. For example, therapists can help parents understand that, although eating too many sweets is not a healthy diet, there

TABLE 10.1. Other Conditions Needing Consideration in the Differential Diagnosis of ADHD

- Normal variations of temperament (most common condition misinterpreted as ADHD).
- Child stress from conflict in family relationships.
- Posttraumatic stress symptoms.
- Conduct disorder.
- Oppositional defiant disorder.
- Early-onset bipolar disorder.
- Pervasive developmental disorder.
- Other medical illness, such as lead poisoning, fetal alcohol syndrome, or traumatic brain injury.

TABLE 10.2. Consequences of Untreated ADHD in Children

- Profound effect on all relationships.
- Child's frustration with self, school, life.
- Lost age-appropriate educational opportunities.
- Possible development of externalizing behavior.
- Adult disapproval and peer rejection, leading to poor self-esteem.
- Depression.
- Frustrated, unhappy, guilt-stricken parents.
- Children at higher risk of abuse than peers.
- Decreased hyperactivity with age, but possible persistence of inattentiveness and impulsivity.
- Approximately one-third of children with ADHD having an Axis I disorder as adults.
- Chronic misunderstanding of medications.

is no objective medical evidence that foods high in sugar or carbohydrates cause hyperactive behavior. On the other hand, there is evidence that fetal exposure to alcohol and exposure to lead (e.g., eating lead-containing paint chips; inhaling lead-containing fumes) can predispose a child to behaviors that can be confused with ADHD. Parents will benefit greatly from information about how they can help their child with hyperactive behaviors, whether the child takes medication or not. Some good sources to recommend can be found on the website of CHADD (Children and Adults with Attention-Deficit/Hyperactivity Disorder; *www.chadd.org*). This website has helpful educational materials for parents, with such titles as "50 Tips on the Classroom Management of Attention Deficit Disorder" and "50 Tips on the Management of Adult Attention Deficit Disorder," among many others. An excellent overview of the diagnosis and treatment of ADHD, titled "Attention-Deficit Hyperactivity Disorder," is available on the website of the National Institute of Mental Health (*https://www.nimh.nih.gov/health/topics/attention-deficit-hyperactivity-disorder-adhd/*). Understandably, parents will look for information on the Internet, and there is a great deal of sensational misinformation out there. Therapists can provide an important service to families by helping them locate high-quality, accurate information.

Medication to treat ADHD should generally be used in concert with behavioral, psychological, and educational interventions and support for the child and family. Medication alone is usually not sufficient. The mainstay of medication treatment continues to be the psychostimulants, such as methylphenidate (trade name Ritalin), dextroamphetamine (trade name Dexedrine), and amphetamine–dextroamphetamine (trade name Adderall).

While psychostimulants can produce notable improvement in symptoms of ADHD, it is important that parents understand that psychostimulants strengthen focused attention and reduce distractibility when given to anyone, regardless of whether they have ADHD. The fact that a child's performance improves with medication does not confirm that ADHD exists. Improvement in focused attention is a universal effect of psychostimulants for either normal individuals or those with diagnosable ADHD, evidenced by the benefit college students report from illicit use of amphetamines during all-night term paper writing sessions or studying for exams. Long-distance truck drivers and airplane pilots both utilize psychostimulants to strengthen vigilant attention when fatigued. A child presenting behavioral problems or poor academic performance still needs a comprehensive diagnostic assessment before being given a trial of psychostimulants.

Psychostimulants are dopamine reuptake inhibitors, bearing kinship with the mechanisms through which SSRIs and norepinephrine reuptake inhibitors ameliorate anxiety and depression. The brain's dopamine system governs the level of activation of the prefrontal cortex. The prefrontal cortex provides the neural infrastructure for executive functions—focusing attention, organizing, prioritizing, conducting multistep problem solving. By moderately increasing activation of the prefrontal cortex, psychostimulant medications can improve a person's capacity for focusing attention on one task while screening out competing distractions. This focusing-in and screening-out can also reduce hyperactivity that is caused by a child constantly alerting to every new event in the environment, rather than staying on task and ignoring competing stimuli.

All psychostimulant medications work through the same mechanism in their effects upon the brain. However, the brands of both tradename and generic psychostimulants have proliferated due to efforts to sustain a therapeutic blood level evenly over the course of a school day. For example, both methylphenidate (trade name Ritalin and others) and generic dextroamphetamine salts (trade name Adderall) are absorbed quickly when swallowed, then show a gradual decline from their peak blood levels. Moreover, the disappearance of the psychostimulant after 4 hours can be followed by a rebound period of hyperactivity, irritability, and distractibility. This combination is intolerable in school classes at the end of the day and sometimes a nightmare for parents receiving an agitated child home after school. Thus, methyphenidate and dextroamphetamine typically require a second dose at lunchtime to stretch effectiveness into the after-school period. Unfortunately, this introduces a new set of social problems around parents sending an FDA-controlled medication to school for teachers to administer: It can subject a child to stigmatization and social exclusion when labeled as "crazy" by class-mates for needing to take a medication.

This compilation of problems has led to different strategies so that a psychostimulant can be personally tailored to a child's unique metabo-lism and behavioral needs. Thus, long-acting formulations were devel-oped so that the medication would be slowly released over the course of a day (trade names Ritalin-SR and Adderall-ER), extending effective duration to 4–6 hours, which is an improvement but still too short for a school day. More recently, sustained-release methylphenidate prepara-tions have been developed that release their medication in two pulses, one immediately, then the remainder slowly, providing an effective 8-hour duration (trade names Ritalin-LA and Metadate-CD). A more sophis-ticated medication (trade name Concerta) utilizes an osmotic pump to slowly release methyphenidate for an effective duration of 12 hours. Generic methylphenidate is a mix of two **isomers,** dextro- and levometh-ylphenidate. Some children seem to respond better to the dextromethy-phenidate alone (trade name Focalin). A mix of dextro- and levoamphet-amine salts (trade name Adderall) is available in both immediate-release and slow-release forms with the same indications, target symptoms, and side effects as methyphenidate. Both methylphenidate and amphetamine salts can contribute to insomnia, appetite loss, irritability, and head-aches as side effects.

It is not necessary for a therapist to have facility with the array of available psychostimulants. However, a therapist can help parents under-stand why their child has a problem, how psychostimulants work, and what therapeutic effects and side effects to monitor. Parents often need to understand that beneficial effects of psychostimulants are limited to improved focus of attention, diminished distractibility, and, sometimes, reduced hyperactivity. They may not correct other academic or behav-ioral problems that require different strategies.

Occasionally, the norepinephrine reuptake inhibitor pemoline (trade name Cylert) is used when a child fails to respond adequately to psychostimulants. It rarely can produce liver damage so requires peri-odic blood tests. The antidepressant bupropion (trade name Wellbutrin) is also sometimes used for children with ADHD, particularly if they also have depression and/or conduct disorder, and bupropion is often the first medication tried in the treatment of ADHD in adolescents and adults. Occasionally, modafinil (trade name Pro-Vigil) is added to an ADHD regimen. Modafanil produces wakefulness but is not a stimulant for the cardiovascular and other body systems. It has few side effects but usu-ally limited effectiveness for ADHD.

While the physician will entirely govern medication selection and monitoring of laboratory tests when psychostimulants are used, the physician has no direct feedback from the child's natural world of school, play, and home life. A therapist plays a vital role in organizing feedback from teachers, parents, and child so that the physician has accurate information about reduction in symptoms and any appearance of side effects. Growth suppression or weight loss are specific side effects to watch for, and some children may experience nervousness, gastrointestinal disturbances, or insomnia. Occasionally, a stimulant is prescribed for a child whom the physician (and perhaps even the parents) did not realize had motor tics, vocal tics, or Tourette's syndrome (the combination of multiple motor tics and vocal tics).

CASE ILLUSTRATION: MICHAEL, ADHD

Mrs. S. made an appointment with her son Michael's pediatrician, Dr. K. During a parent–teacher meeting, Michael's teacher had suggested that Michael have some type of physical and/or academic evaluation. Michael was in fourth grade, a bright boy, a good reader, and a good athlete. Whereas his academic testing showed him to have been above average in the first three grades, Michael now seemed to be struggling with handwriting and punctuation. His writing was not legible, and his papers were messy. Mrs. S. was surprised at the request because the only problems Michael ever had at school were on the playground. He often had trouble with anger and impulsive behaviors during recess. In contrast, in the classroom, Michael seemed spaced out. Michael's teacher, Ms. E., wondered if Michael had some sort of physical limitation that made good handwriting difficult.

Beginning Collaboration

Dr. K. performed a physical examination of Michael but, more importantly, carefully listened to Mrs. S.'s concerns. He gave her a form for the teacher to complete. Dr. K. asked Mrs. S. to talk to the psychologist who works in his office. Although Mrs. S. did not believe that Michael had emotional or learning problems warranting a meeting with a psychologist, she nevertheless consented.

During the meeting with the psychologist, Dr. W., Mr. and Mrs. S. carefully reviewed Michael's physical, social, and academic history. Dr. W. asked Mr. and Mrs. S. if they were willing to consider having Michael tested for learning issues and possibly emotional issues. Again, Michael's parents reluctantly agreed.

Dr. W. tested Michael for intelligence, visual motor skills, academic achievement, and emotional issues. Based on the test results and

Michael's history, Dr. W. and Dr. K. told Mr. and Mrs. S. that Michael had ADHD—inattentive type. They were surprised to hear this finding since Michael had never been "hyper." Dr. K. and Dr. W. scheduled a joint appointment with Mr. and Mrs. S. to go over their questions and concerns.

During the meeting, Dr. K. and Dr. W. focused on the many strengths that Michael displayed during the testing. They recommended several books on ADHD. Dr. W. offered to talk to Michael's teacher and wrote a summary of specific recommendations for Michael that could be given to his teacher. Michael participated in part of the meeting and was given the chance to ask questions and state his perspective. Dr. K. and Dr. W. summarized aids that might help Michael with both his emotional regulation on the playground and his learning challenges in the classroom. Dr. K. gave Mr. and Mrs. S. some information on medications used to treat ADHD and summarized the existing knowledge about both the benefits and the risks of medications. Mr. and Mrs. S. decided to go home and talk over their decisions, and they agreed to meet with Dr. W. the following week to implement a plan.

Ongoing Collaboration

At the meeting the following week, Michael and Mr. and Mrs. S. told Dr. W. that they wanted to try both medication and a learning coach. They also wanted Dr. W. to talk to Ms. E., Michael's teacher. They had many questions and asked Dr. W. if they could return for further follow-up meetings over the coming months. Dr. W. agreed and told them that she and Dr. K. would be working together to monitor Michael's response to both the medications and the behavioral treatments.

As with other patient populations, collaborative practice is essential to the care of children, regardless of the disorder. It is important for the therapist to realize that the scope of the collaborative effort is often expansive, encompassing school staff, pediatricians, and others, and therefore can be more challenging.

Many factors beyond the child's diagnosis influence medication decisions for children. The culture of the clinic where the child is seen in terms of the staff's preference for prescribing psychotropic medications and parents' opinions can be important influences. The availability of therapy and the exhaustion level of the parents and the provider can also influence prescribing trends. Evidence suggests that children in low-income families or foster care get more psychotropic medications than other children, especially for behavior disorders (*The Economist*, 2018).

Vigilance is necessary to ensure that children are afforded appropriate diagnostic assessments and safe treatment regimens. For example, we have witnessed a child being given a stimulant that suppressed hunger at the same time he was in an intensive eating disorder program. Children with behavior challenges can be overmedicated to prevent their behavior from disrupting the people around them. Instead of utilizing behavior management interventions, children can be at risk for polypharmacy that prescribes multiple medications, then additional medications to treat side effects of the initial medications. Children can be given too many medications or be prescribed medication for the convenience of the adults in their lives, while other children who might benefit from medication may not have it available. Further, dilemmas exist about informed consent and age of consent for children who are taking medications.

OLDER ADULTS

Just as midlife brings a new awareness of losses in life, older adults have many ongoing losses, and they may develop major depression. Older patients will develop medical problems, and some of these may mimic symptoms of mental illness. For example, thyroid disease and vitamin B_{12} deficiency are great mimickers of mental illness. The only way to discover them is by medical examination and laboratory testing. Patients who develop psychosis for the first time in their senior years should always be presumed to have a general medical condition or a neurological disorder that explains the psychotic symptoms, until proven otherwise. They should be referred to their physician immediately. Patients may develop neurological problems, and they may become aware of the development of cognitive decline. Older adults will also go through the grief of losing parents, spouses, and many others to whom they have been very close, leading to episodes of bereavement that may run together. The challenge for the patient and the therapist is to discern what is normal developmental and life-phase psychotherapeutic work, and what represents a biological illness that will affect longevity if not treated. Therapists should be sure that all older patients have had a thorough medical evaluation, *and the physician has been informed about the psychiatric target symptoms,* before embarking on therapy. Major depression is an important cause of morbidity in older adults, and studies have shown that untreated depression increases the vulnerability to heart attacks and the probability of dying in the first 6 months after the attack (Frasure-Smith, Lesperance, & Talajic, 1993). Furthermore, studies have demonstrated the safety of antidepressant medication in the time immediately after a heart attack

(Glassman et al., 2002). In addition to the interaction between general medical conditions and depression, seniors are more vulnerable to suicide than many younger depressed patients. Older adults represent about 12% of our population but about 25% of completed suicides. One of the highest risk profiles for successful suicide is an older White or Asian male, widowed, who lives alone, drinks alcohol, has recently developed a serious medical illness, and has a loaded gun in the house. This profile is not rare, and the therapist should be aware of indications for referral of an elderly depressed patient to a doctor with experience in geriatric psychiatry.

If medications are used to treat any disorder in older adults, mental illness or otherwise, there are a few general principles to keep in mind. First, as we age, our ability to metabolize drugs and clear them from our body decreases; that is, the liver and kidneys have gradually diminishing capacity to clear the drugs. Doses of medication that are acceptable in a young adult may be too high for an older patient, and when a starting dose is adjusted upward, the older person will be more sensitive to it and may react to the change more acutely. From this comes the clinical adage: "Start low, go slow." For example, the typical adult dose of the antidepressant paroxetine is 20 mg daily. In an older person, the fully effective dose may turn out to be 10 mg daily, and we might initiate therapy by prescribing the 10 mg tablet and advising the patient to take half a tablet (5 mg) a day to start.

Second, it takes longer to see a therapeutic effect in an older person than in a younger one. Typically, we assume 2–4 weeks of antidepressant medication may be required to see initial antidepressant efficacy in an adult with straightforward major depression. In older adults, 2–3 months may be required before we think that the treatment is clearly not working. The therapist can help the patient understand that it takes longer to see a response and can provide support for the patient to continue medication long enough.

Third, most older adults are taking medications for various general medical conditions, and all psychotropic medications have multiple drug–drug interaction. Some interactions are potentially very serious. The therapist can be helpful in reminding patients to inform their prescribing physicians about *all* of the medications that they take, including OTC (nonprescription) medications and any herbal remedies. Today's mobile phones readily manage drug information through programs, such as Epocrates, that include the ability to check up to 30 simultaneous medications (including herbals) for adverse drug–drug interactions. Most physicians today use these programs, which protect patients from serious consequences *if* they tell their physicians what they take.

Fourth, the side effects of certain psychotropic medications are more worrisome in older patients than in younger patients. For example, the anticholinergic side effects of tricyclic antidepressants can cause cardiac problems, urinary retention, and constipation much more easily in older patients, and the consequences are much more serious. The widespread (and often inappropriate) use of the tricyclic antidepressant amitriptyline is a prominent cause of anticholinergic delirium in older adults and a leading cause of drug-related falls and hip fractures. Now that we have excellent alternatives, amitriptyline is generally contraindicated in older patients.

Bupropion is often regarded as the antidepressant of choice for older patients because it has no cardiovascular or anticholinergic side effects and few drug–drug interactions. SSRI antidepressants as a class are generally well tolerated by older patients.

The benzodiazepines are often used for the treatment of anxiety disorders and for short-term management of insomnia. Different benzodiazepines have different half-lives, and some have **active metabolites** (the metabolic byproducts of the original drug, which are also clinically active compounds in the blood). The best choice is a medication with a relatively short half-life and no active metabolites, especially if the patient (of any age) has liver disease because the liver metabolizes the benzodiazepines. Lorazepam (trade name Ativan) and oxazepam (trade name Serax) have no active metabolites and have comparatively shorter half-lives; hence, they are good choices for older patients. If an older person takes a benzodiazepine, the starting dose usually should be approximately half of the typical adult starting dose. Benzodiazepines least preferred for older adults because of their long half-lives and active metabolites are diazepam (trade name Valium), chlordiazepoxide (trade name Librium), and clonazepam (trade name Klonopin). The problem is that the half-lives of these benzodiazepines, together with their active metabolites, are over 24 hours. If the patient takes these benzodiazepines on a daily basis, the blood levels continue to climb progressively because the drug is more than half-present in the blood when the patient takes the next dose. This leads to risks for falls.

The choice of psychotropic medication is also shaped by one's coincident general medical conditions, and older adults almost always have at least one additional medical problem. For example, depression and anxiety symptoms occur in more than a third of patients with Parkinson's disease (Shulman, Taback, Bean, & Winer, 2001). Antidepressant treatment is often needed, but antidepressants that are anticholinergic, such as tricyclic antidepressants, can both improve motor symptoms and worsen memory problems, requiring finesse in the dosing. As many as 40% of Parkinson's patients experience some degree of psychotic symptoms—hallucinations, delusional thinking, or the sense of a presence. However, most antipsychotic medications worsen parkinsonian motor symptoms, with quetiapine (trade name Seroquel) usually the best choice (Hasnain et al., 2009). Older patients, particularly those with some cognitive impairment, are vulnerable to confusion and memory impairment from benzodiazepines. Falls and hip fractures have been correlated with benzodiazepines, which can impair sense of balance.

WOMEN'S HEALTH AND PSYCHOPHARMACOLOGY

Premenstrual dysphoric disorder (PMDD) is a depressive disorder that affects 1.8–5.8% of women who menstruate (Raffi & Freeman, 2017). The late luteal phase of the menstrual cycle, particularly the week before menstruation begins, is the most vulnerable period. While there can be genetic factors, decreased levels of a metabolite of progesterone (ALLO) during the luteal phase is associated with symptoms. SSRI antidepressants are effective treatment for the irritability, anxiety, and mood symptoms of premenstrual dysphoric disorder, often more quickly than for treatment of major depressive disorder. The MGH Center for Women's Mental Health at *https://womensmentalhealth.org* can provide valuable information for patients with PMDD.

Approximately 20% of women suffer from a mood or anxiety disorder during pregnancy (MGH Center for Women's Mental Health, n.d.). Women who are vulnerable to major depression are especially likely to experience it during their pregnancy and/or postpartum period. For women already taking an antidepressant medication who become pregnant and discontinue the medication, they are five times as likely to relapse compared to those who continue maintenance antidepressant treatment (*https://womensmentalhealth.org*, 2020). Yet many physicians avoid prescribing medications to pregnant women unless absolutely necessary.

These considerations cover three pregnancy-related topics—preterm teratogenic effects of psychotropic medications upon the fetus, breastfeeding and psychotropic medications, and postpartum depression or psychosis. Regarding **teratogenic effects,** or potential for the medication to cause physical deformity in the infant, the medication must be taken during organogenesis (first 3 months), and therefore delay until after the first 3 months of pregnancy is preferred. Regarding the potential toxic effects at the time of birth, including withdrawal syndromes in the infant, the medication must be taken at or near time of delivery for this to occur. Regarding potential behavioral teratogenicity, the long-term effect of the medication on the functioning and behavior of the child many years later is an unknown factor for most medications used today, but no harm in this area is known for the antidepressants commonly prescribed.

Studies have found that women who were given SSRIs during their pregnancy had no increase in fetal malformations, no increase in prematurity, no increase in miscarriage or stillbirths, and no difference in birth weight of the infants, compared to control women who were not given antidepressants (Kulin et al., 1998). Given some of the potential consequences of untreated major depression in the pregnant woman—such as suicide; poor compliance with prenatal care; poor nutrition; sleep problems; increased risk of drug, alcohol, and tobacco use; and the unknown impact of depression on fetal development—the decision to use medication to treat depression in pregnancy, and if so, with which medication, is a complex decision that should be made by each patient and her physician. In this regard, clinicians will find it useful to consult the joint statement produced by the American Psychiatric Association and the American College of Obstetricians and Gynecologists on the management of depression during pregnancy (Yonkers et al., 2009). Whatever is decided, the patient will almost always be advised to continue with psychotherapy; the therapist can monitor the severity of the woman's symptoms and the risk for suicide or behaviors that put the developing baby at risk, as well as alert the physician to the possible need for hospitalization if the pregnant woman's mental health worsens. If a pregnant woman is critically ill with major depression to the extent that her life and her baby's life are at risk, ECT is sometimes safely used in severely ill patients, especially those who continue to be at imminent risk of suicide even while hospitalized.

A majority of women have "baby blues," or transient periods of sadness in the week or two after delivery, and this requires no treatment; the kind support of those whom she loves and trusts is all that is needed. But approximately 10–20% of women will experience postpartum depression, and 0.2% will develop postpartum psychosis. Women who develop postpartum psychosis may be at risk of harming their infants and/or themselves, and deaths of infants and mothers have occurred. Because of these serious potential outcomes, treatment of postpartum mood disorders is recommended, and women may wish to utilize multiple modalities of therapy, including psychotherapy and medication.

Early studies of SSRI use during breastfeeding discouraged mothers from breastfeeding their infants while taking these medications (Baum & Misri, 1996). However, more recent studies on sertraline, for example, showed that very little medication was found in the infant's blood after breastfeeding from a mother taking sertraline, and the tool used to measure the clinical activity of the drug (platelet serotonin levels) showed little to no activity in those infants (Epperson et al., 2001). Nevertheless, the new mother will probably be reluctant to expose her infant to any medication, and she will need support from the therapist for the decision that she and her physician decide upon.

The last women's mental health issue discussed here is menopause. Only a few years ago, women thought that taking **hormone replacement therapy (HRT)** was necessary to prevent every aspect of aging, and the belief that HRT warded off depression in the fifth decade and beyond was just one more element in its assumed panacea. More recent studies have suggested that HRT does not protect against heart disease and dementia, and it does increase the risk for stroke and for certain cancers (Writing Group for the Women's Health Initiative Investigators, 2002). It is unlikely that HRT will provide protection against mental illness, nor does the onset of menopause cause mental illness. Menopause occurs in most women between the ages of 45 and 55, and that age may also be the beginning of losses in a woman's life: childbearing potential; adult children leaving home; parents aging and dying; and one's own aging, bringing with it an altered self-image and an increased awareness of one's own mortality. All of these adult developmental or life-phase issues are very important, and a woman may benefit from psychotherapy at this time if she has symptoms sufficient to cause distress. However, the menopause itself does not cause mental illness or predispose to it, and it is not an indication, in and of itself, for medication.

CONCLUSION

Each of these populations has become its own mental health subspecialty with therapeutic practices that are increasingly evidence based by clinical research. Each population is diverse, which adds complexities to both assessment and interventions for specific patients. This chapter is an overview that should be expanded through further reading of the listed references.

PART III

CREATIVE COLLABORATION

The previous section provides a foundation in the content of psycho-pharmacology and a basic overview of how medications work for a variety of presenting problems and populations.

As most therapists know, a single intervention such as suggesting a medication consultation is only part of the therapeutic process. It is equally, if not more, important to understand how to talk with your patients about medication, how to engage and collaborate with the medical professionals who prescribe your patients' medication, and how to support your patients and their family members after your patient has started medication. We review these process issues in the following chapters.

Patients who need psychotropic medications must have *access* to medical care, and their medications need to be *affordable*. Under many insurance programs, prescription drugs are poorly reimbursed. Medication costs are usually not reimbursed at the same rate as medical procedures, and out-of-pocket costs for medications can be expensive. Thus, a patient might agree to try medication, but when he goes to fill the prescription, decide the cost is beyond his budget—especially if he anticipates refills over many months. So, he simply does not fill the prescription.

In other cases, he fills the prescription, does not feel better after a day or two, or begins to feel negative side effects like dry mouth or poor sexual functioning, and simply stops the medication. No one explained to him that many psychotropic medications take longer than, say, an aspirin or antibiotics, to create positive effects. The patient needs *education and an explanation* about his new medications and needs to know what he might experience. Then he needs to *give consent* to do a trial of a psychotropic medication. Ideally, patients need to be *given the correct medication at the correct dose* for their specific syndrome. Sometimes it takes a few changes to find the best medication and dose.

At times, we've seen cases where the prescriber started a patient on a low dose of a psychotropic medication, but failed to schedule follow-up visits to adjust the dose. Thus, an elderly patient with major depressive disorder who was prescribed a subtherapeutic dose simply gave up and went back to bed after reluctantly seeing her physician one time at the behest of her worried daughter. *Monitoring* is also a critical part of the process for medications to work.

When our patients are taking medication, our ideal goal is to form a multidisciplinary health care team that will work collaboratively with each other, the patient, and the patient's family members. Forming this kind of team is easiest when the professionals are working in the same location. However, we recognize that most therapists do not work in settings that include primary care physicians and psychiatrists. When professionals who care for the same patient work in distant locations, it is often incumbent on the therapist to build the professional relationships and communication system to foster collaboration. The time spent trying to communicate with other distant professionals can sometimes feel like an added burden with little payoff. We hope you will persevere through apparent inequities and continue to reach out to the professionals who are working with your patients and the family members who care for them. As time passes, you will develop a list of excellent referral sources and, we hope, establish some meaningful professional relationships simultaneously.

CHAPTER 11

The Therapeutic Relationship

B., age 65, and his wife, age 66, have been seeing Dr. G., a therapist, for several weeks. Although their marital relationship has been improving, evidenced by better communication and increased intimacy, Mrs. B. continues to worry about Mr. B.'s depressive symptoms, including hypersomnia, little interest in interacting with friends and family, and "grumpiness." When Dr. G. asks Mr. B. for his perspective on Mrs. B.'s concerns, Mr. B. echoes her concerns but explains that he is "used to feeling down and tired." He says that the biggest drawback to feeling down is that he sometimes doesn't feel like spending time with his grandkids. He likes being a grandfather but gets easily irritated when in a bad mood. When Dr. G. asks Mr. B. if he has ever taken medication for these symptoms, Mr. B. says he hasn't given it much thought. Mrs. B. interjects and says, "He doesn't think it would be the manly thing to do." Mr. B. shrugs his shoulders and says, "My dad went through the same stuff and tried to grin and bear it. He worked hard, put food on the table, and would never consider getting any help. I guess I'm using his approach, except he would roll over in his grave if he knew I was seeing a shrink." Between sessions, Dr. G. considers the next steps for addressing Mr. B.'s depressive symptoms.

Mr. and Mrs. B. along with Dr. G. have several options. They can simply continue conjoint therapy and hope that Mr. B.'s depressive symptoms will ameliorate. Mr. B. could be referred for individual therapy for depression, he could be referred for a medication evaluation for his depressive symptoms, or referrals could be made for both treatments. How should they decide which path to take?

HELP FROM EVIDENCE-BASED PRACTICE PRINCIPLES

Principles of evidence-based practice (EBP) can help guide the decision-making process that Dr. G. faces (Patterson, Miller, Carnes, & Wilson, 2004; Williams et al., 2014). EBP is the integration of the *best research evidence* with *clinical expertise* and *patient values* (Sackett, Straus, Richardson, Rosenberg, & Haynes, 2000). In recent years, an expanded definition also includes *the environmental and organizational context* as well (Council for Training in Evidence-Based Behavioral Practice, 2008). Dr. G.'s decision-making process and recommendation is guided by what is already known about depression in older adults based on research. But personal factors such as the patients' preferences, the therapist's experience, and the clinical setting, including available resources, are also forces influencing the decision. A therapist can go through the following steps to make a decision about a medication referral:

1. Identify a common, shared definition of the treatment goals for trying medication, by summarizing the target symptoms and deciding treatment priorities.
2. Offer an initial realistic appraisal of what might be accomplished by using medications and what cannot be accomplished.
3. Remind the patient of additional treatment options—the pluses and minuses of each option based on the scholarly literature and the therapist's professional experiences.
4. Lead a discussion about the best path to take. Give recommendations and explain the reasoning behind each recommendation. If appropriate, make sure each family member can give his or her opinion.
5. Let all stakeholders participate in **shared decision making.** Reach a consensus on the treatment plan. Often this process evolves over several meetings and seldom happens in a neat, stepwise progression (Williams et al., 2014).

Usually a therapist is not making a decision about using or not using medication. He is deciding only whether to make a referral. The therapist leaves the decision to the client and psychopharmacologist. In other situations, the patient may already be taking medications when she comes for her initial therapy session. Perhaps the therapist's physician colleague is referring his patient for therapy after already starting his patient on medication. In many of these situations, the therapist may be interested in learning more. He wants to do **critical appraisal** of the treatment possibilities based on findings in the scholarly literature. What is the standard of care for the problem or diagnosis? What is known about different treatment options?

In these situations, the therapist may want quick information about a specific problem or diagnosis. She wants to give her patients the most current information possible but she has limited time to search for information. For a quick summary, the therapist might turn to **systematic reviews,** such as the summary article by Cipriani and colleagues about how well 21 antidepressants work for acute treatment of depression in adults (Cipriani et al., 2018), or **practice guidelines.** Table 11.1 includes a list of databases that you could search for general questions. Some of these sources are paid subscriptions and some simply summarize the literature, while others give specific recommendations. Once you are familiar with these sites, you can quickly research a treatment question.

SHARED DECISION MAKING

There are many reasons that a therapist or patient will consider a medication evaluation (see Table 11.2). Even when one or more indicators are present, therapists at all levels of experience know that getting a patient on the path toward a medication evaluation is not always easy. A patient's decision to follow through with a referral for a medication evaluation may be a gradual process rather than a single event.

Some researchers have used the transtheoretical model of behavioral change (TTM; Prochaska, DiClemente, & Norcross, 1995) to look at this decision process (see Table 11.3). The authors of the TTM suggest that change is a process that occurs over time. Instead of viewing patients' reluctance or unwillingness to try something new as "resistance" or "noncompliance," their responses are viewed along a continuum of change. Most people weigh the odds of creating change for some time before they actually begin the behaviors necessary to initiate it. Then, once they make the necessary behavioral changes (e.g., exercise, stop smoking, and eat a healthy diet), they probably won't maintain these changes the first time, or even the first several times, they try. Smokers, for example, usually stop several times (and start smoking again) before they finally stop completely, and over half of the people who start a psychotropic medication do not keep using it or do not follow the directions.

Prochaska et al. (1995) defined readiness as the patient's willingness to (1) work with the health care provider to decide if medication is a good treatment choice; (2) discuss any concerns he or she has about taking the medication with the physician; and (3) contact the physician

TABLE 11.1. Databases to Inform Treatment Decisions (Alphabetical)

Agency for Healthcare Research and Quality's Healthcare Cost and Utilization Project

http://hcupnet.ahrq.gov

AHRQ is a federal agency that advances EBP in a number of ways. One of its functions is to support the Healthcare Cost and Utilization Project (HCUP), a free database of health statistics.

Agency for Healthcare Research and Quality's National Guideline Clearinghouse
http://guideline.gov/index.aspx

In addition to HCUP, AHRQ also provides free access to the National Guidelines Clearinghouse, a database of treatment guidelines and expert commentaries on various diagnoses.

American Psychiatric Association Practice Guidelines

www.psychiatry.org/psychiatrists/practice/clinical-practice-guidelines

This website includes evidence-based recommendations for the assessment and treatment of adult psychiatric disorders. These guidelines are free and include information for locating child guidelines.

American Psychological Association Practice Guidelines

www.apa.org/practice/guidelines/index

This website includes several topics that each come with an overview of the literature as well as treatment recommendations. These guidelines are free and do not require membership.

California Evidence-Based Clearinghouse for Child Welfare

www.cebc4cw.org

This website describes a variety of programs aimed at promoting child welfare in different areas, including treating mental illness. In addition to describing each program, the site rates the level of research support for each program. Access to this website is free.

Campbell Collaboration

www.campbellcollaboration.org

The Campbell Collaboration publishes systematic reviews in the areas of education, crime and justice, and social welfare. Access to this website is free.

Center for Evidence-Based Medicine

https://ebm-tools.knowledgetranslation.net

This website serves as a guide for those seeking evidence. It includes educational tools, such as glossaries and search guides, for those that are new to evidence-based medicine. It also includes a list of evidence-based resources. Access to this website is free.

(continued)

TABLE 11.1. *(continued)*

Cochrane Database of Systematic Reviews

www.cochranelibrary.com

The Cochrane Collaboration is a group of providers, patients, advocates, and policy makers. One of the functions of this group is to publish Cochrane Reviews, which are systematic reviews of medical literature. Some people are eligible for free access to these reviews while others need to pay for access. Check the website to see if you are eligible for free access.

EBSCOhost

http://search.ebscohost.com

EBSCOhost is a system that includes access to several different databases, resulting in the ability to cast a broader search that includes several different types of sources. Access to EBSCOhost requires a paid subscription.

Embase

www.embase.com

Embase is a database that includes all of Medline as well as several other sources. It covers biomedical peer-reviewed journals as well as conferences and articles in press. Embase requires a paid subscription.

Evidence-Based Mental Health

http://ebmh.bmj.com

This is a journal that includes the key details from articles published in a wide variety of other biomedical journals. Access to this journal requires a paid subscription.

HighWire

www.highwirepress.com

HighWire is a database hosted by Stanford University that contains publications from journals in medicine, science, and social science. Searching the database is free, and includes links to free full-text for some articles depending upon the journal from which they come.

Medline

www.nlm.nih.gov/medline/index.html

Medline is a database from the U.S. National Library of Medicine containing publications from over 5,600 different journals. Searching the database is free, but most full-text articles require a fee to access.

PsycINFO

www.apa.org/pubs/databases/psycinfo

PsycINFO is the American Psychological Association's database of peer-reviewed articles, books, and dissertations. Searching PsycINFO requires a paid subscription.

(continued)

TABLE 11.1. *(continued)*

PubMed

https://pubmed.ncbi.nlm.nih.gov

PubMed is a database from the U.S. National Library of Medicine that includes all of MedLine as well as some other journals. Searching the database is free and includes links to free full-text articles for some articles depending on which journal they come from.

TRIP

www.tripdatabase.com

This is a database that includes several journals and allows clinicians to locate high-quality research quickly. Searching TRIP is free, but not all of the articles are available in full text for free.

UpToDate

www.wolterskluwer.com/en/solutions/uptodate

UpToDate is a database of literature reviews written by experts in various fields. Full access requires a paid subscription.

Note. From Williams, Patterson, and Edwards (2014). Copyright © 2014 The Guilford Press. Reprinted by permission.

TABLE 11.2. Indications for Referral for Psychotropic Medication Evaluation

- The patient has a serious illness, such as schizophrenia, bipolar disorder, any psychosis, delusions, hallucinations, or any mental illness with suicidal ideation and/or serious impairment of daily life activities.
- The patient has physical symptoms and behaviors suggestive of medical and psychiatric disorders, such as fatigue, concentration and cognitive difficulties, confusion, memory impairment, sleep and appetite disturbance, panic attacks, and ritualistic behaviors.
- The patient is not getting better or perhaps is getting worse, in spite of therapy.
- There is a marked lability in mood or behavior.
- There is a question about diagnosis.
- There is comorbid substance abuse disorder or other multiple conditions.
- There are prominent physical symptoms.
- There is a family history or previous patient history of serious mental illness.
- The patient or family requests consultation.
- A psychopharmacology question arises.
- A second opinion may help the patient to accept diagnosis and comply with psychotherapy and medication treatment.
- It has been a long time since the person has had a medical examination.

TABLE 11.3. Stages of Change

Precontemplation:	No intention to take action in the foreseeable future
Contemplation:	Intention to change in the next 6 months
Preparation:	Intention and plan to change in the next month
Action:	Specific, overt modifications made in the last 6 months
Maintenance:	Working to prevent relapse

Note. Data from *https://sphweb.bumc.bu.edu/otlt/mph-modules/sb/ behavioralchangetheories/behavioralchangetheories6.html.*

if he or she has difficulty in taking the medication. Often, patients are initially only willing to *consider* taking psychotropic medication, not actually to start taking it. A patient's decision to start medication is usually a gradual process. It might begin when the physician mentions the possibility. During the next session, the therapist may offer some reading material or Internet sites for the patient to learn more. Finally, several weeks later, the patient may actually decide to start the medication. Again, this ambivalence is not uncommon. In fact, it is a great opportunity for therapists to continue building the therapeutic relationship with patients and family members as they take the time they need to make a decision. It is generally better to wait for patients to think through their options rather than rush to a premature decision. In fact, it is not uncommon to have patients initially refuse medication and later bring up the possibility of a medication trial.

Of course, waiting for patients to make their own decisions does not mean that the therapist or physician cannot voice an opinion. If the therapist knows that evidence-based literature suggests that the patient's problem is best treated with medication (i.e., bipolar disorder or OCD), that information should be given to patients and their families. Sometimes a simple explanation about how the brain and neurotransmitters work will alleviate the patient's fears. Keeping in mind scope-of-practice issues, the therapist can explain that depression is not about mental weakness or character flaws but often simply the brain's need for more serotonin. Not all patients are interested in biological explanations. But for those who are, a simple explanation and perhaps a drawing of the brain can allay patients' unstated fears.

Patients should have all the necessary information they need to make an informed decision. Family and friends will also influence a patient's initial decision about trying medication, as well as a patient's willingness to comply with the treatment regimen. Therapists should welcome questions from other people in the patient's life. When a question arises that is not within the therapist's scope of practice or knowledge, he or she should help the patient find a physician who can answer the question. Some patients want to do their own research and should be encouraged to do an Internet search, for example.

When a therapist believes a patient would benefit from a medication evaluation, it is not uncommon for the therapist to worry about how the patient will respond to the suggestion. Common responses or beliefs can include such statements as "Even my therapist thinks I'm crazy," "My therapist is going to abandon me," or, as in Mr. B.'s case, "My therapist thinks I'm too weak to handle this problem on my own." Other, more positive responses could be a sense of relief (because the therapy alone has not resulted in enough improvement) or an inference of care and concern from the therapist (because he or she is considering every option available). If a family member or friend suggests medication, that suggestion could have many meanings for the patient. It may feel like a form of control or feel demeaning.

Perhaps a physician started a patient on medication and simultaneously sent the patient to a therapist. In these situations, the patient can view therapy as the requirement to receive the psychotropic medication. Regardless of who suggested medication, it is important to understand the meaning the patient attaches to the suggestion. The following questions are helpful when medication is being considered.

At what point in therapy was the idea of medication first discussed? If the patient is already on medication at the first visit, starts medication shortly after the first visit, or starts medication mid-therapy, the significance to the patient of the medication may vary. For example, if medication begins mid-therapy, the patient may believe that medication is being tried because psychotherapy is not working. If the therapy begins at the same time the medication is started, the patient may credit any positive changes to only the medication or only the therapy.

Has the patient ever been on a psychotropic medication before? What are his or her attitudes about those experiences? Have any family members or friends ever been on psychotropic medications? If so, what medications did they take? What are the patient's views about those experiences? How educated is the patient? How much information does the patient want about the effects—good and bad—of psychotropic medications? It is important to inquire about any previous experiences the patient has had with psychotropic medications because these experiences will influence the initial response and attitude about taking medication. Previous experiences may include the patient's own personal treatment, another person's treatment, or something that the patient read or heard about on the Internet.

Stigma, embarrassment, fear, or shame may influence the patient's views about taking psychotropic medications. Some clients seek therapy but would never take psychotropic medications because they do not want a "mind-altering drug." We have had patients who have a history of substance abuse refuse psychotropic medications because they fear that the medications will change their brains in destructive ways.

The literature on mental illness and stigma discusses **internalized stigma** (Ritsher, Otilingam, & Grajales, 2003). Internalized stigma often involves feelings of alienation, social withdrawal, and discrimination. Patients who consider taking medication may have negative stereotypes about needing medication. Their self-identity changes and they worry about how others perceive them. We often observe patients initially trying to keep their medication usage a secret. Part of the therapist's job is to sort through the beliefs and fears that her patient has regarding using psychotropic medications.

Dr. Patterson had a patient whose wife vehemently opposed her husband taking medication and suggested that he smoke more marijuana instead. He wanted to try medication but hesitated because he worried about his wife's negative views. Eventually he saw a psychiatrist colleague of Dr. Patterson's, who gave him an antidepressant. His response to the medication was uniformly positive. When he saw Dr. Patterson shortly afterward, he explained that it would be his last therapy session. He went on to explain that both therapy and the medication were helpful, but his insurance covered the medication but not the therapy. So, he was making a financial decision to only pursue the treatment that his insurance covered. Finances and insurance coverage can be critical factors influencing decisions about medication.

Does the patient have insurance to pay for a psychiatric evaluation? Patients' financial coverage for medications and therapies vary greatly. Some policies may cover medications that are included on a formulary, but not other medications. In addition, patients may be willing to pay out-of-pocket for some services but not others. Limits or caps may be placed on medication charges or on the number of psychotherapy sessions allowed. Only certain types of providers may be covered by insurance, that is, only a psychiatrist or only certain types of situations, such as "case management" or "crisis intervention." Some services might require a primary care physician's referral, even when that physician knows very little about the patient or the problem. Finally, the deductible can vary, depending on the insurance policy.

Probably the most challenging situation is to provide care for a patient who has no insurance. This often means that the patient is unemployed, between jobs, or has suffered a catastrophic loss. Many ethical issues are embedded in financial decisions about providing care. One way to address these issues is to find out what resources exist in the community for medically indigent patients. If it becomes financially impossible to continue treating a patient, therapists can still remain advocates and consultants in helping the patient find the best possible care he or she can afford—regardless of whether the therapists are compensated for their time. Some examples of this type of financial advocacy include the following:

- Helping an uninsured patient join a clinical trial of a medication so that the care and medication are free (assuming the clinical trial involves medication and/or other treatments that are clinically correct for the patient).
- Keeping a list and business cards of low-fee clinics available in the community.
- Referring a patient to a clinic that provides services for free as long as possible. In the meantime, the therapist educates the patient about obtaining free or low-cost services in the community.

Regardless of the clinic's or practice's financial structure, therapists need to be sensitive to their patients' financial situations. The changing financial landscape of health care and the inequity in reimbursement between physicians and therapists can make this aspect of care challenging. Nevertheless, such care and concern can greatly enhance both the therapeutic relationship and the success of the therapy as a whole.

CONCLUSION

One of the first things beginning therapists learn is that the therapeutic relationship is the foundation for successful therapy. A decision to start medication can be frightening for patients and their family members, which is why a trusting relationship with a therapist is essential. The therapist is not only adding a component to the treatment plan but also introducing the patient and family to new health care professionals who will make specific treatment recommendations.

CHAPTER 12

Effective Referrals

After the therapist and patient have made the decision to pursue a medication evaluation, it is important to understand the medical culture they are attempting to engage (e.g., psychiatrists vs. family physicians vs. nurse practitioners). They will not just be entering medical culture and departing. They will be inviting other professionals into the treatment system and possibly forming lasting relationships. The following description of medical culture begins with an introduction of the key people and continues in the next chapter with a practical guide for engaging them.

WHO PRESCRIBES MEDICATION FOR PSYCHIATRIC DISORDERS?

In the United States, health care providers are licensed to practice medicine by individual states, and it is physicians who typically prescribe medications. As state laws have changed that regulate scope of practice, some psychologists have gained prescriptive authority if they have completed certain training. Some physician assistants can prescribe certain medications. Family and psychiatric nurse practitioners can prescribe medications without physician oversight in many states. Increasingly, therapists may collaborate with a nurse practitioner, rather than a physician, in the role of primary care provider or psychiatric provider. In the overall category of "physicians," there are allopathic physicians with a doctor of medicine, or MD, degree and osteopathic physicians with a doctor of osteopathy, or DO, degree. Although historically they come from different approaches to the practice of medicine, in this era, both MDs and DOs can provide excellent general health care for patients; they often train together, and they both take specialty training in psychiatry in the same manner. MDs, DOs, and many nurse practitioners can prescribe medications for mental health needs. When consulting with any health care provider, it is helpful to understand how he or she relates to others in the larger world of medicine.

CONSULTING WITH PHYSICIANS IN PRIVATE PRACTICE

In private practice, a physician may be in solo or group practice or work for a large health care organization, a health maintenance organization (HMO), or a government agency such as the health department or a public clinic. Who is consulted will probably depend on the patient's health care insurance coverage (or lack thereof). If the patient has HMO coverage, he or she must see the designated physician in that HMO or the cost of care will not be covered. Often, the patient will need to see his or her primary care physician first, and a referral will be given to a psychiatrist only in the case of severe illness. Especially for HMOs and public clinics, cost containment is an ever-present factor, and many patients will not receive psychiatry consultation.

Some health care coverage arrangements **carve out** mental health care coverage so that patients cannot receive their mental health care in the same place as their primary medical care. They must go to another group practice, clinic, or agency, and that agency is often given **capitated** funding. This means that they are paid a fixed number of dollars per month for each patient enrolled, regardless of how many patients are seen or how often. To survive, such groups or agencies may be understaffed, and patients may have to wait for an initial appointment, be seen at longer than desirable intervals, and be seen for short visits.

Because, historically, mental health care is not funded on a par with general health care, it is no surprise that approximately 75% of the antidepressants prescribed in the United States are prescribed by nonpsychiatric physicians. A therapist may be consulting with a psychiatrist, a primary care physician, a nurse practitioner, and perhaps even a psychologist (depending on the state in which one resides), according to the patient's health care insurance and personal preference. The approach may vary slightly, depending on who is consulted.

PSYCHIATRISTS

A psychiatrist has completed 4 years of residency training after medical school (or 5 years for child and adolescent psychiatry or geriatric psychiatry), and the focus of the training is diagnosis and treatment of all mental disorders, including the most complicated, severely ill patients. The psychiatrist should be board eligible or board certified. Board eligible means the psychiatrist has completed all training in a satisfactory manner and is in the process of registering, taking, and waiting for the results of the two-tier board certification examination process. The fastest time in which a newly graduated psychiatrist can complete this process is approximately 2 years, so it is not unusual to see younger psychiatrists listed as board eligible. A psychiatrist is board certified after both part I and part II of the specialty examination have been passed, and he or she must recertify (take another examination) every 10 years. Board certification is a quality standard that most psychiatrists, and in fact most physicians of every specialty, aspire to.

PRIMARY CARE PHYSICIANS

A pediatrician is a specialist physician who provides health care to children. A pediatric residency training program lasts 3 years, and the pediatrician has had training in childhood development and behavior and in the skills of relating to parents. Most pediatricians are comfortable prescribing medication to children who have ADHD, for example, and some will prescribe antidepressants for children with mild to moderate depression. For more serious illnesses, children and adolescents should be referred to a child and adolescent psychiatrist. It is helpful to start with a referral to the pediatrician or family physician to obtain a general medical evaluation prior to the presumption that the child suffers a mental disorder, as well as to obtain that physician's help in locating a child and adolescent psychiatrist if needed.

An internist is a specialist physician who provides health care to adults. Some internists provide a wide range of primary care, and others limit their practice to metabolic disorders and conditions of organs "between the neck and the navel." The internal medicine residency lasts 3 years and does not require training in psychiatry or behavioral health per se; however, many internal medicine residents seek out such training by elective experiences and additional study. Many internists feel comfortable treating their patients who suffer from mild to moderate depression, but most will refer patients with more serious mental health care needs.

Family physicians who are certified by the American Board of Family Medicine and have graduated from a 3-year family medicine residency training program have completed a required curriculum in psychiatry and behavioral health. Most family physicians feel comfortable prescribing most types of psychotropic medications but will refer patients with severe mental illness to a psychiatrist, at least for initial consultation and management direction.

OTHER HEALTH CARE PROFESSIONALS

The physician assistant (PA) has had some graduate school training and has worked in clinical settings under the supervision of a physician. In most states, the PA is licensed as a practice partner with the supervising physician, and whatever the PA does is regarded by the state as an action of the physician, who is fully responsible for the PA's action. A nurse practitioner (NP) is an advanced-practice nurse who has had graduate school training and supervised practice with either NP faculty or physicians. The states vary concerning the autonomy of the NP's practice, and therapists should be familiar with those regulations if they collaborate with a NP in their practice. The NP and the PA can do an excellent job of primary care and health maintenance for many patients. When there is a question of a general medical condition presenting falsely as a mental illness, either may be able to address this problem; however, it is often preferable to consult a physician, as practitioners vary in their interest and skills in this area.

Registered nurses (RNs) are licensed by the state in which they practice, and they have reached their licensing examination through a 2-year associate degree (community college) program, a diploma nurse (hospital-based, usually 3-year) program, or a college/university-based bachelor of nursing (BSN) degree. After initial licensure as an RN, the nurse may take additional graduate training and specialize in an area, such as certified nurse midwife (CNM), family nurse practitioner (FNP), pediatric nurse practitioner (PNP), or mental health nurse practitioner. A nurse who has completed a doctoral degree, as Doctor of Nursing Practice (DNP), practices with a title of doctor.

The licensed vocational nurse (LVN) or licensed practical nurse (LPN) training varies from state to state, but these nurses have often trained in a community college for less than 2 years or in a professional school for health careers. The medical assistant (MA) has typically

trained 1 year or less in a community college or private training program. The MA usually works in a private doctor's office or clinic and is
considered to be acting as an agent of the physician. The certified nursing assistant (CNA) has often trained for one semester in a community
college or private training program and typically works in a hospital or
extended-care facility under the supervision of licensed nurses.

This rather simplistic overview of the hierarchy of health care practitioners should be helpful to the therapist who calls the private physician's office and hears, "This is Dr. Smith's nurse, may I help you?"
That person may be an NP, RN, LVN, or MA. In many offices, the term
nurse is used broadly. How much you rely on that person's advice may be
shaped by your knowledge of his or her training and experience.

Because health care practitioners have varying credentials, experience, and levels of interest in mental health care, it is critical for the therapist to develop a trusting relationship with nearby medical colleagues.
This is essential to meet the patient's needs, but it is also essential for
the therapist to be taken seriously by the medical professionals. Because
in some states, physicians have been held responsible for the therapist's
actions when they share patients, some physicians are reluctant to collaborate with therapists of any discipline. Finding a supportive and psy-
chologically minded primary care physician or psychiatrist and developing a relationship of mutual trust and respect are paramount in the
care of the therapist's seriously ill patients. Building a relationship with
medical colleagues is addressed in more detail in Chapter 13.

HEALTH CARE TEAMS: AN IDEAL MODEL

The Institute of Medicine, a prestigious group that influences health
policy in the United States, has suggested that primary care teams play
a central role in the future of health care. A health care team usually
involves a group of health care professionals from different disciplines
who are committed to enhanced collaboration, a biopsychosocial model,
and continuity of care. They are also committed to sharing care and
learning from each other. Usually, the best teams deemphasize the traditional health care hierarchy and stress shared learning and respect for
multiple perspectives. We have found that the best treatment teams can
be interesting and even inspirational at times.

In a *Journal of the American Medical Association* article, Grumbach and Bodenhemer (2004) suggest that health care teams need to
earn "true team status by demonstrating teamwork" (p. 1246). The
authors identify five characteristics of strong teams:

1. Clear goals with measurable outcomes
2. Clinical and administrative systems
3. Division of labor
4. Training of all team members
5. Effective communication

The authors also point out that health care teams with greater cohesiveness have better clinical outcomes and higher patient satisfaction. On the other hand, if health care teams do not work, it is usually because of problems with relationships and personalities. Thus, it isn't enough to simply find a health care team to join. Therapists have to find a health care team that works, and it helps if they like and respect the team members. Grumbach and Bodenhemer (2004) note that teams may include "initiators, clarifiers, or encouragers," as well as "dominators, blockers, evaders, and recognition seekers" (pp. 2–3). When therapists are looking for colleagues with which to build collaborative relationships, they can consider both their credentials and their interpersonal qualities.

In recent years, health systems and the government have operationalized team-based care by creating the Patient Centered Medical Home (PCMH) in primary care (Agency for Healthcare Quality and Research; *https://pcmh.ahrq.gov/page/defining-pcmh*). The PCMH includes the following goals: comprehensive care, patient-centered care, coordinated care, accessible services, and quality and safety. In this context, the prescriber and the therapist are two parts of comprehensive services.

DECIDING WHERE TO REFER A PATIENT: PSYCHIATRIST OR PRIMARY CARE PHYSICIAN?

Tables 12.1 and 12.2 provide some issues to consider when making a referral. Our general philosophy is that it is important to have contact with the patients' primary care physicians. Should the need arise for a psychiatrist, it is ideal to coordinate this referral with the primary care physician, who will have a vested interest in the overall care that is being provided to his or her patients. Whether consulting with a primary care physician or a psychiatrist, it is helpful and sometimes critical for a patient to be examined by the primary care physician first because many general medical conditions can masquerade as mental illness.

If therapists refer a patient to a new primary care physician or a psychiatrist, they should contact the physician's office before giving the patient the referral information to ensure that the physician accepts the patient's insurance plan, is accepting new patients, and has available

TABLE 12.1. Collaboration with a Primary Care Physician or a Psychiatrist?

Advantages of consulting the primary care physician

- Can do a more thorough evaluation for general medical conditions and/or drugs that may be causing the psychiatric symptoms.
- Might be more readily available to the patient.
- Might already have a treatment relationship with the patient (trust).
- Might carry less stigma than seeing a psychiatrist, so the patient may actually *go* to the appointment.
- Can manage most of the needs of patients with depression, anxiety disorders, and some other mental illnesses.

Advantages of consulting the psychiatrist

- Should always be the consult of first choice when the diagnosis is in question.
- Can manage even the most severely ill patient.
- Usually can readily arrange psychiatric hospitalization when needed.
- Usually a better consult choice for the patient with multiple conditions (comorbidities), especially serious mental illness, personality disorder, and substance abuse.
- Can help the patient who has forensic mental health care needs or disability evaluation because of mental illness.
- Can clarify diagnosis and care for the most severely ill and/or treatment-resistant patients.
- A psychotherapist often understands the therapy goals better than a primary care physician.

appointments in the near future. One could take the position that the patient should assume this responsibility. However, anything a therapist can do to minimize barriers to psychiatric care will increase the likelihood that the patient will follow through with a referral and display a positive attitude about its potential. We have seen many patients become exasperated with stalled referral because of provider unavailability and problems with insurance reimbursement.

The patient's insurance plan will often dictate the referral options. Even if the patient pays out of pocket for the therapist's services, he or she is unlikely to pay privately for medication evaluation and management. Physician charges are usually more expensive than psychotherapy charges, and appointments with physicians—regardless of whether they are psychiatrists or primary care doctors—are usually paid for by the patient's insurance. Thus, a therapist can usually start the referral process by asking whether the patient has previously seen a primary care physician or psychiatrist whose fees are paid by the patient's insurance. If the patient is comfortable with Dr. X., and the therapist is comfortable with Dr. X., the initial referral decision is made.

TABLE 12.2. The Timing of the Referral

Emergent reasons to consult a physician (hospital emergency room, calling 911 for ambulance transport, or calling law enforcement for assistance):

- Patient is suicidal or in danger of harming oneself or others because of mental illness.
- Patient is unable to provide food, clothing, shelter, or safety because of mental illness (in some states, this is called "gravely disabled due to a mental disorder").
- Patient appears very ill and may be medically unstable.

Urgent reasons to consult a physician (same-day or next-day visit):

- Patient's illness is getting significantly worse during therapy.
- Patient has some suicidal thoughts but with no plan or intent.
- Therapist is concerned that a serious metabolic problem is developing (e.g., untreated hypothyroidism, causing depression; untreated diabetes, causing confusion; patient is taking a fluroquinolone antibiotic has developed paranoia and is delusional), and the patient needs urgent medical management of that problem.

Routine reasons to consult a physician (within the next 2 weeks):

- Patient has presented for therapy and has not had a recent physical examination.
- Therapist or patient suspects that medications may be contributing to the mental health problem.
- Therapist or patient suspects that mental symptoms seem to be possibly (or definitely) due to a general medical condition.
- Diagnosis is not clear.
- Patient is improving so slowly with psychotherapy alone that life events are compromised, and medication will probably speed recovery.

Factors that may confound this decision include (1) the match among the patient's preference, the therapist's preference, and the availability of a psychiatrist versus a primary care doctor; (2) differences in the ease of referral, cost, and waiting time for a first appointment; (3) the degree of flexibility of choice the patient's insurance offers; and (4) the influence of preexisting professional relationships that either the therapist or the patient has with specific physicians.

At times, patients want therapists to choose the physician they will see. If their insurance allows that freedom, we are happy to comply. We maintain relationships with different types of physicians, each with different strengths. At times, two psychiatrists may be equally qualified but have different areas of expertise. We hope our patients benefit from our detailed knowledge of possible referral sources. We try to match the patient with the physician by thinking about the personality of the patient and the physician's interview style. In addition, we often offer to call our colleague, to say we are sending a specific patient. We hope this process communicates to the patients that they can expect the same kind of caring, professional behavior from our respected colleague that they have come to expect from us. We find these personal relationships provide a safe, calm context in which patients can consider their treatment options.

WRITING THE REFERRAL EMAIL OR LETTER: THREE DIFFERENT APPROACHES

After confirming the physician's availability, the therapist can then begin to prepare a referral email or letter. The type of note will depend on the audience: a psychiatrist; a primary care physician; or the emergency screening-unit clinician, who may be an MD, nurse, social worker, or psychologist. Regardless of the audience, it is important to use a professional tone when writing a psychopharmacology consultation request.

When writing anything about a patient, always assume two things will happen: First, assume the patient—who has a legal right to do so—will read the email. The written word should contain the truth and be conveyed in a respectful manner, so that if the patient reads it, he or she will not be embarrassed or offended. Second, assume a plaintiff's attorney will ask the therapist to read his or her written record aloud in front of a court, so the notes must be comprehensive and respectful of the patient.

As obvious and unnecessary as this advice may sound, it is not rare to see a note that is too informal for the task. Sample note 1 is such a letter (see Figure 12.1). It is too short, too folksy, and too familiar, with the therapist referring to both the patient and the doctor on a first-name basis. Also, it refers to another patient in the same letter. If the patient reads it, he or she would probably see it as something written by a friend rather than a therapist. If it were ever brought to court for any reason, it would seriously undermine the credibility of the therapist in the eyes of a judge and jury.

Sample note 2 (see Figure 12.2) is written to a family physician, and a similar tone would be appropriate for other primary care physicians. The first paragraph presents an introduction and explains why the referral is coming to Dr. Smith; that is, it explains the relationships. The second paragraph states the target symptoms in sufficient, but not excessive, detail and covers the question of suicide. The third paragraph asks for the consulting note, states support of medication, and offers collaboration. It does not say that the therapist will continue to see the patient,

John Doe, MFT
123 Anywhere Street
Some Town, USA 00000
January 5, 2021

Jane Friend, MD
156 Anywhere Street
Some Town, USA 00000

Dear Jane:

I am sending over Susan Jones for meds. I've seen Suzy a half dozen times or so and I think she's not getting anywhere. I have a release (copy attached). Suzy's depressed and has PTSD, and I'll keep seeing her for therapy. No drugs, no suicidal stuff. She'll probably do well with some Prozac. Let me know if you have any questions.

By the way, I sent Frank to see you last month, and he's doing great!

Thanks.

Johnny

FIGURE 12.1. Sample note 1: Too informal.

as the family physician will assume this to be the case, but it would be a good idea to say it anyway.

Sample note 3 (see Figure 12.3) is written to a psychiatrist. The first paragraph tells how long and for how many sessions the therapist has seen the patient and what psychotherapeutic approach has been used. It also says in the first paragraph that this is a psychopharmacology consultation, and not a referral for the psychiatrist to assume care entirely. The second paragraph provides details, but more concisely than to the family physician. The psychiatrist will be getting these pieces of history from the patient directly, whereas the family physician may not seek all of them herself. The question of suicidal assessment is covered. The third paragraph requests a copy of the consultation note, expresses support for medication, offers collaboration, and also makes it very clear that the therapist intends to continue to see this patient. This is important to state clearly, lest the psychiatrist assume that the referral is intended to transfer psychotherapeutic care, as well as psychopharmacological care.

Sample note 4 (see Figure 12.4) is written to a mental health care professional who is acting as the screening clinician in the psychiatric emergency department of the county mental hospital. There is no

John Doe, MFT
123 Anywhere Street
Some Town, USA 00000
January 5, 2021

Mary Smith, MD
Family Medicine Center
344 Anywhere Street
Some Town, USA 00000

Dear Dr. Smith:

I am the therapist for Ms. Susan Jones, a 34-year-old woman who receives
her primary medical care in your office. Ms. Jones has signed a consent form
to allow us to share information about her care (copy enclosed). I have seen
Ms. Jones for five sessions in the last month, and I have asked her to make an
appointment to see you as soon as possible because I am concerned about her
worsening depression.

Ms. Jones has experienced the following symptoms for the last 3 months:
insomnia (she can get to sleep okay but wakes up at 3 A.M. and cannot get back
to sleep), poor appetite (10-pound weight loss without trying), feels tired all the
time, has difficulty getting work done on time because it's hard to keep focused
on her work, and has lost several work days because of fatigue and tearfulness.
Ms. Jones has a history of a major depressive episode 10 years ago that was
not treated, and she blames it for the loss of her job at the time. She also has a
history of sexual abuse as a child; she has nightmares about it, startles easily, and
sometimes has dissociative episodes when she feels that someone is getting angry
at her. Ms. Jones says that she thinks of suicide occasionally but has no plan to
act on that because she is aware of the pain that would bring to her family. She
has no history of suicide attempts in the past and no history of substance abuse.
My working diagnosis is major depression and PTSD.

I would appreciate receiving a copy of your evaluation note regarding Ms. Jones,
and I would like to know about any medications chosen, as well as the doses
and your follow-up instructions, so that I can help Ms. Jones to comply with the
medication you have prescribed for her. Please feel free to call me if I can provide
any further assistance, and I look forward to collaborating with you in the care of
our mutual patient, Ms. Susan Jones.

Sincerely,

John Doe, MFT

FIGURE 12.2. Sample note 2: To a family physician.

John Doe, MFT
123 Anywhere Street
Some Town, USA 00000
January 5, 2021

John Adams, MD
Psychiatric Associates of Some Town
443 Anywhere Street
Some Town, USA 00000

Dear Dr. Adams:

I am referring to you Ms. Susan Jones, whom I have seen for five cognitive-behavioral therapy sessions in the last month. I believe she will benefit from a psychopharmacology consultation at this time because we have noted that her depression has increased in severity, in spite of therapy. Ms. Jones has signed a consent for us to share information about her care (copy enclosed). I hope that you will be able to see her within the next 3 or 4 days.

Ms. Jones is a 34-year-old divorced woman who has experienced the following symptoms for the last 3 months: insomnia with early morning awakening, poor appetite (10-pound weight loss without trying), fatigue, and difficulty in concentrating on her work; she has lost several work days because of fatigue and tearfulness. Ms. Jones has a history of a major depressive episode 10 years ago that was not treated, and she blames it for the loss of her job at the time. She also has a history of sexual abuse as a child; she has nightmares about it, startles easily, and sometimes has dissociative episodes when she feels that someone is getting angry at her. Ms. Jones says that she thinks of suicide occasionally but has no plan to act on that because she is aware of the pain it would bring to her family. She has no history of suicide attempts in the past and no history of substance abuse. My working diagnosis is major depression and PTSD.

I would appreciate receiving a copy of your consultation note regarding Ms. Jones, and I would like to know about any medications chosen, as well as the doses and your follow-up instructions, so that I can help Ms. Jones to comply with the medication you have prescribed for her. I plan to continue to see her weekly for therapy. Please feel free to call me if I can provide any further information, and I look forward to collaborating with you in the care of our mutual patient, Ms. Susan Jones.

Sincerely,

John Doe, MFT

FIGURE 12.3. Sample note 3: To a psychiatrist.

John Doe, MFT
123 Anywhere Street
Some Town, USA 00000
January 5, 2021

Jane Worker, LCSW
Psychiatric Emergency Department
Some County Psychiatric Hospital
156800 Anywhere Street
Some Town, USA 00000

Dear Ms. Worker:

I am referring to you Ms. Susan Jones, whom I have seen for five therapy sessions in the last month. I believe she is in need of hospitalization today because she has suicidal ideation with a clear plan and intent to carry it out. Ms. Jones is coming to see you voluntarily, but I am so concerned about her risk of suicide that I feel she should be hospitalized on an involuntary basis if she declines care at this time.

Ms. Jones is a 34-year-old married woman who has experienced progressively worsening symptoms for the last 3 months, including insomnia, poor appetite (10-pound weight loss without trying), fatigue, and difficulty in concentrating on her work; she has lost several work days because of fatigue and tearfulness. Ms. Jones has a history of major depression 10 years ago that was not treated; she blames it for the loss of her job at the time, and then she made a serious suicide attempt by drug overdose, resulting in several days in the intensive care unit of the hospital. She also has a history of sexual abuse as a child; she has nightmares about it, startles easily, and sometimes has dissociative episodes when she feels that someone is getting angry at her. Ms. Jones says that she thinks of suicide often and has recently purchased a gun, which she keeps loaded in her bedroom. She states that since the drug overdose did not kill her, she will "be sure to do it right this time." Her husband recently left her, her job is in jeopardy, and she feels that she has nothing to live for. Because of the severity of her symptoms, her recent and pending losses, her prior history of a suicide attempt, and her current clear plans, I feel that Ms. Jones needs emergency psychiatric hospitalization at this time.

I would appreciate receiving a copy of your evaluation note regarding Ms. Jones, and I will resume her care, in collaboration with a psychiatrist, after her hospital discharge. Please feel free to call me if I can provide any further information, and thank you for your urgent attention to the needs of Ms. Susan Jones.

Sincerely,

John Doe, MFT

FIGURE 12.4. Sample note 4: To a screening professional in psychiatric emergency department.

mention of a release of information or consent from the patient, allowing the therapist and screening clinician to speak to each other. It would be good to have consent, of course, but in most states this is not required in such an emergency. In most locales, public hospitals have only a fraction of the number of beds that the community needs to be allocated to the seriously and acutely mentally ill. The staffs are typically hard working, spread too thin, underpaid, and caring for the community's most ill patients. Therefore, unless the screening clinician is convinced that the patient is an imminent danger to oneself and/or others because of the mental disorder, the patient is not seen by the psychiatrist and is not admitted to the hospital. So, if the therapist has a patient who is severely ill and in dire need of admission to a psychiatric hospital, it is essential to convince the screening clinician of the seriousness of the situation—and in one page. Note 4 presents compelling details concisely and offers the opinion that the patient should be involuntarily admitted if necessary, but it does so in a way that does not insult or undermine the decision making of the screening clinician. Also, the letter states that the therapist will be available for follow-up care after hospital discharge. This is important, as many hospitals feel seriously ill patients are "dumped" by therapists when treatment has not gone well.

The detail and style of referral notes should be appropriate to the person to whom they are addressed (e.g., the language for the family physician is a little different from that for the psychiatrist; see Table 12.3). They should be absolutely professional and empathic in tone and,

TABLE 12.3. The Language of the Referral

After you make a referral, the terminology for the timing of the appointment will vary from one community to another. Some examples follow:

- *Routine*—the patient will be seen at the next routinely available appointment, which may be soon or may not occur for 2 months or more.
- *2-week rule*—if mental health clinic patients have to wait more than 2 weeks for their first visit, the probability that they will show up for the appointment approaches zero.
- *Urgent*—should be seen within approximately 72 hours.
- *Emergency/today*—should be seen today; may be referred to a physician's office.
- *Emergency/hospitalize*—often referred to the psychiatric emergency room or community hospital emergency department.
- *Emergency 911*—the patient is severely ill, threatening harm to him- or herself or others and refuses treatment. In many states, the police are called, and they take the patient to a hospital for emergency evaluation and treatment.

if possible, no longer than one page. If the patient is very complex or if there are copious data from psychological testing, for example, then there should be a cover letter of one page and an attached copy of the psychological testing report. A copy of the patient's consent to release information should also be included.

ELECTRONIC MEDICAL RECORDS AND HEALTH TOOLS

The electronic medical record (EMR) has brought numerous changes to doctor–patient communication. While it is still common for two professionals to communicate about a shared patient, patients increasingly initiate their own requests. Many patients have access to a health management tool that allows them to contact their provider from their computer, tablet, or smartphone.

Thus, patients may contact their providers and request an appointment for a medication evaluation. Then, they may send a message a week later describing the symptoms they associate with the medication. Later, they may request refills, even for narcotics, and leave it to the provider to decide whether to refill the prescription without seeing the patient for a follow-up evaluation. In these situations, the therapist may never have direct contact with the provider. We have seen many iterations of doctor–patient communication surrounding psychotropic medications. Prescribing medications can be less expensive, easier and faster than psychotherapy. Responding to a patient email request for a refill can take less time than a follow-up office visit. If the therapist has any concerns about the medication, he should ask his patient to contact the provider who wrote the prescription or obtain written consent to contact the provider himself.

THE MEDICATION EVALUATION

Most physicians today are on a professional treadmill. Their employer requires a certain number of patients to be seen per day, regardless of the nature of the patients' needs. Even if the physician is in private practice, it takes a certain (often large) number of patients per day just to pay the overhead. On average and by specialty, the lowest-paid physicians in the United States are pediatricians, psychiatrists, and family physicians, so there is little room to maneuver more time per patient. Because a patient is probably happy with the pace and generous time allotment for therapy sessions, it is important to prepare him or her for the often chaotic pace of medicine.

The psychiatrist may have anywhere from 30–50 minutes for an initial evaluation, whereas the primary care physician will probably have 15–30 minutes for the first visit. Both of them will probably have about 15 minutes for follow-up visits, sometimes less. Visits are often rushed, and any patient can look like *anything* for an hour. Patients can look healthy when they are psychotic, they can look happy when they are depressed and suicidal, they can successfully sublimate personality-disordered behavior, and they can (and usually do) hide substance abuse disorders. Whoever is chosen for a referral, it is critical to communicate the reasons for it; never assume the presenting problem or diagnosis will be obvious in the visit with the physician.

The physician will take a medical history and perform a physical examination. The details of the mental status examination will be greater from a psychiatrist than a primary care physician, and the primary care physician will probably conduct a more thorough physical examination than most psychiatrists. In common, their consultations will usually include the elements in Table 12.4.

Ideally, the therapist will receive a consultation note from the physician, and, if not, he or she should request one if the patient consents. This note is likely to contain the elements listed in Table 12.4 for the first visit only. Follow-up psychotropic medication visits should usually include the following:

- Patient education regarding illness
- Medication benefits and side effects, including informed consent
- Information regarding therapy options, including no medication
- Planning, adjustments, encouragement
- Tracking efficacy/necessity of treatment (target symptoms/behaviors)
- "Support"

During both the initial and follow-up visits, the physician's priorities in the crush of the time allowed for the visit include the following:

- Is this patient going to die before he or she even gets back here?
- What medical conditions does this patient have that, although not fatal before the next visit, are critical to manage now?
- What health maintenance matters need to be taken care of (for the patient's benefit and/or to avoid penalty from the HMO)?
- Does the reason for referral fit into one of the first two categories? If it does not, and if there are pressing needs in those areas, then the reason for referral may be only partly addressed.

TABLE 12.4. Elements of a Basic Medical Initial Diagnostic Evaluation

- **Chief complaint (CC):** the presenting problem that brings the patient to care.

- **History of present illness (HPI):** "The patient was in his or her usual state of health until . . ."; the rest of this paragraph describes the onset of the presenting problem.

- **Past psychiatric history (PPH):** a listing of prior episodes of mental illness, treatment, hospitalizations.

- **Past medical history (PMH):** a listing of significant medical conditions, treatment, hospitalizations.

- **Current medications (meds):** a listing of names, doses, duration of treatment, reason for their use—for example, "HCTZ 25 mg qd [once a day] × 5 years for HTN [hypertension]."

- **Allergies:** particularly to medications.

- **Substances used:** smoking, alcohol, recreational drugs.

- **Family history:** medical and psychiatric.

- **Social history:** living situation, occupation, education, recreational activities, and so on.

- **Review of systems (ROS):** questions asked about each organ system of the body, head to toe.

- **Mental status exam (MSE):** extent of detail varies from psychiatrist to primary care physician.

- Other medical examinations and report of diagnostic test results, if appropriate.

- Psychiatrists may obtain additional or a more detailed history regarding development, relationships, sexual and legal issues, disruptive behavior, and other psychiatric issues.

- **Plan:** usually includes diagnostic tests as indicated, medications prescribed, referrals written, and follow-up plans; if medication is prescribed, this section often refers to the informed consent that was obtained.

How Does the Physician Decide Which Medication to Use within a Class?

Psychiatric diagnosis is occasionally obvious, but it is always a work in progress. Some patients clearly have psychosis, and their behavior may indicate that they are suffering from schizophrenia—until the urine drug screen comes back positive for amphetamines, revealing that the underlying problem is amphetamine-induced psychosis. Some people have such obvious depression that everyone around them knows that the diagnosis is major depression. But then, the major depression is only major depression until the patient's first manic episode, which prompts the therapist or the physician to change the diagnosis to bipolar disorder. We have to make the best diagnoses we can make, given the information we have. However, the diagnosis does not dictate what the treatment will be. Treatment is based on many interwoven factors, some of which are described in Table 12.5.

What Are the Criteria for an Adequate Trial of a Psychotropic Medication?

Criteria for an adequate trial of a psychotropic medication include the following:

- Accurate diagnosis and/or tracking of target symptoms
- Appropriate medication class for the target symptom
- Adequate dose and duration—with particular attention to the variations in the dose and the longer duration of treatment typically required for seniors
- Monitoring plasma and blood levels of the drug, if indicated, to ensure therapeutic levels and compliance with medication
- Supporting the patient's adherence with treatment; anticipating and asking about side effects since this is a major reason that patients stop medications, often without discussing it with their physician or therapist. Patients rarely volunteer information about sexual side effects, a major reason for stopping medication prematurely.

AFTER THE PATIENT STARTS MEDICATION

The research literature on adherence to treatment suggests that the degree to which a patient agrees with a health care decision strongly influences his or her adherence to the treatment regimen. The patient's agreement is especially important when there are challenges and difficulties along the way. Patients often experience the negative side effects of medications before they experience the symptom relief that the medications offer. In addition, there is a black box warning on all antidepressant medications prescribed in the United Sates (as well as on some other psychotropic medications) that warns the patient about the possibility of emerging suicidal ideation, especially during the early days of treatment. Patients should be followed very closely during those early days of treatment, to monitor for this very rare but critically important issue. If a therapist has allowed the patients to make the decision about medication themselves in their own time, they are more likely to persevere during this early period.

TABLE 12.5. Some of the Interwoven Factors That Dictate Which Medication within a Class Will Be Used to Treat a Patient for a Given Illness

• *What are the target symptoms and problems that are interfering with the person's life?* Hallucinations may be a target symptom and also one of the elements of the diagnosis; but even if the diagnosis changes from schizophrenia to drug-induced psychosis or to psychosis due to a general medical condition, the target symptom remains the same—hallucinations. Other examples of target symptoms include crying spells, poor concentration, poor appetite, insomnia, anger outbursts, and threatening behavior. The target symptoms are what we want to treat and follow, regardless of the diagnosis.

• *What other medical conditions does the patient have?* Choosing an antidepressant for a healthy young adult may lead to a different choice than an antidepressant for a man in his 60s with diabetes, hypertension, glaucoma, and prostatism. Some psychotropic medications can make the symptoms of other medical conditions worse.

• *What other illness might the patient have that has not yet been diagnosed and may be causing the target symptoms?* For example, thyroid disease more often presents for the first time in a mental health clinic than in primary care, usually as depression or an anxiety disorder. Severe vitamin B_{12} deficiency can cause serious neurological symptoms, including depression, psychosis, and dementia. (This is not due to a poor diet, and vitamin tablets will not help.) A person who has unknowingly been infected with syphilis for decades can present with mental symptoms, and a significant minority of HIV-infected patients (human immunodeficiency, or AIDS, virus) will present with mental symptoms as the very first manifestation of illness. There are many other medical disorders that can masquerade as a mental illness.

• *What medications must the patient take for other medical conditions?* Psychotropic drugs very often have interactions with other medications. Physicians must check for adverse drug–drug interactions before prescribing. When it looks as if an adverse interaction might occur, the physician must change some medication in order to avoid the problem. Also, the prescribing physician must be ready to manage the consequences of unforeseen adverse interactions, which are not rare.

• *What medications have worked for this patient (or for family members with a similar condition) in the past?*

• *What side-effect profile is most desirable for this patient?* All medications have side effects. If the patient is having trouble sleeping, a medication that causes drowsiness and is taken at bedtime might be preferred.

• *If the first medication did not work or was not tolerated, what were the problems?* Knowing the problems with the first medication will help dictate the next one to be tried.

• *Does the patient have a preference for a particular medication?* Media advertisements for medications may convince the patient that a particular drug is the only one that will work. Although this is rarely if ever the case, going against that conviction may doom the treatment to failure.

(continued)

TABLE 12.5. *(continued)*

⚬ *Is the patient restricted to a particular formulary (list of drugs) by his or her insurance plan or HMO?* Prescribing outside of the formulary can sometimes occur, but it may require the patient to pay full cost for the drug. When many medications cost at least $1.00–$2.00 per pill (and some psychotropic medications cost $8.00 or more per pill), and one might take several pills per day, the cost may be prohibitive; thus staying within the formulary may be the only treatment available.

⚬ *How does the patient respond to the informed consent procedure?* All medications have risks and benefits. The only reason to use them is if the benefits outweigh the risks, and this requires predicting the outcome when the drug is first started. Some patients cannot tolerate the uncertainty; they become too anxious and are not able to proceed with a medication trial.

⚬ *Is the patient taking the medication voluntarily or under the order of a guardian/conservator or court?* States have different laws concerning involuntary treatment of those who have a serious mental illness, often presenting a danger to themselves and others, but refuse treatment. The therapist should become familiar with the laws in his or her state. Often the choice of medication is shaped by the degree of cooperation from the patient. For example, a psychotic patient who is being treated voluntarily may be given risperidone pills or oral solution, a modern antipsychotic with relatively fewer side effects. However, a patient who refuses to take medication orally might be cared for by administering long-acting, intramuscular injections of antipsychotic medication (e.g., haldol decanoate, fluphenazine decanoate, Risperdal Consta, or paliperidone (Invega Sustenna), even if these may have more potential adverse effects.

Often, the therapist is seeing the patient more frequently than the physician. The therapist may be the first to hear about positive or negative effects. In addition, the patient may look to the therapist to answer questions about the medications. Scope of practice concerns can arise for therapists during this tenuous period where the benefits of medication for a particular patient are yet unknown. The therapist can use the trust he has built with his patient to lead the patient back to the prescribing physician for questions about the medication effects.

At the same time, the physician may have her own unstated questions about the therapist. Is this someone I would like to share patients with in the future? Will the therapist have appropriate boundaries? Are we a team? Will the therapist let me know about any risk such as suicidal thoughts that the patient describes to the therapist? Does the therapist demonstrate respect for my time and expertise in our interactions?

If we view the decision to take medications as a process, we will not be surprised if, after having decided to begin medication, the patient or a member of the family complains or questions the value of the medication during the first few weeks of treatment. Because it often takes up to 6 weeks for the positive effects of medications to be felt, this early period is a critical time. The patient is waiting for symptom relief but is experiencing some *negative* effects. Patients may complain of feeling dizzy or "spacey," being tired, having trouble sleeping, and having no appetite.

They may wonder aloud whether it is worth the time and expense to take the medication. They may be fearful about how the medication is affecting their bodies. They also worry that they will have to be on medication their entire lives or that they will be the exceptions for whom the medications won't work. If they have kept their decision to try medication a secret, they may worry that their families and friends may find the medication bottles.

It is common for patients initially to experience a change in self-identity. Our culture values the "rugged individual" who can "pull himself up by his bootstraps." Patients may worry that it is a sign of weakness or disability to try medication for an invisible problem. Other patients may express concerns about the cost of medication and wonder how they can afford to pay for it.

CONTINUING MEDICATIONS DURING THERAPY

The decision to start medication is only the first step. Issues and questions about the medications often arise in the course of therapy. The therapist's response to these questions may vary, depending on (1) the therapist's scope of knowledge, (2) the proximity and frequency of interaction that the therapist has with the prescribing physician, (3) the severity of the patient's symptoms or responses to medications, and (4) the patient's wishes and attitudes.

In Chapter 13, we discuss how to collaborate with physicians when they are treating patients who are taking psychotropic medications. Therapists face many of these challenging situations because they often see their shared patients more often than the physician sees them. In addition, it is sometimes easier to get an appointment or have a phone conversation with a therapist than with a physician—simply because the physician often has double or even triple the number of patients that a typical therapist sees in a day. Nevertheless, even when it is difficult for the patient (or the therapist) to reach the physician, the therapist must continue to affirm, both verbally and by his or her behavior, that the physician is in charge of prescribing medications and that the patient must consult the physician about treatment changes, including evaluating side effects, changing doses, or discontinuing medication.

CONCLUSION

We listen carefully as our patients talk about their medications. They seldom want to spend more than 5 or 10 minutes discussing medication issues. Instead, they want to continue working on their therapeutic issues. However, our support and willingness to answer the appropriate questions, find answers to other questions, and help contact their physician for their biomedical questions can make the difference in whether they maintain their medications during the first few difficult weeks or stop taking them before they have experienced the positive and healing effects.

A therapist's relationships with the medication providers and a therapist's knowledge about the providers' knowledge and training can help the therapist facilitate her patients' adherence to medication trials.

CHAPTER 13

Sharing Care

Dr. R., a family physician, is seeing a patient, Mrs. C., who complains of depressed mood, low energy, and decreased appetite. Dr. R. prescribed an SSRI, but Mrs. C. stopped it after only 2 weeks because she felt "too jittery." Dr. R. decides to refer Mrs. C. to Dr. W., a family therapist, for further assessment and treatment. Mrs. C. had been diagnosed with bipolar disorder many years ago and had seen a psychiatrist, who prescribed medication for the bipolar disorder. She had stopped taking the medication when her symptoms seemed to improve. Mrs. C. has not seen a psychiatrist in 2 years. Dr. W.'s assessment of Mrs. C.'s depression uncovers a clear pattern: Her bouts with depression typically occur between December and May, followed by manic-like symptoms between June and November. This initial interview is taking place in April, and Mrs. C. predicts that her depression will lift in a few weeks. In the second interview, Mrs. C.'s husband provides another perspective on this cycle of depression and mania: Although he worries about her during the depression cycle, she is more predictable then than during the manic cycle. As predicted, when Mr. and Mrs. C. arrive for their third meeting in May with Dr. R., the depression has lifted. Mrs. C. reports feeling energetic and enthusiastic about reconnecting with friends and family she has been distancing herself from during her depression. Although Mrs. C. is relieved that the depression has dissipated, both Mr. C. and Dr. W. are concerned about what appears to be mania, evidenced by little sleep, spending binges at the mall, and a general anxious appearance. Dr. W. wants to discuss these concerns with Dr. R. and ask if a referral to a psychiatrist is warranted, considering the history of her illness and current disconnection from a psychiatrist.

239

Dr. W., who is afraid Dr. R. might take offense by the inclusion of a specialist, asks the question about a psychiatric evaluation with some trepidation. Will Dr. R. think Dr. W. is disrespectfully questioning her ability to offer ongoing mental health care to Mrs. C.? If Dr. R. agrees to a psychiatric evaluation, Dr. W. wonders, will the three health care professionals be able to work together in an effective way, or will there be disagreements? How will the professionals communicate, with Drs. W. and R. in one location and the psychiatrist in another? Will Mr. and Mrs. C. be overwhelmed by the addition of another physician?

THE NEW ROLE OF COLLABORATOR: ESSENTIAL SKILLS

In our roles as educators, we have noticed that there is little guidance for therapists interested in answering the questions above. Instead, most students are busy learning the language, skills, and paradigm of their own discipline. To collaborate successfully with physicians, including psychiatric physicians, most therapists will have to relinquish some ideas they learned in training and embrace new ideas and skills. However, many skills that therapists already possess in their work with patients can be transferred to their collaborative work with other professionals. This chapter identifies the essential skills for collaboration (Ivbijaro, 2012; McDaniel, Doherty, & Hepworth, 2014; Seaburn, Lorenz, Gunn, Gawinski, & Mauksch, 1996).

Redefine the Role

Successful collaboration often demands a shift in attitude. Patterson, Peek, Heinrich, Bischoff, and Scherger (2002) summarize the differences between viewing oneself as a traditional mental health specialist and viewing oneself as a member of a collaborative team (see Table 13.1). In general, the therapist relinquishes the role of expert on the mental health and emotions of a shared patient and instead embraces a more holistic view of the patient's problems—medical and mental health. In this model, the therapist acknowledges that all areas related to health are inextricably intertwined. In redefining one's role as a therapist who collaborates with other professionals, a therapist will probably have to make some basic changes in the way he or she works. Some possible changes are listed in Table 13.2.

We realize the process implied in these changes can take more time, thought, and energy than simply telling the patient to "go see your

TABLE 13.1. Traditional and Integrated Behavioral Health: A Contrast in Focus and Purpose

Behavioral health as a specialty (traditional mental health)	Behavioral health integrated into medical care (integrated mental health)

Professional model

Behavioral health as a specialty service for referral and consultation.	Behavioral health services integrated into medical care (mental health provider as a member of a medical team).

Clinical focus

Mental health care	Medical and all health care

Mental health care
* Separate mental health problems.
* Considered the mental health care plan.
* Care of mental illnesses and conditions such as
  o Major mental illness and chemical dependency
  o Diagnosable mental health conditions
  o Specialty treatment groups and programs
  o Hospital, day treatment
  o Psychiatric emergency, triage
  o Evaluation for any mental health–related complaint
  o Coordination with medical care, nursing homes, other venues for care

Medical and all health care
* Intertwined medical and mental health problems.
* Considered part of medical care plan.
* Psychological aspects of care for any illness or complaint, such as
  o Common depression and anxiety, comorbidity
  o Somatic symptoms, psychophysiological symptoms
  o Rehabilitation, back to work
  o Complex cases, "thick charts," difficult patients
  o Family distress that complicates medical care
  o Chronic illnesses of all kinds
  o Adjustment to illness, adherence to treatment
  o Evaluation and referral for any mental health–related complaint, even if not appropriate for follow-up care in medical setting
  o Coordination with specialty mental health care, hospital, nursing homes, other care venues

Patient view

* Patient sees it as "mental health care."
* Patient expects exclusive relationship with little coordination or information sharing.
* Patient self-refers for mental health care or comes to treatment via a referral.

* Patient sees it as "health care."
* Patient expects team-based medical coordination and information sharing.
* Patient can call in for medical and mental health care.

(continued)

TABLE 13.1. *(continued)*

Behavioral health as a specialty (traditional mental health)	Behavioral health integrated into medical care (integrated mental health)
Offices and working culture	
• Mental health clinic space and therapy offices. • Mental health chart. • Mental health clinic systems and support staff. • Culture of traditional mental health clinic and professions.	• Medical clinic space and exam rooms. • Medical chart or quick access to therapist notes. • Medical clinic systems and support staff. • Culture of medical clinic and professions.
Covered benefits and financing	
• Care limited to diagnosable and covered mental health conditions, as per patient's mental health insurance coverage. • Considered part of mental health costs; another referral specialty.	• Care of any covered health care condition, regardless of mental health insurance coverage. • Considered a part of medical costs; a member of the in-house medical team.

Note. Reprinted from Patterson et al. (2002). Copyright © 2002 by Norton. Reprinted by permission.

TABLE 13.2. Tips for Working with Physicians

- Become more succinct, use less theoretical jargon, and talk about your patients' symptoms such as loss of sleep or change in appetite.
- Respond quickly to any initiatives to communicate that the physician makes and initiate the exchange of information with the physician (within the confines of medical confidentiality).
- Accept all "comers." We have noticed that physicians often enthusiastically refer their most difficult, challenging patients to us once they have confidence in our work.
- Accept the patient's and physician's conceptualization of the problem and the referral. Try to use the patient's language when you are describing the problem, not your traditional mental health language.
- Align with the patients' strengths, including their reasons for not needing therapy or medication.
- Help the patient identify social support. Think about the patient's social system, not just the patient. Enlist the family, friends, or medical team in the treatment.
- If you work in an integrated, on-site system, put yourself in the traffic pattern of the clinic, where staff and physicians are constantly running into you.
- Understand and accept the fact that the financial constraints and administrative concerns are as important and influential as the clinical concerns. For example, if the patients' potential medication is not on their formulary they may not be able to obtain it.

Note. Physicians also have to make changes to effectively collaborate. But here our focus is on the changes that therapists must make. Data from Patterson et al. (2002).

doctor for medication." But we believe this initial extra time can lead to better patient care and more fulfilling clinical work. It also gives the therapist the chance to learn knowledge outside of the usual discipline. To that end, it is important to reiterate that effective collaboration often requires concise, specific, and to-the-point communication with the physician. Furthermore, consultations are often brief (e.g., communications via an electronic medical record, hallway discussions between patients), in keeping with the often fast-paced primary care setting and contrary to the more traditional consultation parameters to which many therapists are accustomed. Ultimately, working collaboratively will save time because of the streamlined process established with the physician.

Become Culturally Competent

Therapists train and practice in a world that is different from that of physicians. Because therapists' contact with physicians is often limited, they rarely have opportunities to immerse themselves in the culture of medicine in order to learn about the roles, customs, and beliefs of its members. Just as it is important to be culturally competent with patients from ethnically diverse backgrounds, knowledge of and appreciation for medical culture is also helpful and can strengthen collaborative relationships (Edwards & Patterson, 2006).

Therapists are sometimes discouraged from pursuing collaboration with primary care physicians who are intimidating or unresponsive (e.g., by failing to return a phone call). Therapists' negative beliefs about physicians and medication can also contribute to a lack of collaboration. These negative beliefs are formed by stereotypes of physicians, particularly psychiatrists, as "controlling," "egotistical," and "reductionistic." Physicians carry their own stereotypes of therapists, viewing them as too "touchy-feely," "flaky," and "cerebral" (McDaniel, Campbell, & Seaburn, 1995). Although there may be a grain of truth in these stereotypes, believing them will interfere with your ability to form a relationship with other professionals.

The Culture of Primary Care

There are differences between the medical cultures of mental health and primary care. As mentioned in the previous chapter, physicians are under severe time constraints, which should be respected. For example, telephone conversations with physicians rarely last longer than 5 minutes without interfering with the physician's responsibilities for patient care. A physician may appreciate a two- or three-sentence note or email, providing a brief update on a patient, rather than having to find time to return a phone call.

Another cultural difference is how the law, therapists, and primary physicians view patient responsibility. Because physicians' greatest fear is missing something potentially life threatening, they are loyal to the adage "Don't just stand there, do something" (Bray & Rogers, 1997). Physicians take a tremendous amount of responsibility for their patients' well-being and in facilitating change in their patients' behavior. For example, the federal government may "incentivize" or offer payments to physicians who influence their diabetic patients' behavior choices. The depressed, diabetic patient who eats poorly and risks his health is at least partially the physician's responsibility. In addition, the legal system places great responsibility on physicians for any harm that might happen to their patients. A physician prescribed a sleeping medication for a patient. After taking the dose past midnight the first night, the patient drove to work early the next morning and had a terrible accident in which she and the other driver were seriously injured. The patient's attorney urged her to sue the physician because he had not explicitly told her to take the medication early in the evening.

The opioid crisis has heightened physicians' legal culpability. While overprescribing opioids may be largely to blame for the current crisis, the current legal solution is to hold physicians responsible for their opioid-addicted patients' choices. Physicians risk legal liability each time they prescribe an opioid. As a result, physicians make patients sign contracts about usage and withhold opioids from a pain patient who might have easily obtained all the pain medications she wanted in earlier years.

In contrast, therapists are often trained in the adage "Don't just do something, stand there" (Bray & Rogers, 1997). That is, therapists often place responsibility for change on the shoulders of their patients. This difference can create conflict between therapists and physicians when, for example, physicians expect therapists to intervene more aggressively with patients or when therapists expect physicians to listen to their patients concerns about medication side effects rather than just changing the medication. Recognizing and appreciating the different roles therapists and physicians play can be a helpful step in working collaboratively.

Finally, therapists and primary care physicians have different approaches to confidentiality. Sometimes there are signs in the elevators of hospitals or medical offices reminding physicians to maintain patient confidentiality. Whereas primary care physicians routinely and informally discuss patients with one another, therapists view patient information as sacred. One of the biggest complaints physicians have about therapists is their protectiveness of information, which at times can dramatically impede collaboration.

If a therapist and physician are located in different settings, a signed release of information will allow them to communicate. In addition, a conversation about the boundaries of disclosure with the patient and the family avoids misunderstandings that could later lead to problems. For example, a patient may not want a history of sexual abuse to be discussed with other members of the treatment team.

For professionals who work in the same setting, the rules around confidentiality are less clear, particularly when patient charts contain both medical and mental health notes. Treatment teams in the same setting could assume that a free exchange of information is allowed and necessary. We agree, but we also believe that making this policy explicit to the patient and family is important. Case notes are especially vulnerable to mishandling. For example, there is always a chance that mental health notes that are part of the medical record could be unintentionally released to a third party. If expectations are communicated and understood among the patient, family, therapist, and physicians, confidentiality need not impede collaboration (see Tables 13.3 and 13.4). Furthermore, collaboration need not violate confidentiality.

TABLE 13.3. What the Physician Needs from the Therapist

- Obtain proper release of information and consent to share information from patient prior to contact (unless dire emergency).
- Present patient history with appropriate degree of detail . . . and *target symptoms.*
- Present specific questions or problems that prompted the consultation request.
- Leave the practice of medicine to the physician. Most physicians do not appreciate a referral such as "I'm sending you this patient to get him started on Prozac . . ." (or any other named medication). However, some physicians, especially those who have had limited training in mental health care, do appreciate the therapist's suggestion. Learn who does and does not.
- Keep apprised of medication treatment and support it.

TABLE 13.4. What the Therapist Should Receive from the Physician

- Access/availability—especially emergency contact procedure.
- Consultation/collaboration.
- Information about medications used (to support treatment and help the patient understand and cope with side effects).

The Culture of Psychiatry

Much said about primary care applies as well to the culture of psychiatry. Psychiatrists complete 4 years of medical school, then 4 years of specialty training in psychiatry, the first year of which largely consists of internal medicine, neurology, and emergency medicine. During residency, psychiatrists train broadly in diagnostic methods, treatment, and prevention of psychiatric disorders in a range of inpatient, outpatient, and community agency settings. The best residencies provide balanced training in psychopharmacological and psychotherapeutic therapies, although only the former are provided by less well-equipped residencies.

However, much of the culture of psychiatry is shaped by the structure and practices of our health care systems, rather than the teaching of psychiatry as a scientific or academic discipline. Physicians, both psychiatrists and primary care physicians, are typically the most expensive health care professionals in the budget of health care systems. In addition, there are too few psychiatrists nationwide, particularly child and adolescent psychiatrists, to meet the needs of our health care systems. Both workforce and economic forces have led health care systems to press psychiatrists "to practice at the top of your licenses." Health care systems press psychiatrists to limit their clinical encounters to skill sets that cannot be shifted to less costly mental health professionals, particular diagnostic assessments of complex cases, such as patients with comorbid medical illnesses, forensic assessments, and psychopharmacological treatment focused upon patients with severe psychotic, mood, cognitive, or anxiety disorders. Although a psychiatrist may have received excellent psychotherapy training during residency, there may be no opportunities to practice psychotherapy in a health care system organized around 15- to 20-minute patient appointments with psychiatrists. Psychiatric patient populations who have severe, chronic disorders are also ones at greatest risk for suicide or acts of violence. Psychiatric practices thus more commonly include patients for whom safety is a question.

This shaping of psychiatric practices has impacts upon the content of clinical encounters. A brief interview may provide a sufficient description of signs and symptoms for the psychiatrist to make a diagnosis of a psychiatric disorder. However, a narrative account of the patient's experience cannot be elicited in 15 minutes; it can in fact require multiple 45- to 60-minute sessions to unfold. As a consequence, psychiatrists often focus primarily upon symptom reduction, while therapists work more broadly with the patient's life as a whole person. Psychiatrists rely upon accounts of the patient's pattern of symptoms and their intensity. Therapists rely upon stories of the patient's experiences, utilizing extensive discussion of the patient's feelings, motivations, choices, and actions. The psychiatrist's symptom-focused assessment can be adequate for guiding psychopharmacological treatment, but often insufficient for guiding psychotherapy. The therapist's understanding of the patient's experience and life story may be adequate for guiding psychotherapy, yet insufficient for guiding treatment with medication. Through collaboration, the patient can benefit from each of these portals that together can construct a more complex, in-depth understanding of the patient's suffering, revealing pathways toward relief. This bicultural lens greatly improves the likelihood of adherence to a treatment regimen that includes both psychotherapy and medication (Frank, 1997).

Build a Relationship

A good relationship with the physician paves the way to effective collaboration (Seaburn et al., 1996). As in work with a new patient, "joining" is the most critical task in building a good relationship. Minuchin and Fishman (1981) define joining as "the glue that holds the therapeutic system together" (p. 32). This is equally true for the professionals in the therapeutic system. Collaboration is much easier if professionals respect one another and have confidence in one another's abilities.

It is easy to move too fast through this relationship-building phase or to neglect it because contacts with physicians take place in formats—referral letters, communications via an electronic medical record, and hallway chats—that therapists may not associate with the process of joining. This is a mistake. Basic joining skills—such as listening; expressing empathy, respect, and concern; and asking questions for better understanding—will make all communications with the physician more effective. Using joining skills allows therapists to understand more fully unique clinical perspectives, as well as the needs and hopes of other professionals.

However, the relationship-building phase often contains two inequalities. The first, described earlier, is a sense that collaboration is more important to the therapist than to the physician, which means that the therapist works harder to make contact with the physician than vice versa. The second inequality is related to decision making about medications because the physician has the final say about treatment. Both of these inequalities are related to hierarchies that exist between different disciplines, which collaboration does not change. These contrasting positions demand that professionals in collaborative relationships become familiar with each other's role in patient care and respect the validity of each other's opinions and ideas. Although the physician may still have decision-making power, the therapist should offer diagnostic observations and medication inquiries without fear. Respect for the hierarchy and respect for perspective are the key features in building a relationship.

Clarify Frequency and Form of Communication

After release-of-information forms are signed and there is agreement with the patient and family about what can and cannot be told to other professionals, it is important to contact the involved health care providers as soon as possible (Seaburn et al., 1996). During the initial contact, preferably in person or over the phone, the therapist should introduce him- or herself and ask the physician about his or her goals for the shared patient. In addition to the initial impressions and preliminary goals, it is helpful to clarify the frequency and form of future communications.

The frequency of communication often depends on the seriousness of the patient's problem. For example, a patient may be suicidal or have complex medical concerns that require more frequent contact, which will benefit all professionals. At the very least, the therapist should make contact with the physician at the time of referral and the time of termination (Seaburn et al., 1996).

Face-to-face communication is ideal, but such an expectation is unrealistic if professionals work in different locations. Most communication between professionals takes place on the phone. Email is convenient and provides greater flexibility for responding, but it also raises serious questions about confidentiality (Seaburn et al., 1996). If used to provide brief updates, ask questions, or plan a meeting, we endorse the use of email. However, we strongly suggest that any sensitive information be communicated in person or over the phone and that lengthy reports be sent in sealed envelopes through the mail. As electronic medical records become more common and security is improved, electronic communications may provide greater options.

Clarify Boundaries

Boundary clarification is a requirement to successful collaboration (McDaniel et al., 2014), particularly when multiple mental health providers participate in one case. Regardless of the degree one has earned, patients and family members may refer to all health care professionals as "doctor" and have skewed expectations about who is responsible for what. For example, patients commonly discuss medication with their nonprescribing therapist and occasionally solicit advice on how much medication to take, when to take it, and whether to discontinue its use.

Similarly, patients report the progress of a therapy intervention with their psychiatrist or family physician.

Avoid Triangulation

As with any triad, avoiding triangulation can be a bit like avoiding breathing. A physician, therapist, and patient can form a natural triangle that can be functional and healthy. Our patients are often willing to try medication or at least talk to a physician about medication because they want to help us. They know we are trying to provide good care. In essence, they are willing to try anything we think might help because they trust us. The goodwill they feel toward us spills over into their initial visit with the physician. The respect and goodwill that a particular physician and therapist have for each other facilitates the care of a mutual patient. Such a triangle of patient care can be quite effective.

However, this triangle is not without its risks. Because of their trust of one another, a physician and therapist may become more lax about evaluating or continually assessing a shared patient. For example, Dr. Patterson asked a close colleague to provide medication to a patient during the session with the patient. She felt the patient needed medication immediately and knew there were no openings in the doctor's schedule for several days. Catching the doctor in the hall, she asked him to talk to the patient for a few minutes. In less than 5 minutes, the physician asked a few brief questions and gave the patient some medication samples to start. The physician told the patient to make an appointment for a full evaluation and mentioned that he would start a patient chart later in the day. By providing only medication samples, he felt he could ensure the patient's quick return for an office visit.

This situation was full of good intentions and full of ethical and legal risks. Dr. Patterson was trying to be an advocate for the patient and obtain access to care as quickly as possible. The physician was trying to please his colleague and respond to her request. The patient was trying to please the therapist by responding to the therapist's suggestions. However, the patient could not get an appointment for several weeks because the physician had no openings. At the end of his overwhelmingly busy day, the physician forgot to start a chart for Dr. Patterson's patient. There was no documentation of the visit or of the physician providing medication samples to the patient. In this situation, the lack of openings in the physician's schedule and his demanding caseload led to compromised patient care.

Sometimes patients and their family members recruit therapists or physicians into an alignment against other professionals. For example, patients may tell the therapist that the psychiatrist does not spend enough time with them and is not as caring as the therapist. Then the patients might ask the therapist for advice on whether to fire the psychiatrist. The therapist could feel flattered by such a comparison and agree with the description of the uncaring psychiatrist. Such a move would damage the collaborative relationship between the therapist and psychiatrist and would be therapeutically counterproductive for many reasons.

Triangulation comes in many different forms. Avoiding this trap is easier with strong, unified, collaborative relationships. With that aim, it may prove beneficial to have an initial joint session with the physician and/or patient to prevent triangulation and cultivate communication. Fostering the collaborative relationship allows a therapist or physician to respond to triangulation attempts with a restatement of the treatment mission, a recommendation to the patient to direct concerns to the appropriate person, or in the above example, education about the differences between psychiatric evaluation and therapy.

COLLABORATION IN ACTION

To illustrate these collaborative skills, we return to the case presented at the beginning of this chapter. Mrs. C.'s case is a common example of a therapist and physician who are working together in a family medicine setting and seeking consultation from a psychiatrist in a different setting. Although it would be more challenging, a similar process and outcome could be achieved with each professional working in a different setting.

> Dr. W. decides to inform Dr. R. about the changes in Mrs. C.'s mood. Although both express relief that the depression has lifted, they also express concern about her current manic symptoms. Since Mrs. C. has experienced similar cycles over the years, Dr. W. wonders aloud if it might be helpful to get the input of a psychiatrist, who could offer another perspective on Mrs. C. and the long-held diagnosis of bipolar disorder. Since she has not been in touch with a psychiatrist in many years, Dr. W. suggests it might be time for a checkup to make sure they are on the right track. Dr. R. agrees that such an evaluation will be helpful. Dr. W. meets Mr. and Mrs. C. to discuss a referral to a psychiatrist concerning her current manic symptoms. Mr. C. states that this manic cycle is familiar and often worries him more than the depression cycle because of Mrs. C.'s unpredictability. Mrs. C. agrees to the referral and is given the name and number of a reputable psychiatrist. A release-of-information form is signed,

giving Drs. W. and R. permission to speak to the psychiatrist. Drs. W. and R. write a letter to the psychiatrist, Dr. O., before Mrs. C.'s appointment to provide a brief history of her illness and their current questions. Following the evaluation, Dr. O. sends Dr. R. a written summary, which includes his treatment recommendations. Because of Mrs. C.'s clear descriptions of her mood cycle and attention to detail in her yearly calendar, it is not a surprise that Dr. O. changes her diagnosis from bipolar disorder to seasonal affective disorder. Consistent with this diagnosis, Dr. O. stops Mrs. C.'s medication and recommends light treatment, which serves as a preventive measure in preparation for the shorter days of winter. In a therapy session after the evaluation, Mr. and Mrs. C. are cautiously optimistic and ready to begin the light treatment. During a routine medical visit 3 months after the evaluation, Dr. R. notices symptoms that appear consistent with mania. Dr. R. consults with Dr. W., and both agree that Mrs. C. needs to see Dr. O. again. Dr. O. decides to start her on 600 mg of lithium and schedules regular monthly appointments to monitor her progress. The combination of medication, light treatment, and individual and family therapy significantly improve Mrs. C.'s mood disorder. Although she experiences a reemergence of depression as the winter months approach, the depression arrives late in the year and is much less severe. Mrs. C. says, "I feel so blessed to have the three of you working together on my behalf!"

This case is a common scenario for therapists: A patient is referred who is currently on medication or needs medication and multiple professionals become involved, usually a family physician and a psychiatrist. When therapists refer to a physician for assistance with the care of their patients, they are influencing the treatment plan in significant ways. First, and most obvious, is the possible addition of medication. Second, and equally important, is the expansion of the treatment system to include other professionals, who will have some say in the care of a particular patient and family. If the patient was already taking medication when therapy started, the therapist is in the position of a newcomer to the treatment system. It is not uncommon for a patient and physician to have a long-standing relationship, which will continue after the therapist discontinues work with the patient and family.

CONCLUSION

In summary, therapists serve critical roles in successful collaborative care:

1. A therapist can help a patient to understand the meaning and significance of a psychiatric diagnosis, the treatment recommendations, and expectations for treatment outcome. It is important that the therapist knows how to monitor symptoms for early detection of relapse, as well as for medication side effects.

2. A therapist can help a patient to accept the need to follow all elements of a recovery program, in addition to taking the prescribed medication. These include healthy diet and exercise, resolving relationship stressors, and adopting daily practices that strengthen emotion regulation (e.g., mindfulness practices, yoga, spiritual practices).

3. Contact time for follow-up visits with the prescribing physician, other than the initial diagnostic session, are typically brief, infrequent, and focused upon state of remission of depression symptoms. The therapist has more regular and in-depth contact with a patient's daily life in all its richness. Information about the patient's quality of life, including but in addition to specific symptoms, needs to be reported back to the physician, particularly if it suggests that treatment is falling short.

4. The therapist can help a patient to voice concerns during meetings with their physician by helping a patient to organize his or her thoughts or to write down questions to ask as a reminder.

5. The therapist is best positioned to note when stigma hinders treatment adherence. Patients who are too embarrassed to complain about sexual side effects may simply stop taking their antidepressant. Patients who feel a loss of respect from family members, employers, or coworkers for seeking psychiatric treatment may simply drop out of care. A therapist can not only alert the prescribing physician but also work with the patient in practicing what to say to whom in their lives about taking an antidepressant, and who has no business knowing.

These contributions can be most effective when there is a comfortable, collaborative relationship between therapist and physician. The physician values the roles that the therapist can serve, and the therapist appreciates the diagnostic and medical expertise of the physician.

CHAPTER 14

Strengthening Bonds

Mrs. J. has been coming to see Ms. T., a family therapist, for treatment of depression for the last 6 weeks. Ms. T. understands the current life stressors that Mrs. J. faces. She also knows Mrs. J. has struggled with depression on and off for many years and that Mrs. J.'s mother also struggled with depression. Ms. T. has come to believe Mrs. J. might benefit from medication and wants to send her for a medication consultation.

When Ms. T. broaches the subject of medication as a possible treatment, Mrs. J. reacts strongly. She explains that she is already concerned about the dissipating intimacy in her marriage and that medication could make it worse. Mrs. J. explains that her cousin Sally, who also suffers from depression, had tried medication. Her cousin's husband did not support his wife's decision because he believed she should be emotionally stronger. He did not want her to try medication that might "change her personality and mess with her head." In spite of her husband's objections, Sally tried an antidepressant. About 6 weeks later she felt much better, but she also gained 5 pounds, needed more sleep, and became anorgasmic. Although she was feeling better, her husband was increasingly distant and angry about the changes in their sex life. He was also angry that he had to get up earlier to care for their two small children so Sally could get the extra sleep she now needed. According to Sally's husband, "Sally might be feeling better, but I'm feeling worse every day." Mrs. J. told Ms. T. that she would rather live with her depression than risk further disrupting her already strained marital relationship. She saw how "medication affected my cousin's marriage and I don't need those problems."

There is little information to guide Ms. T.'s next move. She could try to talk Mrs. J. into trying the medication, but doing so risks creating another area of conflict for her patient. She could ask Mrs. J. to bring in her husband so Ms. T. can talk to him about psychotropic medications, but he may be unwilling to come. She could try to find a medication that does not affect sex, sleep, and weight, but she knows that all medications have some side effects. Finally, she could give up on the idea of medication even though she thinks drug therapy will help her patient. Although Mrs. J. is the individual patient who takes the pills and experiences the side effects, the implications of the medication extend to her family, which will be affected by the changes, positive or negative, that the medication creates.

> Ms. T.'s next patients are a father and stepmother, Mr. and Mrs. H., of a 9-year-old boy, Tommy. Mr. and Mrs. H. have demanding jobs as attorneys and have been married only a year. Tommy lives with them full-time and spends a lot of time alone in his room, playing video games on his computer. He has gotten in trouble at school for aggressive behavior on the playground, leaves his room a mess, easily loses his homework, and fails to do his chores unless he has multiple reminders. Mrs. H. is clearly frustrated and angry about Tommy's disruptive behavior, and Mr. H. is sympathetic to his wife's frustrations. They bring Ms. T. a list of Tommy's infractions during the previous week. After reciting each problem, they conclude by saying that the therapy isn't working and that a friend said her son with attention-deficit disorder got better with Ritalin. Mr. and Mrs. H. want to try Ritalin or some other drug that will calm Tommy down and make him behave.

Ms. T. is again unsure about what to do next. She has not even considered medication for Tommy and had ruled out the diagnosis of attention-deficit disorder several weeks earlier. What Ms. T. does know is that Mrs. H. is ambivalent about caring for Tommy and would prefer more time alone with her new husband and a more orderly, calm household. In addition, Tommy does not go to bed until almost midnight many nights, and the exhausted parents have been unwilling to enforce Ms. T.'s recommendation of an earlier bedtime. Tommy is angry with his dad for getting married when he thought their living situation was fine with just the two of them, especially after the painful adjustment to his mother's departure. Tommy is completely uninterested in his schoolwork, and his main source of pleasure is playing his video games, which he does for 3 or 4 hours per day.

Scientific literature about the biochemical impact of medications, their positive and negative effects, and basic neuroscience may be of little value to Ms. T. in these situations. It may also be of little use to Tommy because someone else in the family is going to make the decision about medication use. For Mrs. J., her husband's fear of the unknown will ultimately determine her medication question, and for Tommy, Mrs. H.'s difficulties in adjusting to a new life might lead to his inappropriate use of medication.

We have seen situations like these many times, but there is little discussion in the literature of the family's impact on an individual psychotropic medication decision or the impact of the medication on the family. In a study on practice patterns of marriage and family therapists, Hernandez and Doherty (2005) reported that 24% of cases involving medication included a spouse or partner, and 8.5% included other family members. In a similar manner, physicians prescribe medication for an individual patient and target individual symptoms. It may seem irrelevant to most physicians to consider the impact of the medication on the family and vice versa. But most patients live in families, and they are concerned about their family members' responses to their choices.

MENTAL ILLNESS, MEDICATION, AND FAMILIES

We involve family members early and consult with them as often as possible because they have an enormous impact on health and illness and on how the patient relates to health care providers (McDaniel et al., 1995). All family members are impacted by the strains of living with mental illness, including the immediate emotional and practical needs of the patient, as well as guilt, shame, helplessness, and conflict around illness decision making (Berman et al., 2008). Families adjust their behaviors to accommodate and change the course of the illness, often in the face of volatility and unpredictability. Regardless of possible dysfunction within a family, they provide important information about medications and treatment compliance and may keep patients safe between appointments. Unfortunately, families have been historically blamed for the presence of mental illness.

In the mid-20th century, some psychiatrists and family therapists conceptualized schizophrenia as emerging from unhealthy family communication, child-rearing practices, and the mother–child relationship (Weinstein, 2013). Murray Bowen, for example, hospitalized multiple family members to treat family disruptions hypothesized to cause schizophrenia.

Medication was not viewed as a primary treatment method, but rather as a palliative measure to sooth anxieties (Weinstein, 2013). This extreme systemic view of mental illness eventually gave way to a more nuanced biopsychosocial perspective that views mental illness as biological and influenced by multiple systems, including family relationships.

Unhealthy family interactions can complicate the lives of patients suffering from mental illness. Since most mental disorders begin in childhood and adolescence and the first symptoms are often insidious, damaging family behaviors may emerge gradually and continue for many years. At the beginning of the illness, family members often rally to support their loved one. But, over time, the family can become exhausted due to their perceived inability to help and wariness of the ongoing needs of the ill family member. The interactional patterns that plague families are not solely internal; they can be influenced by stigma in the larger community leading to ostracization. The long-term costs become burdensome and family members begin to criticize the ill member. This pattern of overinvolvement, criticism, and hostility has been labeled **expressed emotion (EE)** in the family literature (Hooley, 2007; Miklowitz, 2019). A high level of EE has been associated with more frequent relapses and more severe symptoms (Miklowitz, 2004).

Developmental Differences

The age of the patient plays a key role in the level of involvement of family members and the treatment they seek. Often other family members make decisions, including medication decisions, for the very young and the very old, as can be seen in the literature concerning the increase of antipsychotic medications for older patients with dementia or agitation. At the opposite end of the life cycle, an alarming trend may be occurring: Very young children are increasingly prescribed psychotropic medications, especially children from poor families (Coyne, 2000; Pennap et al., 2018). Using psychotropic medications to treat problems of childhood has increased over the past 30 years (Ninan, Stewart, Theall, Katuwapitiya, & Kam, 2014). Children, particularly boys under 8, are given diagnoses indicating behavioral disorders and then given medication to treat behaviors such as impulsiveness and uncooperativeness. Other common childhood diagnoses that often lead to psychotropic medications include anxiety and learning disorders. Many of these children do not receive any type of psychotherapy.

Coyne (2000) laments that one cause of this trend is the lack of collaboration between mental health professionals and physicians. Recent initiatives to offer integrated care or collaborative care in primary care clinics may improve this situation. If front-line primary care providers have access to therapists and other mental health professionals, they may refer their young patients and families for therapy and psychoeducation instead of pulling out their prescription pad.

A CLINICAL GUIDE TO COLLABORATING WITH FAMILIES

Although there are few studies of the interaction between families and psychotropic medications, and the existing studies focus on severe mental illness, we can still glean clinical wisdom from the literature. It makes sense that families would be concerned about their ill family member and that they would be affected by his or her behavior. Although inclusion of the family seems to be a simple guideline, we have been surprised at how seldom families are consulted about treatment decisions or educated about the illness. We have also been surprised by how infrequently therapists and physicians utilize family members as sources of information about the patient's history and progress. Finally, we are often surprised to find that some therapists and physicians are treating seriously ill adult parents, often single parents, and failing to inquire about the welfare of their dependent children.

If we know a collaborative approach that includes family members works best, why aren't we using it? Our best guess is that family work takes more time, is more complicated, and can provoke more anxiety in therapists and physicians. If we are already feeling pressed for time, it is easy to overlook family members' input. Below are suggestions for therapists who want to practice in a collaborative care context and simultaneously expand the scope of care to the patient and family.

Ask Family-Oriented Questions

Systems theory provides a lens both to understand the relational context of patients' lives and to predict issues that might arise during the course of treatment. Cole-Kelly and Seaburn (1999) suggested the following family-oriented questions to better understand a patient's illness:

- Has anyone else in the family had this problem?
- What do family members believe caused the problem or could treat the problem?
- Who in the family is most concerned about the problem?

- Along with the illness and symptoms, have there been any other recent changes in the family?
- How can the family be helpful in dealing with this problem?

Additional questions to consider include the following:

- How is decision making balanced in the family? Who will make the decisions for the ill family member if the patient cannot?
- Who in the family wants the patient to try psychotropic medication? Who opposes the medication option? Why? Try to obtain a family history of medication issues.
- What are the effects of the member's illness on the family? The more the family is affected by stressors such as financial costs, time demands, or the patient's inability to contribute to family tasks, the more the family members might want to influence medication decisions.
- Are there influences from outside the family to be considered? The family may experience some pressure to create change in a member's behavior. For example, an employer or school official might notify a family that there are problems with a family member's behavior. The family may be expected to solve these problems. Also, are income, insurance status, or other financial factors likely to influence medication decisions?
- Are any dependent family members strongly influenced by the ill member's functioning, for example, dependent children or dependent older adults? Does anything need to be done to ensure their care as well?

These are just a few questions a therapist can consider in understanding the family structure, particularly the interactional patterns that help shape it. For example, an overfunctioning spouse may be attempting to make a treatment decision for an underfunctioning patient. In such a case, a therapist would not want to alienate the spouse or support the patient's sense of powerlessness in the relationship. The therapist would want to acknowledge the spouse's efforts to be helpful and attempt to give the patient a voice in his or her own care.

The responsibility of caring for a patient usually falls on members of the family. Thus, they are not simply uninvolved bystanders. For example, it is not unusual for family members to prompt the patient to make the initial appointment with the therapist or physician. Because of the stigma of mental illness and the patient's worries about burdening family members, the family may not be fully informed on the health status of the patient. This lack of knowledge may be related to conflictual relationships in the family and a patient's preference to keep family members uninformed.

Address the Family's Belief System

Family members come to treatment with a variety of beliefs about mental illness and medication. These beliefs play a significant role in shaping a family's response to illness and their willingness to support a treatment regimen that has been recommended by a team of professionals (Rolland, 2018). For example, family members may come to therapy with one of the following beliefs:

- "Mental illness is a character flaw."
- "Everyone gets depressed; why should he receive special attention?"
- "Medication is only for crazy people."
- "Medication doesn't work. My mother took several medications for depression and each medication made it worse."

These beliefs often develop over many years and can be influenced by many ethnic, cultural, and religious traditions. Stigma and shame are associated with mental illness in many countries, and families may choose to hide a family member's illness or prevent him or her from seeking treatment because the family would be perceived as inadequate or responsible for the illness (Thornicroft, 2006). For treatment to move forward successfully, it is important to explore these effects.

Often the family's beliefs about the medication are as important in the treatment as its actual effects. Medicine has long recognized this fact, as seen in the discussions of the "placebo effect." Thus, a therapist is juggling multiple meanings about the purpose, effects, and risks of medications. At times, the therapist won't recognize family members' beliefs or hidden agendas concerning psychotropic medications. In addition, the therapist needs to be aware of his or her own beliefs about the role of medications. Is medication essential? Optional? Dangerous? Demeaning? Redemptive? There are as many possibilities for the beliefs about psychotropic medications in the family–therapist–doctor–patient system as there are medications. It is hoped that the skilled therapist can make the covert beliefs overt. People's fears and concerns can be addressed. When there is scientific evidence to guide a decision, that evidence can be related and applied to the unique situation. When there is little evidence, the therapist can be frank about the limits of our knowledge and help the family, the patient, and the physician make as informed a decision as possible.

Elicit the Goals of Each Family Member

In clinical practice, one caveat in considering the applicability of the outcome research is the question of whose goals are being measured. Different members of the treatment system may have different goals. The family may want specific symptom amelioration. For example, family members may want the patient to be less agitated or more able to perform the daily tasks of family life. The physician may want better medication compliance or major clinical outcomes such as reductions in psychopathology and increases in functioning. The patient may just want to be left alone.

These numerous and often unspoken agendas about the goals and impact of medications have to be considered; otherwise, disappointment when the expectations are not met could overshadow other positive effects. For example, in one study of the effects of a psychoeducational intervention for married patients with bipolar disorder and their spouses, medication *plus* a marital intervention led to better overall functioning and better medication compliance but not ultimately to better overall symptom reduction (Clarkin, Carpenter, Hull, Wilner, & Glick, 1998). Depending on each participant's goals, the marital intervention may or may not have been viewed as a success.

FAMILY-BASED INTERVENTION

Intervention studies focused on severe mental illness provide helpful direction for therapists working with patients and their family members coping with mental illness. **Family psychoeducation (FPE),** also called "family intervention" in some countries (National Institute for Health and Clinical Excellence, 2009), has been shown to be effective in the treatment of schizophrenia and is now deemed an evidence-based practice for reducing relapse and hospitalizations (Jewell, Downing, & McFarlane, 2009). FPE is a collection of programs aimed at providing information about the illness, medication management, and treatment planning to family members as they cope with their family member's symptoms and the effects of illness on the family (Lucksted, McFarlane, Downing, Dixon, & Adams, 2012). These programs assume (1) the actions of family members impact the person coping with illness and his or her treatment and (2) family members need information and support in caring for a family member with severe mental illness. FPE is increasingly offered in a group format, where families join together to decrease social isolation and stigmatization and reap the benefits of mutual support (Jewell et al., 2009). Below are examples of interventions in FPE (McFarlane, Dixon, Lukens, & Lucksted, 2003):

- Assess the family's strengths and limitations in their ability to support the patient.
- Help resolve family conflict through sensitive response to emotional distress.
- Address feelings of loss.
- Provide an explicit crisis plan and professional response.
- Help improve communication among family members.
- Encourage the family to expand their social support networks.
- Be flexible in meeting the needs of the family.

Research has demonstrated decreased relapse and rehospitalization rates for schizophrenic patients whose families received psychoeducation (McFarlane, 2016). Family interventions led to improvements not only in the patients' symptoms but also in the relationships between patients and family members. In a study on the impact of medication on the families of schizophrenic patients, the authors concluded that all family members interviewed felt that their relative had responded positively to the medication (Najarian, 1995). Family members also stated that their relationships improved as a result of the patient's positive response to the medication. The patient could relate better to other family members and had increased interest and ability to participate in social activities.

Another study interviewed families of schizophrenic patients, asking specific questions about the families' responses to the medications and the medications' effects on the families. Families hope that the medications will lessen their relatives' suffering and ease the burden of care (Stebbin, 1995). In a similar study, the researchers concluded that medication had a small but significant effect on the patients' families (Rosenheck et al., 2000). The primary impact was to help reduce negative symptoms in the patient and thus reduce the family's burden. However, the schizophrenic patient who has reduced symptoms may then be released from the hospital and placed in the care of the family, thus transferring the responsibility for the patient from the hospital to the family.

What can we learn from this research? When we expand our target patient to include the family, how do our treatment goals change? Table 14.1 summarizes answers to these questions.

TABLE 14.1. A Summary of Family Research

- Psychoeducation for family members can increase the patient's compliance with taking the medications.

- Even when the family interventions or therapy are not specifically focused on the medications, one effect of the therapy can be increased adherence to medication regimens.

- Medication adherence decreases as the complexity, cost, and duration of the regimen increases, even with supportive families that encourage compliance.

- Families with members with serious mental illnesses, such as schizophrenia, may be more pleased with the effects of medication because it can lessen the family's burden.

- Families' hidden agendas or expectations about the medications can vary widely. Family members may hope that the medication "cures" the troubled family member and rescues the family from the overwhelming caretaking burden.

- Power struggles and conflicts in the family can erupt over the individual member's decision about taking medication and his or her compliance.

- Both therapy and medication compliance can improve when the family therapist and physician have a collaborative alliance with the family, not simply the patient, and can manage the varying responses of family members over time to the patient, the illness, and the medication.

- Interdisciplinary communication and more consistent patient care, including frequent communication with the family, make the burden of caring for the troubled family member easier. One study concludes by stating, "An alliance between professionals and families holds great potential for maximizing the positive effects of [medication] therapy" (Stebbin, 1995).

Note. Data from Coldham, Addington, and Addington (2002); Dickson, Williams, and Dalby (1995); Haynes, McDonald, and Garg (2002); Kotcher and Smith (1993); McDonald, Garg, and Haynes (2002); Olfson et al. (2000); Ran and Xiang (1995); Smith, Barzam, and Pristach (1997); Stebbin (1995); and Wysocki, Greceo, Harris, Bubb, and White (2001).

CONCLUSION

The explosion of knowledge in biology, neuroscience, and technology means that therapists of the future cannot work in the same ways we have worked in the past decade. Our scope of knowledge has to expand, and we have to work more closely with health professionals from other fields who have different expertise.

As we train new therapists, we are aware that many of our students chose the mental health field because they wanted to help people and found themselves at home in the social sciences (and, often, did not feel comfortable in their biology, physics, and chemistry classes). They knew a career in mental health seldom offers fame, glory, and wealth, and they accepted these limitations. What they did expect from their careers was a sense of personal satisfaction and pride in helping people change their lives for the better.

When they began their graduate training programs, they immersed themselves in the knowledge, culture, and clinical work of their specific disciplines. They became experts in cognitive-behavioral therapy, family systems work, or developmental psychopathology. For the most part, their training occurred in settings where they would be exposed to other students and faculty who were similar in training and clinical practice. But new forms of practice require that we all begin to learn and communicate across the boundaries of our various disciplines.

We hope this book has filled an important gap by making the scientific information user-friendly and by pointing out the strengths and pleasures of working with colleagues from other disciplines. In addition, we hope this book has made you think more about your patients' families and their impact on treatment.

Although this book has focused on imparting to therapists scientific information about psychotropic medications and practical guidelines for collaboration with families and other professionals, we are aware that for a collaborative care model to work, other changes must be made. Ideally, physicians need to know more about psychotherapy so they can have a better appreciation for what a therapist can offer to shared patients—and what the therapist cannot supply.

In this book we have focused treatment discussions on psychotropic medications. But bear in mind that however remarkable the advances in drug therapy may be, the traditional knowledge and skills of psychotherapy practice remain vitally important. In fact, research suggests that an ideal treatment often occurs when both psychotherapy and psychotropic medications are part of the treatment plan. In addition, services and interventions that enhance social support, such as group therapy, family psychoeducation, and Internet chat groups, are often critical to the success of the therapy.

We have suggested that therapists must expand their interests and influence to other factors that have an impact on clinical care: the patient's family, the clinic's organizational structure, the finances of therapy, and the physician–therapist–patient relationships. These factors can influence the outcome of therapy as much as the specific medication or specific psychotherapy techniques used.

Our overall goal in writing this book is to improve the clinical care of patients with mental health problems. We encourage the reader to stay focused on this goal and to measure every new intervention, idea, or technique by asking, "How will this information help me provide better care for my patients?" If better care is our ultimate outcome and measure of success, therapists will continue to learn and to adapt the way they practice as new knowledge is added. We will learn from our colleagues in different disciplines. We will consider the multitude of influences on our patients' care. In the end, not only will patients prosper, but also the therapist's attitude of curiosity and openness will lead to a more rewarding career.

Glossary

Absorption—the process of putting drugs into the bloodstream.

Abuse—the maladaptive pattern over at least a 12-month period of substance use, leading to impairment or distress, but this does not include substance dependence, tolerance, or withdrawal.

Acamprosate—a drug for the treatment of alcohol dependence that mimics the neurochemical effects of alcohol.

Active metabolites—an active form of a drug after it has been processed by the body.

Agnosia—the inability to recognize the nature of sensory input such as objects, voices, faces, and environments.

Agranulocytosis—a severe drop in white blood cell count that can potentially be fatal.

Alcohol use disorder—a diagnosis given to a person if they continue to drink despite awareness that continued use will lead to adverse consequences in health, employment, relationships, or the law.

Allodynia—pain elicited by a non-noxious stimulus; for example, the touch of clothing causes pain, or air movement causes a burning sensation on the skin.

Amantadine—a medication that is an agonist at dopamine receptors and can ameliorate extrapyramidal side effects of antipsychotic medications.

Amitriptyline—a tricyclic antidepressant used to treat anxiety and depression.

Amnestic disorder—disorders that are marked by problems with memory.

Amygdala—emotion processing part of the limbic system; located in the medial temporal lobe.

Antagonist—something that works against something else.

Aphasia—a defect or loss of the power of communication by, or comprehension of, speech, writing, and signs.

Apoptotic pathway—two types of apoptotic pathways: intrinsic and extrinsic. Intrinsic pathways are activated by cellular stresses where a cell receives a signal to destroy itself from one of its own genes or proteins due to the detection of DNA damage. Extrinsic pathways are where a cell receives a signal to start apoptosis from other cells in the organism.

Apraxia—the inability to perform goal-oriented movements or to use objects properly.

Atypical antipsychotic—a drug used to treat psychotic disorders that produces fewer side effects than typical antipsychotics.

Atypical depression—a subtype of depression that involves symptoms such as increased appetite, increased weight gain, sleepiness (hypersomnia), fatigue, and sensitivity to rejection.

Augmentation—the process whereby the addition of a second medication enhances the effect of the first.

Autonomic nervous system—the part of the nervous system that controls and regulates bodily functions such as heart rate, digestion, respiratory rate, sexual arousal, pupillary response, and urination.

Axon—the part of the neuron that carries the electrical impulse away from the body.

Benzodiazepines—a type of medication that works in the central nervous system and acts on the $GABA_A$ receptors; used for anxiety, panic symptoms, and other medical conditions.

Benztropine—an anticholinergic medication used to relieve symptoms such as tremor, muscle rigidity, loss of balance, and stooped posture.

Bipolar depression—a disorder associated with episodes of mood swings ranging from depressive lows to manic highs.

Blood alcohol level (BAL)—the percent of ethyl alcohol or ethanol in a person's bloodstream (see Table 8.1 for levels of cognitive/behavioral impairment).

Bottom-up information processing—analysis that begins with processing the smallest pieces of sensory information from the five senses.

Brain-derived neurotrophic factor (BDNF)—a protein growth factor that serves a key role in memory and resilience by stimulating neurogenesis in the hippocampus and repair of neurons injured by stress.

Buprenorphine—a medication used to treat opioid use disorder that stimulates opioid receptors and also blocks their activation by other opioids.

CAGE questions—four simple screening questions to identify problems with alcohol.

Capitated—a fixed amount of funding for a particular provider (such as a practice, agency, or clinic) for each patient enrolled in a particular insurance policy, regardless of how many patients are seen or how often.

Carve out—an insurance policy such that one health provider (such as a primary care provider) is excluded from coverage for a particular condition or treatment while another provider (such as a clinic or agency) is covered, often for a flat fee.

Catatonia—a state of abnormality in mobility and behavior that is often accompanied by an underlying neurological, psychiatric, or physical illness.

Chlorpromazine—an antipsychotic medication in a group of drugs called phenothiazines used to treat disorders of schizophrenia.

Chronic pain—a pain state that is persistent and for which the cause cannot be removed or otherwise treated even after reasonable efforts.

Chronological Assessment of Suicide Events—also known as the CASE approach, a flexible interviewing strategy designed to efficiently uncover suicidal ideation, planning, behaviors, and intent in a patient.

Clomipramine—a tricyclic antidepressant used to treat obsessive–compulsive disorder (OCD), major depressive disorder, and other conditions. It is the only TCA with a serotonin reuptake mechanism robust enough to treat OCD.

Collaborative care—also referred to as integrated care; combines primary health care and mental health care in one setting.

Comorbidity—the state of having one or more diagnosable conditions.

Concentration—the amount of medication dissolved in the blood.

Conners Comprehensive Behavior Rating Scale—a tool used to assess and measure an array of behaviors, emotions, and problems for children between ages 6 and 18 years.

Continuation phase—the phase of treatment that follows the remission of symptoms after the acute phase and may be followed by the maintenance phase.

Critical appraisal—a systemic evaluation of the best course of treatment based on scholarly evidence.

D_2 dopamine receptor—the main receptor blocked by many antipsychotic drugs.

Delirium—a global impairment of cognitive processes due to metabolic derangements, such as low blood glucose inflammation from bacteria, or some other medical cause.

Delirium tremens—severe alcohol withdrawal symptoms such as shaking, confusion, and hallucinations.

Dendrite—the portion of the neuron that carries the electrical impulse toward the body.

Dependence—any one or the combination of cognitive, behavioral, and physical symptoms that indicate that the individual continues to use the substance in spite of significant harm or life problems.

Depot—an administration method in which a drug is released consistently over an extended period (days or weeks).

Discontinuation syndrome—a condition that can occur after changing, discontinuing, or interrupting an antidepressant.

Distribution—the process by which drugs are transported throughout the body and brain (the bloodstream).

Disulfiram (Antabuse)—a drug that interferes with the metabolism of alcohol, leading to the accumulation of acetaldehyde and its attendant unpleasant symptoms.

Dopamine—a hormone and neurotransmitter that plays many important roles in the brain and body, including reward-motivated behavior.

Dorsal cingulate cortex—a part of the brain that promotes cognition and motor control.

Dorsal column stimulator—a device used to treat certain pain conditions by sending electrical signals to select areas of the spinal cord.

Dysregulation—the inability of a person to control or regulate their emotional responses.

ECT (electroconvulsive therapy)—a medical treatment most commonly used in patients with severe major depression or bipolar disorder who have not responded to other treatments.

Emotion regulation—the ability to manage one's emotional state.

Endogenous opiate system—an innate pain-relieving system consisting of widely scattered neurons that produce opioids.

Ethnopharmacology—the study of drug behavior in different ethnic groups.

Excretion—the elimination of a drug from the body, through a pathway such as the kidney or liver.

Executive function—a set of mental skills that are necessary for cognitive control of behavior, including working memory, flexible thinking, and self-control.

Expressed emotion (EE)—how the family members of an identified patient talk about the patient voluntarily; high expressed emotion includes hostility, a high level of criticism, and intolerance.

Family psychoeducation (FPE)—programs and information for families about the illness, medication management, and treatment planning, delivered to assist in coping and managing the effects of the illness on the whole family.

Fluoxetine—a selective serotonin reuptake inhibitor used to treat depression, panic, anxiety, and obsessive–compulsive symptoms.

Functional brain circuit—a neural circuit that consists of neurons that are interconnected by synapses and carry a specific function.

Gabapentin—a medication that reduces anxiety by augmenting the efficiency of the brain's GABA systems. It is also used to prevent seizures and the pain caused by seizures.

Gamma-aminobutyric acid (GABA)—the brain's major inhibitory neurotransmitter, it attenuates the salience network's capability for generating fear. It is also used recreationally and as a date-rape drug.

Glial cells—the "supporting cells" of the nervous system; surround neurons and hold them in place, supply nutrients and oxygen to neurons, insulate one neuron from another, and destroy and remove the dead neurons.

Half-life—the time required for a medication to decrease its concentration by 50% in relation to its peak level.

Hamilton Depression Scale (HAM-D)—a measurement tool used to determine a patient's level of depression.

Hedonia—a condition of pleasure and cheerfulness.

Heterocyclic—refers to a compound whose molecule contains a ring of atoms of at least two elements, where one is generally carbon.

Hormone replacement therapy—a treatment for the common symptoms of menopause and to ameliorate long-term biological changes caused by declining levels of estrogen and progesterone.

Hyperalgesia—a heightened perception of pain.

Hyperglycemia—elevated blood sugar; it can be caused by an underlying disease, high carbohydrate meals, or side effects from medication.

Hyperlipidemia—elevated blood fats, which can be caused by foods that have cholesterol, saturated fats, and trans fats. It is diagnosed by blood tests and often doesn't cause any symptoms.

Hypomania—an emotional state characterized by elevated mood (euphoria), but not so extreme to cause impairment.

Imipramine—a tricyclic antidepressant used to treat depression, anxiety, panic disorder, and in some cases, bedwetting.

Insula—small region of the cerebral cortex located deep within the brain between the frontal and temporal lobes.

Insulin resistance—when cells in the muscles, body fat, and liver start resisting or ignoring the signal that the hormone insulin sends out—which is to grab the glucose out of the bloodstream and put it in your cells.

Integrated care—also referred to as collaborative care; combines primary health care and mental health care in one setting.

Internalized stigma—feelings of alienation, social withdrawal, discrimination, and changes in self-identity as a result of receiving a mental health diagnosis or treatment.

Intramuscular—inside the muscle.

Intrinsic connectivity networks (ICN)—the set of large-scale functionally connected brain networks.

Isomers—ions or molecules with the same formulas but different structures.

K-2—synthetic cannabinoids that often contain other drugs, such as methamphetamine.

Lamotrigine—an anticonvulsant medication that is also used as a mood stabilizer. It's used to treat seizures in adults and children and delay mood episodes in adults with bipolar disorder.

Lithium carbonate—an antimanic agent used to treat bipolar disorder and prevent cluster headaches.

Lithium toxicity—also known as lithium overdose; occurs when a person takes too much of a lithium generally taken as a mood-stabilizing medication for bipolar disorder and major depressive disorder.

Maintenance phase—the final stage of recovery where the person learns to successfully avoid triggers and temptations that can lead to a relapse.

Major depression with psychotic features—a serious mental disorder where the person experiences a combination of depressed mood and psychosis.

Mania—a state of elevated mood with abnormally elevated arousal, affect, and energy level usually associated with bipolar disorder.

Medication-assisted treatment—treatment that combines behavioral therapy and medication to assist in substance abuse.

Melancholic depression—a form of major depressive disorder characterized by melancholic features.

Mentalization—ability to understand the mental state, of oneself or others, that controls observable behavior.

Metabolic syndrome—a set of conditions that occur together and increase the risk of heart disease, stroke, and type 2 diabetes.

Metabolism—the process of the body's elimination or transformation of a drug.

Methadone—long-lasting opioid medication used in medication-assisted treatment of opioid addiction to prevent withdrawal symptoms that would otherwise prompt drug craving.

Mild cognitive impairment—the intermediate stage between age-related cognitive decline and dementia.

Mini-Mental Status Exam—a standardized exam used to measure cognitive impairment.

Mirror neuron system—a group of specialized neurons that mimics the actions and behaviors of others.

Monoamine—a neurotransmitter part of a chemical group that is composed of one amino group.

Monoamine oxidase inhibitors (MAOIs)—a class of antidepressant medications whose action is to deactivate the enzyme monoamine-oxidase, which normally would degrade norepinephrine, serotonin, and dopamine released by axon terminals into synaptic clefts. Deactivation causes these neurotransmitters to accumulate in the synaptic cleft.

Monoamine systems—the primary target of psychostimulant activity, which includes dopamine, noradrenaline, and serotonin neurotransmitters.

Monotherapy—the use of one type of treatment or drug to treat a disease or condition.

Naloxone—medication designed to rapidly reverse an opioid overdose.

Naltrexone—opioid-antagonist drug for the treatment of alcohol dependence.

Negative symptoms—defined by the absence of something, such as enthusiasm (apathy) and desire for social interaction (social withdrawal).

Neural tube defects—birth defects of the brain and spinal cord.

Neurodegenerative—the breakdown of neurons and the nervous system.

Neurogenesis—the process by which nerve cells are generated in the brain.

Neuroleptic malignant syndrome—a rare but potentially fatal condition that can develop in patients treated with conventional antipsychotics, it is caused by blockage of dopamine receptors.

Neurons—nerve cells.

Neurotransmission—the process by which neurotransmitters are released by the axon terminal of a neuron and bind to and react with the receptors on the dendrites of another neuron.

Neurotransmitters—chemicals within a neuron that allow one neuron to transmit an impulse to another.

NMDA glutaminergic receptors—a glutamate receptor and ion channel protein found in nerve cells.

Nociception—the physical transmission of danger signals from sensory organs.

Noradrenergic pathways—a system that creates elevated arousal in stress.

Norepinephrine—a neurotransmitter primarily secreted by the sympathetic nervous system.

Normal syndrome of distress—disorders that produce normal levels of distress and are not considered psychiatric.

Obesity—a state of excessive fat tissue in the body, defined by a body mass index of 30 or more.

Oxycontin—slow-release form of the opioid oxycodone.

Parasympathetic nervous system—the part of the nervous system that causes a focused response of a particular organ and prevents the body from overworking by restoring it to a calm state.

Parenterally—the administration of a drug by a route other than the digestive system.

Patient navigator—a person who helps patients and families learn how systems of care operate and how to solicit system resources, such as financial and legal support.

Peak concentration—the time required for a drug to go from ingestion to its maximum concentration in the bloodstream.

Pharmacodynamics—the mechanism of drug action and the relationship between drug concentration and the effects (positive and negative) that it has.

Pharmacokinetics—the processes and rates of absorption, metabolism, half-lives, distribution, and elimination of medications in the body.

Phenelzine—a monoamine oxidase inhibitor (MAOI) that increases chemicals in the brain to treat symptoms of depression.

Plasma levels—the concentration of a drug in the plasma.

Polydrug—use of more than one type of drug, either at the same time or at different times.

Polysomnogram—known as a sleep study, a test used to diagnose sleep disorders by recording brain waves, heart rate, and other physiological metrics.

Positive symptoms—defined by the presence of something, such as hallucinations, delusions, jumbled thoughts, and strange behavior.

Practice guidelines—documents aimed to optimize treatment by systematic analysis of treatment options, including the potential risks and benefits of each option.

Prefrontal cortex—the cerebral cortex that covers the front part of the frontal lobe; implicated in planning, personality expression, decision making, and moderating social behavior.

Pregabalin—a medication that reduces anxiety by augmenting the efficiency of the brain's GABA systems. It is also an antiepileptic drug.

Psychomotor retardation—consists of slowed speech, movement, and cognition.

Psychotropic medication—a drug that affects the mind, behavior, and emotions by adjusting levels of brain chemicals, or neurotransmitters.

Rapid cycling—indicates the particular speed of mood swings in bipolar disorder, defined by four or more mood swings (depression, mania, or hypomania) within a year.

Rapid metabolizers—individuals who metabolize medications too quickly to experience relief from symptoms.

Recovery Movement—a consumer-driven movement that affirms that patients with chronic psychotic disorders are able to achieve significant degrees of life satisfaction and that these patients ought to become partners with mental health professionals in the delivery of care (providing peer expertise to other patients for instance).

Refractory—difficult to control and resistant to treatment.

Remission—complete resolution of illness or symptoms.

Reuptake—the process of extra neurotransmitters in the synapse being taken back into the presynaptic neuron.

Risk–benefit ratio—the process of selecting a medication that will produce the strongest possible therapeutic effect with the fewest possible side effects.

Salience network—a collection of regions in the brain that detect and filter stimuli.

Seasonal depression—depression that occurs at the same time every year.

Selegiline—a monoamine oxidase inhibitor MAOI that can be absorbed via a transdermal patch directly through the skin into the bloodstream without entering the gastrointestinal tract.

Serotonergic pathways—involved in the regulation of mood, eating, sleep, nociception, body temperature, vomiting, and emotional behaviors.

Serotonin—a monoamine neurotransmitter that serves a variety of biological functions and physiological processes, including feelings of well-being and happiness.

Serotonin syndrome—a very dangerous syndrome caused by high levels of serotonin, a severe form can be lethal if not treated quickly. Other symptoms include hyperthermia, coma, and seizures.

Shame attenuation—a technique to reframe suicidal thoughts as a response to stressful events.

Shared decision making—the process of reaching a consensus on a treatment plan by allowing all stakeholders to participate.

Signaling pathway—a group of molecules in a cell that work together to control one or more cell functions, such as cell division or cell death.

Sleep logs—a systematic recording of a patient's sleep, including bedtime, time falling asleep, number of awakenings during the night, awakening time, and the number of naps during the day.

Slow metabolizers—individuals who metabolize medications too slowly, which makes side effects more pronounced.

SNRI (serotonin–norepinephrine reuptake inhibitors)—inhibit the reuptake of serotonin and norepinephrine after they have been released into the synaptic cleft. They are used to treat a number of symptoms and disorders, including major depressive disorder, anxiety disorders, obsessive–compulsive disorder (OCD), menopausal symptoms, and others.

Social cognition—the part of social psychology that studies how people store, process, apply information about other people or social situations.

Soma—a cell body that contains the nucleus.

Somnolence—marked by a powerful desire to sleep, or the act of sleeping for excessive amounts of time.

Spina bifida—a type of neural tube defect in which a portion of the spine or spinal cord don't develop normally.

Split care—collocated care where physicians treat only the biological part of patients by prescribing medication, leaving therapists to treat the rest.

SSRI (selective serotonin reuptake inhibitor)—inhibit the reuptake of serotonin after it has been released into the synaptic cleft; they are typically used in the treatment of major depressive, anxiety, and obsessive–compulsive disorders.

STAR*D—Sequenced Treatment Alternatives to Relieve Depression, a large, important study conducted by the National Institute of Mental Health to study the treatment of depression; it revealed helpful information about the benefits and limitations of a sequence of treatment strategies as well as the minimum duration and dosages of such treatments.

Steady state—the amount of time required for a drug to reach a balanced concentration level in the bloodstream.

Subcallosal cingulate gyrus—the portion of the cingulum that includes cortical structures, the limbic system, thalamus, hypothalamus, and brainstem nuclei.

Sympathetic nervous system—the part of the autonomic nervous system that has multiorgan impact, such as the fight-or-flight response.

Synapse—the tiny space between two neurons.

Systematic reviews—a literature review that assesses, condenses, and synthesizes the findings of multiple controlled studies to provide a high level of evidence for the best course of treatment.

T3 (Cytomel)—a synthetic thyroid hormone used to augment an antidepressant.

T4 (thyroxine)—a thyroid hormone used to augment an antidepressant.

Tardive dyskinesia—the abnormal involuntary movements, especially of the tongue, mouth, and face, can occur after long-term use of antipsychotic medications.

Teratogenic effects—causing harm or deformity to a developing fetus.

Therapeutic index—the difference in doses of medication between a dose that produces serious side effects and the dose needed for therapeutic effectiveness.

Therapeutic window—the blood level below and above which a drug does not work well.

TMS (transcranial magnetic stimulation)—a noninvasive neuromodulation treatment in which an electromagnetic field is used to generate small electrical currents within the prefrontal cortex of a patient's brain.

Tolerance—the need to consume progressively larger quantities of the substance (e.g., alcohol, benzodiazepines, or opiates) to achieve intoxication or the desired effect, or the state of needing a progressively increasing dose in order to maintain a sense of normality.

Top-down regulation—a set of mechanisms through which the brain can be damped or suppressing incoming nociceptive information, tempering any behavioral responses to it.

Transcutaneous nerve stimulator—a device that uses low-voltage electric currents to treat pain.

Tranylcypromine—a monoamine oxidase inhibitor (MAOI) and antidepressant available as a tablet for oral ingestion.

Tricyclic—antidepressant medications that have three rings in their chemical structure.

Trough levels—the point at which the concentration of a medication in the bloodstream is at its lowest just before the ingestion of the next scheduled dose.

Unipolar depression—depression without mania.

Vagus nerve—a long, cranial nerve that interacts with the parasympathetic control of many organs in the body.

Valproic acid—one of only a few drugs to be approved by the U.S. Food and Drug Administration for treating acute mania.

Venlafaxine—known by the brand name Effexor, a selective serotonin-norepinephrine reuptake inhibitor (SSNRI).

Ventral anterior cingulate gyrus—involved when effort is needed to carry out a task, such as in early learning or problem solving.

Withdrawal—a syndrome of very unpleasant cognitive, psychological, and physical symptoms that occurs when the amount of the substance declines in the bloodstream.

Yale–Brown Obsessive Compulsive Rating Scale (Y-BOCS)—a measure designed to assess the severity of obsessive–compulsive disorder (OCD) symptoms and to detect changes during treatment.

References

Abramowicz, M. (2000). Rivastigmine (Exelon) for Alzheimer's disease. *Medical Letter on Drugs and Therapeutics, 42,* 93–94.

Abramowicz, M. (2001). Galantamine (Reminyl) for Alzheimer's disease. *Medical Letter on Drugs and Therapeutics, 43,* 53–54.

Abramowicz, M. (2003). Memantine for Alzheimer's disease. *Medical Letter on Drugs and Therapeutics, 45,* 73–74.

Adler, L., Slootsky, V., Griffith, J. L., & Khin Khin, E. (2016). Teaching the fundamentals of the risk assessment interview to clinicians. *Psychiatric Annals, 46,* 293–297.

American Psychiatric Association. (2013). *Diagnostic and statistical manual of mental disorders* (5th ed.). Arlington, VA: Author.

Anderson, R. J., Frye, M. A., Abulseoud, O. A., Lee, K. H., McGillivray, J. A., Berk, M., et al. (2012). Deep brain stimulation for treatment-resistant depression: Efficacy, safety and mechanisms of action. *Neuroscience and Biobehavioral Reviews, 36*(8), 1920–1933.

Andre, C. (2011). *Looking at mindfulness.* New York: Blue Rider Press.

Bagge, C. L., Glenn, C. R., & Lee, H. J. (2013). Quantifying the impact of recent negative life events on suicide attempts. *Journal of Abnormal Psychology, 122,* 359–368.

Bajor, L. A., Ticlea, A. N., & Osser, D. N. (2011). The psychopharmacology algorithm project at the Harvard south shore program: An update on post-traumatic stress disorder. *Harvard Review of Psychiatry, 19*(5), 240–258.

Baldwin, D. S., Anderson, I. M., & Nutt, D. J. (2014). Evidence-based pharmacological treatment of anxiety disorders, post-traumatic stress disorder, and obsessive-compulsive disorder: A revision of the 2005 guidelines from the British Association of Psychopharmacology. *Journal of Psychopharmacology, 28,* 403–439.

Balon, R., & Segraves, R. T. (2008). Survey of treatment practices for sexual dysfunction(s) associated with antidepressants. *Journal of Sex and Marital Therapy, 34,* 353.

Barlow, D. H. (2002). *Anxiety and its disorders: The nature and treatment of anxiety and panic* (2nd ed.). New York: Guilford Press.

Barlow, D. H., & Craske, M. G. (2006). *Mastery of your anxiety and panic* (4th ed.). New York: Oxford University Press.

Barsaglini, A., Sartori, G., Benetti, S., Pettersson-Yeo, W., & Mechelli, A. (2014). The effects of psychotherapy on brain function: A systematic and critical review. *Progress in Neurobiology, 114,* 1–14.

Bauer, M., & Dopfmer, S. (1999). Lithium augmentation in treatment-resistant depression: Meta-analysis of placebo-controlled studies. *Journal of Clinical Psychopharmacology, 19,* 427–434.

Baum, A. L., & Misri, S. (1996). Selective serotonin-reuptake inhibitors in pregnancy and lactation. *Harvard Review of Psychiatry, 4*(3), 117–125.

Beitman, B. D., Blinder, B. J., Thase, M. E., Riba, M., & Safer, D. L. (2003). *Integrating psychotherapy and pharmacotherapy: Dissolving the mind–brain barrier.* New York: Norton.

Berlant, J. (2006). Topiramate as a therapy for chronic posttraumatic stress disorder. *Psychiatry (Edgmont), 3,* 40–45.

Berman, E. M., Heru, A., Grunebaum, H., Rolland, J., Sargent, J., Wamboldt, M., et al. (2008). Family-oriented patient care through the residency training cycle. *Academic Psychiatry, 32,* 111–118.

Bianchi, M. T., Smallwood, P., Quinn, D. K., & Stern, T. A. (2018). Patients with disordered sleep. In T. A. Stern, O. Freudenreich, F. A. Smith, G. I. Fricchione, & J. F. Rosenbaum (Eds.), *Massachusetts General Hospital handbook of General Hospital psychiatry* (7th ed., pp. 267–278). New York: Elsevier.

Bjorkholm, C., & Monteggia, L. M. (2016). BDNF—a key transducer of antidepressant effects. *Neuropharmacology, 102,* 72–79.

Blendy, J. A. (2006). The role of CREB in depression and antidepressant treatment. *Biological Psychiatry, 59,* 1144–1150.

Boisen, A. T. (1936/1962). *The exploration of the inner world: A study of mental disorder and religious experience.* New York: Harper & Brothers.

Bray, J. H., & Rogers, J. C. (1997). The linkages project: Training behavioral health professionals for collaborative practice with primary care physicians. *Families, Systems, and Health, 15*(1), 55–63.

Busch, K. A., Fawcett, J., & Jacobs, D. G. (2003). Clinical correlates of inpatient suicide. *Journal of Clinical Psychiatry, 64,* 14–19.

Cameron, R. P., & Schatzberg, A. F. (2002). Mixed anxiety-depressive disorder. In D. J. Stein & E. Hollander (Eds.), *Textbook of anxiety disorders,* (pp. 159–172). Washington, DC: American Psychiatric Publishing.

Caplan, J. P. (2018). Delirious patients. In T. A. Stern, O. Freudenreich, F. A. Smith, G .L. Fricchione, & J. F. Rosenbaum (Eds.), *Massachusetts General Hospital handbook of General Hospital psychiatry* (7th ed., pp. 83–94). New York: Elsevier.

Chadwick, P. K. (2009). *Schizophrenia: The positive perspective.* New York: Routledge.

Cipriani, A., Furukawa, T. A., Salanti, G., Chaimani, A., Atkinson, L. Z., Ogawa, Y., et al. (2018). Comparative efficacy and acceptability of 21 antidepressant drugs for the acute treatment of adults with major depressive disorder: A systematic review and network meta-analysis. *Lancet, 391,* 1357–1366.

Citrome, L. (2014). Treatment of bipolar depression: Making sensible decisions. *CNS Spectrums, 19,* 4–12.

Clark, C. M., Sheppard, L., Fillenbaum, G. G., Galasko, D., Morris, J. C., Koss, E., et al. (1999). Variability in annual Mini-Mental State Examination score in patients with probable Alzheimer's disease: A clinical perspective of data from the Consortium to Establish a Registry for Alzheimer's Disease. *Archives of Neurology, 56*(7), 857–862.

Clarkin, J., Carpenter, D., Hull, J., Wilner, P., & Glick, I. (1998). Effects of psychoeducational intervention for married patients with bipolar disorder and their spouses. *Psychiatric Services, 49*(4), 531–533.

Clomipramine Collaborative Study Group. (1991). Clomipramine in the treatment of patients with obsessive–compulsive disorder. *Archives of General Psychiatry, 48*(8), 730–738.

Coldham, E., Addington, J., & Addington, D. (2002). Medication adherence of individuals with a first episode of psychosis. *Acta Psychiatrica Scandinavica, 106*(4), 286–290.

Cole-Kelly, K., & Seaburn, D. (1999). Five areas of questioning to promote a family-oriented approach in primary care. *Families, Systems, and Health, 17,* 341–348.

Consensus Development Conference on Antipsychotic Drugs and Obesity and Diabetes. (2004). *Diabetes Care, 27*(2), 596–601.

Cook, S. R., & Evans, K. A. (2018). Obesity. In O. J. Z. Sahler, J. E. Carr, J. B. Frank, & J. V. Nunes (Eds.), *The behavioral sciences and healthcare* (4th ed., pp. 197–203). Boston: Hogrefe.

Council for Training in Evidence-Based Behavioral Practice. (2008, July). Definition and competencies for evidence-based behavioral practice (EBBP). Retrieved May 19, 2020, from *https://ebbp.org/home/competencies.*

Coyne, J. (2000). Psychotropic drug use in very young children. *Journal of the American Medical Association, 283*(8), 1059–1060.

Curtiss, C. P. (2001). JCAHO meeting the standards for pain management. *Orthopaedic Nursing, 20,* 27–30.

Davidson, J. R. T. (2003). Pharmacotherapy of social phobia *Acta Psychiatrica Scandinavica, 108*(417), 65–71.

De Figueiredo, J. M., & Griffith, J. (2016). Chronic pain, chronic demoralization, and the role of psychotherapy. *Journal of Contemporary Psychotherapy, 46,* 167–177.

Depression Guideline Panel. (1993). *Depression in primary care: Vol. 2. Treatment of major depression* (Clinical Practice Guideline No. 5; AHCPR Publication No. 93-0551). Rockville, MD: U.S. Department of Health and Human Services, Public Health Service, Agency for Health Care Policy and Research.

Dickson, R., Williams, R., & Dalby, J. (1995). The clozapine experience from a family perspective. *Canadian Journal of Psychiatry, 40,* 627–629.

Edwards, T. M., & Patterson, J. (2006). Supervising family therapy trainees in primary care medical settings: Context matters. *Journal of Marital and Family Therapy, 32,* 33–43.

Eisen, J. L., Sibrava N. J., Boisseau, C. L., Mancebo, M. C., Stout, R. L., Pinto, A., et al. (2013). Five-year course of obsessive–compulsive disorder: Predictors of remission and relapse. *Journal of Clinical Psychiatry, 74*(3), 233–239.

El-Mallakh, R. S., Vohringer, P. A., Ostacher, M. M., Baldassano, C. F., Holtzman, N. S., Whitlam, E. A., et al. (2015). Antidepressants worsen rapid-cycling course in bipolar disorder: A STEP-BD randomized control trial. *Journal of Affective Disorders, 184,* 318–321.

Engel, G. L. (1980). The clinical application of the biopsychosocial model. *American Journal of Psychiatry, 137*(5), 535–544.

Epperson, N., Czarkowski, K. A., Ward-O'Brien, D., Weiss, E., Gueorguieva, R., Jatlow, P., et al. (2001). Maternal sertraline treatment and serotonin transport in breast-feeding mother–infant pairs. *American Journal of Psychiatry, 158*(10), 1631–1637.

Erickson, M. H. (1980). On the nature of hypnosis. In E. Rossi (Ed.), *The collected works of Milton H. Erickson on Hypnosis: Vol. I. The nature of hypnosis and suggestion* (pp. 1–132). New York: Irvington.

Erickson, M. H., & Erickson, E. M. (1980). The hypnotic induction of hallucinatory color vision followed by pseudonegative afterimages. In E. Rossi (Ed.), *The collected works of Milton H. Erickson on hypnosis: Vol. II. Hypnotic alteration of sensory, perceptual and psychophysiological processes* (pp. 5–32). New York: Irvington.

Fava, M., & Davidson, K. G. (1996). Definition and epidemiology of treatment-resistant depression. *Psychiatric Clinic of North America, 19*(2), 179–200.

Fawcett, J., Scheftner, W. A., Fogg, L., Clark, D. C., Young, M. A., Hedeker, D., et al. (1990). Time-related predictors of suicide in major affective disorders. *American Journal of Psychiatry, 147,* 1189–1194.

Fazel, S., & Runeson, B. (2020). Suicide. *New England Journal of Medicine, 382*(3), 266–274.

Flier, J. S. (2001). Obesity. In E. Braunwald, A. C. Fauci, D. L. Kasper, S. L. Hauser, D. L. Longo, & J. L. Jameson (Eds.), *Harrison's principles of internal medicine* (15th ed.). New York: McGraw-Hill.

Foa, E. B., & Yadin, E. (2012). *Exposure and response (ritual) prevention for obsessive–compulsive disorder: Therapist guide* (2nd ed.). New York: Oxford University Press.

Folstein, M. F., Folstein, S. E., & McHugh, P. R. (1975). "Mini-mental state": A practical method for grading the cognitive state of patients for the clinician. *Journal of Psychiatry Research, 12*(3), 189–198.

Fox-Rawlings, S., & Zuckerman, D. (2018). Is TMS proven effective for depression? *National Center for Health Research.* Retrieved from *www.center4research.org/wp-content/uploads/201811/NCHR-Analysis-of-TMS-Effectiveness.pdf.*

Frank, E. (1997). Enhancing patient outcomes: Treatment adherence. *Journal of Clinical Psychiatry, 58*(Suppl. 1), 11–14.

Frank, E., Kupfer, D. J., Perel, J. M., Cornes, C., Jarrett, D. B., Mallinger, A. G., et al. (1990). Three-year outcomes for maintenance therapies in recurrent depression. *Archives of General Psychiatry, 47,* 1093–1099.

Frank, J. D., & Frank, J. B. (1991). *Persuasion and healing: A comparative study of psychotherapy* (3rd ed.). Baltimore, MD: Johns Hopkins Press.

Frasure-Smith, N., Lesperance, F., & Talajic, M. (1993). Depression following myocardial infarction: Impact on 6-month survival. *Journal of the American Medical Association, 270,* 1819–1825.

Geddes, J. R., Carney, S. M., Davies, C., Furukawa, T. A., Kupfer, D. J., Frank, E., et al. (2003). Relapse prevention with antidepressant drug treatment in depressive disorders: A systematic review. *Lancet, 361,* 653–661.

Gitlin, M. J. (1996). *The psychotherapist's guide to psychopharmacology* (2nd ed.). New York: Free Press.

Glassman, A. H., O'Connor, C. M., Califf, R. M., Swedberg, K., Schwartz, O., Bigger, J. T. (2002). Sertraline treatment of major depression in patients with acute MI or unstable angina. *JAMA, 288,* 701–709.

Goebel-Fabbri, A., Musen, G., & Levenson, J. L. (2010). Endocrine and metabolic disorders. In J. L. Levenson (Ed.), *Textbook of psychosomatic medicine: Psychiatric care of the medically ill* (2nd ed., pp. 503–524). Washington, DC: American Psychiatric Publishing.

Gonzalez, S., Steinglass, P., & Reiss, D. (1989). Putting the illness in its place: Discussion groups for families with chronic medical illnesses. *Family Process, 28,* 69–87.

Goodwin, F. K., & Jamison, K. R. (2007). *Manic–depressive illness: Bipolar disorders and recurrent depression.* New York: Oxford University Press.

Griffith, J. L. (2010). *Religion that heals, religion that harms.* New York: Guilford Press.

Griffith, J. L. (2018). Hope modules: Brief psychotherapeutic interventions to counter demoralization from daily stressors of chronic illness. *Academic Psychiatry, 42,* 135–145.

Griffith, J. L., & Gaby, L. (2005). Brief psychotherapy at the bedside: Countering demoralization from medical illness. *Psychosomatics, 46,* 109–116.

Griffith, J. L., & Norris, L. (2012). Distinguishing spiritual, psychological, and psychiatric issues in palliative care: Their overlap and differences. *Progress in Palliative Care, 20,* 79–85.

Groopman, J. (2004). The anatomy of hope: How people prevail in the face of illness. New York: Random House.

Gross, J. J. (Ed.). (2007). *Handbook of emotion regulation.* New York: Guilford Press.

Grumbach, K., & Bodenheimer, T. (2004). Can health care teams improve primary care practice? *Journal of the American Medical Association, 291*(10), 1246–1251.

Hall, R. C., Platt, D. E., & Hall, R. C. (1999). Suicide risk assessment: A review of risk factors for suicide in 100 patients who made severe suicide attempts: Evaluation of suicide risk in a time of managed care. *Psychosomatics, 40,* 18–27.

Hamilton, M. (1960). A rating scale for depression. *Journal of Neurology, Neurosurgery, and Psychiatry, 23,* 56–62.

Hans-Ulrich W., & Hoyer, J. (2001). Generalized anxiety disorder: Nature and course. *Journal of Clinical Psychiatry, 62*(Suppl. 11), 15–19.

Hansen, B. (2005). The dodo manifesto. *Australian and New Zealand Journal of Family Therapy, 26,* 210–218.

Hasnain, M., Vieweg, V. R., Baron, M. S., Beatty-Brooks, M., Fernandez, A., & Pandurangi, A. K. (2009). Pharmacological management of psychosis in elderly patients with Parkinsonism. *American Journal of Medicine, 122,* 614–622.

Haynes, R. B., McDonald, H. P., & Garg, A. X. (2002). Helping patients follow prescribed treatment: Clinical applications. *Journal of the American Medical Association, 288,* 2880–2883.

Health, B., & Beller, J. (2019). *Dementia types, risk factors, and symptoms.* Authors.

Hernandez, B. C., & Doherty, W. J. (2005). Marriage and family therapists and psychotropic medications: Practice patterns from a national study. *Journal of Marital and Family Therapy, 31*(3), 177–189.

Hooley, J. M. (2007). Expressed emotion and relapse of psychopathology. *Annual Review of Clinical Psychology, 3,* 329–352.

Horwitz, A. V., & Wakefield, J. C. (2007). *The loss of sadness: How psychiatry transformed normal sadness into depressive disorder.* New York: Oxford University Press.

Horwitz, A. V., & Wakefield, J. C. (2012). *All we have to fear: Psychiatry's transformation of normal anxieties into mental disorders.* New York: Oxford University Press.

Horwitz, S., Higham, S., Bennett, D., & Kornfield, M. (2019, December 9). Inside the industry's marketing machine. *The Washington Post,* pp. A1–A16.

Insel, T. (2012, February 24). NIMH spotlight on eating disorders. Retrieved from *www.nimh.nih.gov.*

Inskip, H. M., Harris, E. C., & Barraclough, B. (1998). Lifetime risk of suicide for affective disorder, alcoholism and schizophrenia. *British Journal of Psychiatry, 172,* 35–37.

Institute of Medicine. (2012). *Best care at lower cost: The path to continuously learning health care in America.* Washington, DC: National Academies Press.

Ivbijaro, G. (2012). *Companion to primary care mental health.* London: Radcliffe.

Jamison, K. R. (1993). *Touched with fire: Manic-depressive illness and the artistic temperament.* New York: Free Press.

Jamison, K. R. (2009). *Nothing was the same: A memoir.* New York: Knopf.

Jewell, T. C., Downing, D., & McFarlane, W. R. (2009). Partnering with families: Multiple family group psychoeducation for schizophrenia. *Journal of Clinical Psychology, 65,* 868–878.

Joiner, T. (2005). *Why people die by suicide.* Cambridge, MA: Harvard University Press.

Joynt, K. E., & O'Connor, C. M. (2005). Lessons from SADHART, ENRICHD, and other trials. *Psychosomatic Medicine, 67,* S63–S66.

Kampman, K., & Jarvis, M. (2015). American Society of Addiction Medicine (ASAM) National Practice Guideline for the use of medications in the treatment of addiction involving opioid use. *Journal of Addiction Medicine, 9,* 358–367.

Kandel, E. R. (1995). Neuropeptides, adenylyl cyclase, and memory storage. *Science, 268,* 825–826.

Kandel, E. R. (1998). A new intellectual framework for psychiatry. *American Journal of Psychiatry, 155,* 457–469.

Kandel, E. R. (2006). *In search of memory.* New York: Norton.

Kane, J. M., Marder, S. R., Schooler, N. R., Wirshing, W. C., Umbricht, D., Baker, R. W., et al. (2001). Clozapine and haloperidol in moderately refractory schizophrenia: A 6-month randomized and double-blind comparison. *Archives of General Psychiatry, 58*(10), 965–972.

Kavan, M. G., Elsasser, G. N., & Barone, E. J. (2009). Generalized anxiety disorder: Practical assessment and management. *American Family Physician, 79,* 785–791.

Kessler, R. C., McGonagle, K. A., Zhao, S., Nelson, C. B., Hughes, M., Eshleman, S., et al. (1994). Lifetime and 12-month prevalence of DSM-III-R psychiatric disorders in the United States: Results from the national comorbidity survey. *Archives of General Psychiatry, 51*(1), 8–19.

Kessler, R. C., Sonnega, A., Bromet, E., Hughes, M., & Nelson, C. B. (1995). Post-traumatic stress disorder in the National Comorbidity Survey. *Archives of General Psychiatry, 52*(12), 1048–1060.

Kessler, R. C., Stein, M. B., & Berglund, P. (1998). Social phobia subtypes in the National Comorbidity Survey. *American Journal of Psychiatry, 155,* 613–619.

Kinney, J. (Ed.). (1989). *The busy physician's five-minute guide to the management of alcohol problems.* Chicago: American Medical Association.

Kirsch, I., Moore, T. J., Scoboria, A., & Nicholls, S. S. (2002). The emperor's new drugs: An analysis of antidepressant medication data submitted to the U.S. Food and Drug Administration. *Prevention and Treatment, 5*(1), Article 23.

Kissling, W. (1991). The current unsatisfactory state of relapse prevention in schizophrenic psychoses—Suggestions for improvement. *Clinical Neuropharmacology, 14*(Suppl. 2), 33–44.

Kohrt, B., Griffith, J. L., & Patel, V. (2018). Chronic pain and mental health: Integrated solutions for global problems. *Pain, 159,* S85–S90.

Kotcher, M., & Smith, T. (1993). Three phases of clozapine treatment and phase-specific issues for patients and families. *Hospital and Community Psychiatry, 44*(8), 744–747.

Kraepelin, E. (1971). *Dementia praecox and paraphrenia.* Huntington, NY: Krieger. (Original work published 1919)

Kraepelin, E. (1976). *Manic-depressive insanity and paranoia* (reprint ed.). New York: Arno Press.

Kramer, P. (2005). *Against depression.* New York: Viking.

Kroger, W. S. (1977). *Clinical and experimental hypnosis* (2nd ed.). Philadelphia: Lippincott.

Kulin, N. A., Pastuszak, A., Sage, S. R., Schick-Boschetto, B., Spivey, G., Feldkamp, M., et al. (1998). Pregnancy outcome following maternal use of the new selective serotonin reuptake inhibitors: A prospective controlled multicenter study. *Journal of the American Medical Association, 279*(8), 609–610.

Kupfer, D. J. (1991). Long-term treatment of depression. *Journal of Clinical Psychiatry, 52*(Suppl. 5), 28–34.

Kupfer, D. J. (2005). The increasing medical burden in bipolar disorder. *Journal of the American Medical Association, 293*(20), 2528–2530.

Laird, A. R., Fox, P. M., Eickhoff, S. B., Turner, J. A., Ray, K. L., McKay, D. R., et al. (2011). Behavioral interpretations of intrinsic connectivity networks. *Journal of Cognitive Neuroscience, 23,* 4022–4037.

Lebowitz, B., Shores-Wilson, K. S., Rush, A. J., & STAR*D Study Team. (2006). A comparison of lithium and T3 augmentation following two failed medication treatments for depression: A STAR*D report. *American Journal of Psychiatry, 163,* 1519–1530.

Levine, P. A. (2010). *In an unspoken voice: How the body releases trauma and restores goodness.* Berkeley, CA: North Atlantic Books.

Lewis, G., Duffy, L., Ades, A., Amos, R., Araya, R., Brabyn, S., et al. (2019). The clinical effectiveness of sertraline in primary care and the role of depression severity and duration (PANDA): A pragmatic double-blind, placebo-controlled randomized trial. *The Lancet Psychiatry, 6,* 903–914.

Liebowitz, M. R., Hollander, E., Schneier, F., Campeas, R., Fallon, B., Welkowitz, L., et al. (1990). Anxiety and depression: Discrete diagnostic entities? *Journal of Clinical Psychopharmacology, 10*(3, Suppl.), 61S–66S.

Lindh, A. U., Dahlin, M., Beckman, K., Stromsten, L., Jokinen, J., Wiktorsson, S., et al. (2019). A comparison of suicide risk scales in predicting repeat suicide attempt and suicide: A clinical cohort study. *Journal of Clinical Psychiatry, 80*(6), 18m12707.

Loo, C. K., Sachdev, P., Martin, D., Pigot, M., Alonzo, A., Malhi, G. S., et al. (2010). A double-blind, sham-controlled trial of transcranial direct current stimulation for treatment of depression. *International Journal of Neuropsychopharmacology, 13,* 61–69.

Lucksted, A., McFarlane, W., Downing, D., Dixon, L., & Adams, C. (2012). Recent developments in family psychoeducation as an evidence-based practice. *Journal of Marital and Family Therapy, 38,* 101–121.

Luhrmann, T. M. (2000). *Of 2 minds: The growing disorder in American psychiatry.* New York: Knopf.

Lukoff, D. (2007). Visionary spiritual experiences. *Southern Medical Journal, 100,* 635–641.

Luukinen, H., Viramo, P., Koski, K., Laippala, P., & Kivela, S. L. (1999). Head injuries and cognitive decline among older adults: A population-based study. *Neurology, 52*(3), 557–562.

Marder, S. R., Essock, S. M., Miller, A. L., Buchanan, R. W., Casey, D. E., Davis, J. M., et al. (2004). Physical health monitoring of patients with schizophrenia. *American Journal of Psychiatry, 161*(8), 1334–1349.

Mathew, S. J., Hoffman, E. J., & Charney, D. S. (2009). Pharmacotherapy of anxiety disorders. In D. S. Charney & E. F. Nestler (Eds.), *Neurobiology of mental illness* (3rd ed., pp. 731–754). New York: Oxford University Press.

McCourt, F. (1996). *Angela's ashes.* New York: Scribner.

McCutcheon, R. A., Marques, T. R., & Howes, O. D. (2020). Schizophrenia—an overview. *JAMA Psychiatry, 77*(2), 201–210.

McDaniel, S. H., Campbell, T. L., & Seaburn, D. B. (1995). Principles for collaboration between health and mental health providers in primary care. *Family Systems Medicine, 13*(3–4), 283–298.

McDaniel, S. H., Doherty, W. J., & Hepworth, J. (2014). *Medical family therapy and integrated care* (2nd ed.). Washington, DC: American Psychological Association.

McDonald, H., Garg, A., & Haynes, R. (2002). Interventions to enhance patient adherence to medication prescriptions: Scientific review. *Journal of the American Medical Association, 288*(22), 2868–2879.

McFarlane, W. R. (2009). Chapter 24: Family intervention for psychotic and severe mood disorder. In G. O. Gabbard (Ed.), *Textbook of psychotherapeutic treatments* (pp. 641–671). Washington, DC: American Psychiatric Publishing,

McFarlane, W. R. (2016). Family interventions for schizophrenia and the psychoses: A review. *Family Process, 55,* 460–482.

McFarlane, W. R., Dixon, L., Lukens, E., & Lucksted, A. (2003). Family psychoeducation and schizophrenia: A review of literature. *Journal of Marital and Family Therapy, 29,* 223–246.

McRae, K., Misra, S., Prasad, A. K., Pereira, S. C., & Gross, J. J. (2012). Bottom-up and top-down emotion generation: Implications for emotion generation. *SCAN, 7,* 253–262.

MGH Center for Women's Mental Health. (n.d.). Psychiatric disorders during pregnancy.

Miklowitz, D. J. (2004). The role of family systems in severe and recurrent psychiatric disorders: A developmental psychopathology view. *Developmental Psychopathology, 16*(3), 667–688.

Miklowitz, D. J. (2008). *Bipolar disorder: A family-focused treatment approach* (2nd ed.) New York: Guilford Press.

Miklowitz, D. J. (2019). *The bipolar disorder survival guide: What you and your family need to know* (3rd ed.). New York: Guilford Press.

Miklowitz, D. J., & Gitlin, M. J. (2014). *Clinician's guide to bipolar disorder: Integrating pharmacology and psychotherapy.* New York: Guilford Press.

Miklowitz, D. J., Schneck, C. D., Singh, M. K., Taylor, D. O., George, E. L., Howe, M. E., et al. (2013). Early intervention for symptomatic youth at risk for bipolar disorder: A randomized trial of family-focused therapy. *Journal of the American Academy of Child and Adolescent Psychiatry, 52,* 121–131.

Minuchin, S., & Fishman, H. C. (1981). *Family therapy techniques.* Cambridge, MA: Harvard University Press.

Mithen, S. (1996). *The prehistory of the mind: A search for the origins of art, religion, and science.* London: Thames & Hudson.

Moltz, D. (1993). Bipolar disorder and the family: An integrative model. *Family Process, 32,* 409–423.

Montgomery, S. A., & Asberg, M. (1979). A new depression scale designed to be sensitive to change. *British Journal of Psychiatry, 134,* 382–389.

Myers, N. L. (2010). Culture, stress and recovery from schizophrenia: Lessons from the field for global mental health. *Culture, Medicine, and Psychiatry, 34,* 500–528.

Najarian, S. (1995). Family experience with positive patient response to clozapine. *Archives of Psychiatric Nursing, 9*(1), 11–21.

National Institute for Health and Clinical Excellence. (2009). *Core interventions in the treatment and management of schizophrenia in adults: Clinical guideline 82, updated edition.* London: Author.

National Institute on Alcohol Abuse and Alcoholism. (2019). What's at-risk drinking?: Re-thinking drinking. Retrieved from *www.rethinkingdrinking.niaaa.nih.gov.*

Ninan, A., Stewart, S. L., Theall, L. A., Katuwapitiya, S., & Kam, C. (2014). Adverse effects of psychotropic medications in children: Predictive factors. *Journal of the Canadian Academy of Child and Adolescent Psychiatry, 23*(3), 218–225.

Nisavic, M., & Nejad, S. H. (2018a). Patients with alcohol use disorder. In T. A. Stern, O. Freudenreich, F. A. Smith, G. I. Fricchione, & J. F. Rosenbaum (Eds.), *Massachusetts General Hospital handbook of General Hospital psychiatry* (7th ed., pp. 141–148). New York: Elsevier.

Nisavic, M., & Nejad, S. H. (2018b). Patients with substance use disorders. In T. A. Stern, O. Freudenreich, F. A. Smith, G. I. Fricchione, & J. F. Rosenbaum (Eds.), *Massachusetts General Hospital handbook of General Hospital psychiatry* (7th ed., pp. 149–159). New York: Elsevier.

Nurnberg, H. G., Hensley, P. L., Gelenberg, A. J., Fava, M., Lauriello, J., & Paine, S. (2003). Treatment of antidepressant associated sexual dysfunction with sildenafil: A randomized controlled trial. *JAMA, 289,* 56–64.

Olfson, M., Mechanic, D., Hansell, S., Boyer, C., Walkup, J., & Weiden, P. (2000). Predicting medication noncompliance after hospital discharge among patients with schizophrenia. *Psychiatric Services, 52*(2), 216–222.

O'Reardon, J. P., Cristancho, P., & Peshek, A. D. (2006). Vagus nerve stimulation (VNS) and treatment of depression: To the brainstem and beyond. *Psychiatry (Edgment), 3*(5), 54–63.

Parthvi, R., Agrawal, A., Khanijo, S., Tsegare, A., & Talwar, A. (2019). Acute opiate overdose: An update on management strategies in emergency department and critical care unit. *American Journal of Therapeutics, 26,* e380–e387.

Patten, S. B., & Barbui, C. (2004). Drug-induced depression: A systematic review to inform clinical practice. *Psychotherapy Psychosomatics, 73,* 207–215.

Patterson, J., Miller, R., Carnes, S., & Wilson, S. (2004). Evidence-based therapies for marriage and family therapists. *Journal of Marital and Family Therapy, 30*(2), 183–195.

Patterson, J. E., & Magulac, M. (1994). The family therapist's guide to psychopharmacology: A graduate level course. *Journal of Marital and Family Therapy, 20*(2), 151–173.

Patterson, J. E., Peek, C. J., Heinrich, R. L., Bischoff, R. J., & Scherger, J. (2002). *Mental health professionals in medical settings: A primer.* New York: Norton.

Peebles, S. A., Mabe, P. A., Davidson, L., Fricks, L., Buckley, P. F., & Fenley, G. (2007). Recovery and systems transformation for schizophrenia. *Psychiatric Clinic of North America, 30,* 567–583.

Pennap, D., Zito, J. M., Santosh, P. J., Tom, S. E., Onukwugha, E., & Magder, L. S. (2018). Patterns of early mental health diagnosis and medication treatment in a Medicaid-insured birth cohort. *JAMA Pediatrics, 172*(6), 576–584.

Petersen, R. C., Doody, R., Kurz, A., Mohs, R. C., Morris, J. C., & Rabins, P. V. (2001). Current concepts in mild cognitive impairment. *Archives of Neurology, 58,* 1985–1992.

Petrides, G., Fink, M., Husain, M. M., Knapp, R. G., Rush, A. J., Mueller, M., et al. (2001). ECT remission rates in psychotic versus nonpsychotic depressed patients: A report from CORE. *Journal of ECT, 17*(4), 244–253.

Pitman, R. K., Sanders, K. M., Zusman, R. M., Healy, A. R., Cheema, F., Lasko, N. B., et al. (2002). Pilot study of secondary prevention of posttraumatic stress disorder with propranolol. *Biological Psychiatry, 51*(2), 189–192.

Porges, S., & Dana, D. (2018). *Clinical applications of the polyvagal theory: The emergence of polyvagal-informed therapies.* New York: Norton.

Preskorn, S. H., Feighner, J. P., Stanga, C. Y., & Ross, R. (Eds.). (2004). *Antidepressants: Past, present, and future.* New York: Springer.

Prochaska, J. O., DiClemente, C. C., & Norcross, J. C. (1995). *Changing for good.* New York: Morrow.

Raffi, E. R., & Freeman, M. P. (2017). The etiology of premenstrual dysphoric disorder: 5 interwoven pieces. *Current Psychiatry, 16,* 20–28.

Ran, M., & Xiang, M. (1995). A study of schizophrenic patients' treatment compliance in a rural community. *Journal of Mental Health, 4*(1), 85–89.

Rappaport, M. H. (2007). Dietary restrictions and drug interactions with monoamine oxidase inhibitors: The state of the art. *Journal of Clinical Psychiatry, 68*(8), 42–46.

Ravindran, L. N., & Stein, M. B. (2010). The pharmacologic treatment of anxiety disorders. *Journal of Clinical Psychiatry, 71,* 839–854.

Resnick, S. G., Fontana, A., Lehman, A. F., & Rosenhack, R. (2005). An empirical conceptualization of the recovery orientation. *Schizophrenia Research, 75,* 119–128.

Rhee, T. G., Olfson, M., Sint, K., & Wilkinson, S. T. (2020). Characterization of the quality of electroconvulsive therapy among older Medicare beneficiaries. *Journal of Clinical Psychiatry, 81*(4), 19m13186.

Riba, M. B., & Balon, R. (1999). *Psychopharmacology and psychotherapy: A collaborative approach.* Washington, DC: American Psychiatric Association.

Ritsher, J., Otilingam, P. G., & Grajales, M. (2003). Internalized stigma of mental illnesss: Psychometric properties of a new measure. *Psychiatry Research, 121*(1), 31–49.

Robinson, D. G., Woerner, M. G., Alvir, J. M., Geisler, S., Koreen, A., Sheitman, B., et al. (1999). Predictors of treatment response from a first episode of schizophrenia or schizoaffective disorder. *American Journal of Psychiatry, 156*(4), 544–549.

Roesler, T. A., Gavin, L. A., & Brenner, A. M. (1995). *Family Systems Medicine, 13*(3–4), 313–318.

Rolland, J. S. (2018). *Helping couples and families navigate illness and disability: An integrated approach.* New York: Guilford Press.

Rosenheck, R., Cramer, J., Jurgis, G., Perlick, D., Xu, W., Thomas, J., et al. (2000). Clinical and psychopharmacologic factors influencing family burden in refractory schizophrenia: The Department of Veterans Affairs Cooperative Study Group on Clozapine in Refractory Schizophrenia. *Journal of Clinical Psychiatry, 61*(9), 671–676.

Rothbaum, B. O., Davidson, J. R., Stein, D. J., Pedersen, R., Musgnung, J., Tian, X. W., et al. (2008). A pooled analysis of gender and trauma-type effects on responsiveness to treatment of PTSD with venlafaxine extended release or placebo. *Journal of Clinical Psychiatry, 69,* 1529–1539.

Rotheneichner, P., Lange, S., O'Sullivan, A., Marschallinger, J., Zaunmair, P., Geretsegger, C., et al. (2014). Hippocampal neurogenesis and antidepressant therapy: Shocking relations. *Neural Plasticity, 2014,* 723915.

Rothschild, B. (2017). *The body remembers: Vol. 2. Revolutionizing trauma treatment.* New York: Norton.

Royal College of Psychiatrists. (2017). *Statement on electroconvulsive therapy (ECT).* London: Author.

Rush, A. J., Trivedi, M. H., Wisniewski, S. R., Stewart, J. W., Nierenberg, A. A., Thase, M. F., et al. (2006). Bupropion-SR, sertraline, or venlafaxine-XR after failure of SSRIs for depression. *New England Journal of Medicine, 354,* 1231–1242.

Sackett, D. L., Straus, S., Richardson, S. W., Rosenberg, W., & Haynes, B. R. (2000). *Evidence based medicine: How to practice and teach EBM* (2nd ed.). New York: Churchill Livingstone.

Safire, W. (1997). *Lend me your ears: Great speeches in history.* New York: Norton.

Sammons, M. T., & Schmidt, N. B. (2001). *Combined treatment for mental disorders: A guide to psychological and pharmacological interventions.* Washington, DC: American Psychological Association.

Sanacora, G., Frye, M. A., McDonald, W., Mathew, S., Turner, M. S., Schatzberg, A. F., et al. (2017). A consensus statement on the use of ketamine in the treatment of mood disorders. *JAMA Psychiatry, 74*(4), 399–405.

Schatzberg, A. F., & DeBattista, C. D. (2015). *Manual of clinical psychopharmacology* (8th ed.). Washington, DC: American Psychiatric Publishing.

Schoeyen, H. K., Kessler, U., Andreassen O. A., Auestad, B. H., Bergsholm, P., Malt, U. F., et al. (2015). Treatment-resistant bipolar depression: A randomized controlled trial of electroconvulsive therapy versus algorithm-based pharmacological treatment. *American Journal of Psychiatry, 172,* 41–51.

Schuckit, M. A. (1994). Low level of response to alcohol as a predictor of future alcoholism. *American Journal of Psychiatry, 151,* 184–189.

Schuckit, M. A. (1995). Alcohol-related disorders. In H. I. Kaplan & B. J. Sadock (Eds.), *Comprehensive textbook of psychiatry/VI* (6th ed.). Baltimore: Williams & Wilkins.

Schuckit, M. A. (2001). Alcohol and alcoholism. In E. Braunwald, A. C. Fauci, D. L. Kasper, S. L. Hauser, D. L. Longo, & J. L. Jameson (Eds.), *Harrison's principles of internal medicine* (15th ed.). New York: McGraw-Hill.

Schuckit, M. A. (2003). Alcohol and alcoholism. In E. Braunwald, A. S. Fauci,

K. J. Isselbacher, D. L. Kasper, S. L. Hauser, D. L. Longo, et al. (Eds.), *Harrison's online*. New York: McGraw-Hill.

Schuckit, M. A., & Smith, T. L. (1996). An 8-year follow-up of 450 sons of alcoholic and control subjects. *Archives of General Psychiatry, 53*(3), 202–210.

Seaburn, D. B., Lorenz, A. D., Gunn, W. B., Jr., Gawinski, B. A., & Mauksch, L. B. (1996). *Models of collaboration: A guide for mental health professionals working with health care practitioners*. New York: Basic Books.

Shea, S. C. (2002). *The practical art of suicide assessment*. Hoboken, NJ: Wiley.

Shulman, L. M., Taback, R. L., Bean, J., & Weiner, W. J. (2001). Comorbidity of the nonmotor symptoms of Parkinson's disease. *Movement Disorders, 16*, 507–510.

Simeon, D., & Abugel, J. (2006). *Feeling unreal: Depersonalization disorder and the loss of the self*. New York: Oxford University Press.

Slavney, P. R. (1999). Diagnosing demoralization in consultation psychiatry. *Psychosomatics, 40*, 325–329.

Smith, C., Barzam, D., & Pristach, C. (1997). Effect of patient and family insight on compliance of schizophrenic patients. *Journal of Clinical Pharmacology, 37*, 147–154.

Snyder, C. R. (2000). Chapter 1: Hypothesis: There is hope. In C. R. Snyder (Ed.), *Handbook of hope: Theory, measures, and applications* (pp. 3–21). New York: Academic Press.

Sparks, J. A., Duncan, B. L., Cohen, D., & Antonuccio, D. O. (2011). Psychiatric drugs and common factors: An evaluation of risks and benefits for clinical practice. In B. L. Duncan, S. D. Miller, B. E. Wampold, & M. A. Hubble (Eds.), *The heart and soul of change* (2nd ed., pp. 199–236). Washington, DC: American Psychological Association.

Stebbin, H. (1995) Families' perspective of clozapine treatment. *Perspectives in Psychiatric Care, 31*(4), 14–18.

Steeg, S., Haigh, M., Webb, R. T., Kapur, N., Awenat, Y., Gooding, P., et al. (2015). The exacerbating influence of hopelessness on other known risk factors for repeat self-harm and suicide. *Journal of Affective Disorders, 190*, 522–528.

Stein, M. B., Torgrud, L. J., & Walker, J. R. (2000). Social phobia symptoms, subtypes, and severity: Findings from a community survey. *Archives of General Psychiatry, 57*, 1047–1052.

Stein, M. B., Walker, J. R., & Forde, D. R. (1996). Public-speaking fears in a community sample: Prevalence, impact on functioning, and diagnostic classification. *Archives of General Psychiatry, 53*, 169–174.

Taylor, F., & Raskind, M. A. (2002). The alpha1-adrenergic antagonist prazosin improves sleep and nightmares in civilian trauma posttraumatic stress disorder. *Journal of Clinical Psychopharmacology, 22*, 82–85.

The Economist. (2018, May 10). Too often, poverty is treated with pills. Retrieved from *www.economist.com/united-states/2018/05/10/too-often-poverty-is-treated-withpills*.

The Washington Post. (2020, January 24). Executive sentenced in opioid scheme, p. 2.

Thornicroft, G. (2006). *Shunned: Discrimination against people with mental illness*. Oxford, UK: Oxford University Press.

Thurman, H. (2010). Session 5 (7): Joy over pain [CD recording of reading]. *The Living Wisdom of Howard Thurman: A Visionary for our Time*. Sounds True and the Howard Thurman Family.

Trivedi, M. H., Fava, M., Wisniewski, S. R., Thase, M. E., Quitkin, F., Warden, D., et al. (2006). Medication augmentation after the failure of SSRIs for depression. *New England Journal of Medicine, 354,* 1243–1252.

Trivedi, M. H., Rush, A. J., Wisniewski, S. R., Nierenberg, A. A., Warden, D., Ritz, L., et al. (2006). Evaluation of outcomes with citalopram for depression using measurement-based care in STAR*D: Implications for clinical practice. *American Journal of Psychiatry, 163,* 28–40.

Turner, R. S. (2012). Alzheimer's disease: Clinical aspects. In R. D. Wegrzyn & A. S. Rudolph (Eds.), *Alzheimer's disease: Targets for new clinical diagnostic and therapeutic strategies* (pp. 211–230). Boca Raton, FL: CRC Press.

Twain, M., Fishkin, S. F., Doctorow, E. L., & Stone, A. E. (1997). *The adventures of Tom Sawyer (1876)*. New York: Oxford University Press.

Unutzer, J., & Park, M. (2012). Older adults with severe, treatment-resistant depression: "I got my mother back." *JAMA, 308,* 909–918.

VA/DoD Working Group. (2010). *VA/DoD clinical practice guideline for the management of post-traumatic stress update 2010*. Washington, DC: Department of Veterans Affairs.

van der Kolk, B. (2014). *The body keeps the score*. New York: Viking.

van Dis., E. A. M., van Veen, S. C., Hagenaars, M. A., Batelaan, N. M., Bockting, C. L. H., van den Heuvel, R. M., et al. (2020). Long-term outcomes of cognitive behavioral therapy for anxiety disorders: A systematic review and meta-analysis. *JAMA Psychiatry, 77*(3), 265–273.

Velez-Ruiz, N. J., & Meador, K. J. (2015). Neurodevelopmental effects of fetal antiepileptic drug exposure. *Drug Safety, 38,* 271–278.

Volkow, N. D., Koob, G. F., & McLellan, A. T. (2016). Neurologic advances from the brain disease model of addition. *New England Journal of Medicine, 374,* 363–371.

Weinstein, D. (2013). *The pathological family: Postwar America and the rise of family therapy*. Ithaca, NY: Cornell University Press.

Weissman, A. D., & Worden, J. W. (1972). Risk-rescue rating in suicide assessment. *Archives of General Psychiatry, 26,* 553–560.

Weissman, M. M., Klerman, G. I., Markowitz, J. S., & Ouellette, R. (1989). Suicidal ideation and suicide attempts in panic disorder and attacks. *New England Journal of Medicine, 321,* 1209–1214.

Williams, L., Patterson, J., & Edwards, T. (2014). *The clinician's guide to research methods in family therapy: Foundations of evidence-based practice*. New York: Guilford Press.

Wittchen, H. U., Schuster, P., & Lieb, R. (2001). Comorbidity and mixed anxiety-depressive disorder: Clinical curiosity or pathophysiological need? *Human Psychopharmacology, 16*(S1), S21–S30.

World Health Organization. (2019). *International statistical classification of diseases and related health problems, 11th revision: Vol. 2. Instruction manual.* Geneva, Switzerland: Author.

Writing Group for the Women's Health Initiative Investigators. (2002). Risks and benefits of estrogen plus progestin in healthy postmenopausal women: Principal results from the Women's Health Initiative Randomized Controlled Trial. *Journal of the American Medical Association, 288,* 321–333.

Wysocki, T., Greceo, P., Harris, M. A., Bubb, J., & White, N. H. (2001). Behavior therapy for families of adolescents with diabetes: Maintenance of treatment effects. *Diabetes Care, 24*(3), 441–446.

Xie, J., Yuanhao, Z., Alkhatib, A., Pham, T. T., Gill, F., Jang, A., et al. (2020). Metabolic syndrome and COVID-19 mortality among adult black patients in New Orleans. *Diabetes Care, 44*(1), 188–193.

Yonkers, K. A., Wisner, K. L., Stewart, D. E., Oberlander, T. F., Dell, D. L., Stotland, N., et al. (2009). The management of depression during pregnancy: A report from the American Psychiatric Association and the American College of Obstetricians and Gynecologists. *Obstetrics and Gynecology, 114*(3), 703–714.

Zajecka, J. (2001). Strategies for the treatment of antidepressant-related sexual dysfunction. *Journal of Clinical Psychiatry, 62*(Suppl. 3), 35–43.

Index

Page references in **bold** indicate glossary entries; *f* indicates a figure; *t* indicates a table.

Information processing. *See* Bottom-up
    information processing
Inhalation administration, 18–19
Inpatient treatment, 158, 229f. *See also*
    Hospitalization
Insomnia, 146t, 172–176, 173t, 174t. *See also*
    Health conditions; Sleep problems
Insula, 3, 5f, **270**
Insulin resistance, 74–75, 74t, **270**
Insurance issues
    medication evaluation and, 236t
    physicians in private practice and, 218
    shared decision making and, 215–216
    where to refer a patient and, 222–223
Integrated care, 240–250, 241t–242t, 245t,
    270. *See also* Collaborative care; Health
    care team
Interactions between medications. *See* Drug–
    drug interactions
Interferon alpha, 171t
Interleukin-2, 171t
Internalized stigma, 215, **270**
Internists, 219–220. *See also* Collaborative
    care; Physicians
Interpersonal psychotherapies, 63
Intramuscular, 18, **270**
Intravenous injection, 18
Intrinsic connectivity networks (ICN), 11, **270**
Isomers, 196, **270**

Joining, 247

K-2, 163, **271**. *See also* Substance abuse
Ketamine, 51–52

Lamotrigine, 73, 74, **271**
Language systems, 186f, 187, 187f
Late onset, 65
L-dopa, 171t
Levofloxacin (Levaquin), 172
Levomethylphenidate, 196
Lewy body dementia, 137, 141t. *See also*
    Dementia
Licensed practical nurse (LPN), 220
Licensed vocational nurse (LVN), 220
Lifestyle changes, 90–91
Lithium carbonate
    acute mania/hypomania and, 70–72, 70t,
        71t
    combining medication and, 75
    defined, **271**
    lithium augmentation, 56
    side effects of, 71–72, 72t, 73t
Lithium toxicity, 72, 73t, **271**. *See also*
    Toxicity

Lorazepam (Ativan). *See also* Benzodiazepines
    alcoholism and, 159
    dementia and, 146t
    older adults and, 201
    panic disorder and, 96
    sleep problems and, 175
LSD (lysergic acid diethylamide) abuse, 163,
    164t. *See also* Substance abuse
Lurasidone (Latuda), 74t, 76

Maintenance phase of treatment
    bipolar disorders and, 76–77
    defined, **271**
    psychotic disorders and, 120–121
    treating depression as a chronic illness and,
        62, 62t
Major depression with psychotic features, 53,
    271
Major depressive disorder (MDD). *See also*
    Depression
    antidepressants and, 36–38, 37t
    case illustrations, 32–36
    depression as a chronic illness and, 61–63,
        62t
    distinguishing normal distress from, 28–36,
        32t
    panic disorder and, 94
    threat of suicide and, 78–79
Mania. *See also* Bipolar disorders; Hypomania
    case illustrations, 66–68
    defined, **271**
    overview, 65–66, 69, 84
    threat of suicide and, 79
    treatment and, 70–75, 70t, 71t, 72t, 73t, 74t
Marijuana abuse, 163, 164t. *See also* Substance
    abuse
Medical assistant (MA), 220–221
Medical illness. *See* Health conditions; Illness
Medication referrals. *See* Referral for
    medication
Medication-assisted treatment, 161–162, **271**
Medications that produce psychiatric
    symptoms, 169–172, 171t. *See also*
    Health conditions
Mefloquine, 171t
Melancholic depression, 49, **271**
Melatonin, 175
Memantine (Namenda), 143, 145t
Memory impairment, 134–137, 201–202
Menopause, 204
Mentalization, **271**
Meperidine (Demerol), 50
Meprobamate, 157
Metabolic syndrome, 74–75, 127–128, 127t,
    271